INDUSTRIAL RESPIRATORY PROTECTION

MICHAEL F. TERESINSKI
PAUL N. CHEREMISINOFF

PREFACE

Respiratory protection is the interdisciplinary science comprised of human physiology, anatomy, toxicology, biomechanical engineering and plant engineering. It has evolved from man's desire to explore the unknown depths of the oceans and the earth's mineral resources to become a prime factor in space exploration. However, development has been hampered continually by an imbalance in equipment design, materials of construction, human physiology, medical testing and general lack of knowledge. With a rise in the number of compensable respiratory diseases and corresponding employment compensation awards, it is not cost-effective to provide services or products that could cause impairment to the user or manufacturer.

The objective of this book is to provide a basic overview of respiratory protection in the industrial sector. Further, it is intended to give the reader a methodology by which to approach the many and varied aspects of industrial respiratory protection.

By its content and structure, this book is intended to be useful as a complete work or for its individual components. It discusses the major technical aspects of respiratory protection that the industrial plant engineer should know, and is intended to be used as a guide. The authors have condensed a large volume of technical data into this book and it includes their own personal experiences in the field. The origin of figures, tables and other material is given wherever possible so that readers may further evaluate the data.

A successful respiratory protection program can be achieved only by combining the talents of the equipment manufacturer with selection of the appropriate equipment based on measurement of hazards, and proper care, use and maintenance.

Michael F. Teresinski
Paul N. Cheremisinoff

ABOUT THE AUTHORS

MICHAEL F. TERESINSKI is Safety Engineer with the U.S. Department of Labor, Occupational Safety and Health Administration (OSHA), and is a registered Professional Engineer. In his work with OSHA, he has inspected major industries, construction projects and maritime facilities for compliance with federal safety and health standards. He has participated in OSHA's foundry, grain dust and special programs and has served as an expert witness in federal hearings and as an instructor at the OSHA Training Institute, Chicago, Illinois. Prior to his OSHA position, he was responsible for design and installation of ventilation, pollution and mechanical systems for plant engineering projects in the textile and rubber industries. A mechanical engineering graduate of Marquette University, he is a member of the American Society of Mechanical Engineers; American Society of Heating, Ventilating and Air Conditioning Engineers and the American Conference of Governmental Industrial Hygienists.

PAUL N. CHEREMISINOFF is Professor of Civil and Environmental Engineering at the New Jersey Institute of Technology. He is a licensed Professional Engineer with more than 40 years of engineering experience in a broad range of industries, and is a consultant to many major organizations on engineering design, process and pollution control. An internationally known scholar and researcher, he holds engineering degrees from Pratt Institute and Stevens Institute of Technology, and is a Fellow of the New York Academy of Sciences, member of Sigma Xi and Tau Beta Pi. He is the author/editor of many publications and as a result of his work in the area of in-plant environmental control, he has joined with Michael Teresinski to author INDUSTRIAL RESPIRATORY PROTECTION.

CONTENTS

xi

CHAPTER 1

INTRODUCTION AND EARLY HISTORY

Almost 2000 years have elapsed since the Romans constructed the first crude respirator from animal entrails. Yet each year millions of dollars are paid out in compensation to black lung victims, employees occupationally disabled or impaired in their respiratory function and to firemen injured by smoke inhalation. If a country can send a man to the moon, why should respiratory protection continue to be a problem?

Consider respiratory protection in terms of the U.S. space program:

1. **Cost.** The U.S. space program was the best and most expensive.
2. **Design.** All equipment was designed specifically for the purpose of survival in a hostile environment.
3. **Training.** All astronauts were well trained in the use of the equipment and were highly motivated.
4. **Physical Condition.** The astronauts were in ideal physiological condition.
5. **Consequence.** To not wear the equipment in space would mean certain death.

This book is a guide for potential users to the concept of teamwork required to achieve respiratory protection, which is complete coordination among supplier, buyer and user. The required protection can be achieved only if the supplier has the proper equipment for the required use. The proper equipment must be specified for the operations that exist, and these must be surveyed accurately by the buyer or potential user. Once the proper protection is selected, the fitting of the equipment to the person, training and maintenance must be conducted as required for the existing conditions. The user not only must wear the equipment but must learn how to use it properly, and be fully aware of its limitations or pay the price of improper use. Its failure to perform increases the user's chances of succumbing to physical disease, impairment or injury.

Since 1910 the U.S. Bureau of Mines, Mine Enforcement Safety Administration (MESA) and, currently, the Mine Safety and Health Administration (MSHA) [1,2], have sought to specify and improve the best possible respiratory equipment by devising rigid regulations about the design and certification of the different types of apparatus marketed in the United States. These regulations have been a worldwide benchmark of such safety and protection practice.

Since the passage of the 1970 Occupational Safety & Health Act (OSHA), the employer has been responsible for a safe workplace, free from recognized hazards, through *engineering control methods,* such as general and local ventilation. When these methods are not feasible or being instituted, appropriate respirator protection is required. Since OSHA was passed, the subject of respiratory protection has been a tug-of-war with labor unions and management. Management either would not admit to the hazard or would pass out respirators like paper towels, only to have them thrown into a pile at the end of the day. The union claimed that the respirators never fit, but workers would not shave their beards when requested.

In the opinion of the authors the workplace is a much different place now than in past years, and union and management must unite to achieve their common goal of productivity. The common enemies of both sides are inflation, hazardous materials, improper training, attitude, lack of motivation, insurance compensation–medical liability rates and special interest groups.

HISTORY

Most engineers and general industrial users know little about respirators. America was introduced to the respirator during the poisonous gas attacks of World War I, but its history is fairly extensive.

Drinker and Hatch [3] published a history of the early use of respirators in 1936. Most industrial health texts on respirators generally attribute the first use to Pliny the Elder (23–79 A.D.) [4]. He tried to use loose-fitting animal bladders in Roman mines to protect against various harmful materials, such as lead and mercury. A century later, Julius Pollex (124–192 A.D.) described a respirator made from a bladder, with a sack cloth filter for protection against dusts in mines.

In the early 1500s, Leonardo da Vinci worked on respiratory protection and recommended the use of a wet cloth as protection against chemical warfare agents. Also, he designed a "snorkel" [4], which consisted of a breathing tube with an attached float; a soldier thus could sneak up on his enemy under water. Meanwhile, Bernadino Ramazzini, generally acknowledged as the father of industrial hygiene, was concerned about the hazards faced by miners, gypsum workers, bakers and stone cutters. In England, at about the same time, military diving came into practice to recover sunken treasure and military hardware. For example, if the brass cannons could be recovered from a 100-gun ship, they would be worth more than $50,000 in the money of that day [5]. This developed a strong incentive for a diving dress design that would increase efficiency, considering that 1000 new military and civilian wrecks littered the shores of England every year. The forerunner of the hard hat diving suit was "Deanes Diving Suit" [5]. Later, August Siebe modified it by sealing the helmet to the rest of the suit. With the installation of an exhaust valve, it became the direct ancestor to the standard deep seas diving dress in use today or the air-supplied respirator (Figure 1).

In 1825 John Roberts developed a "smoke filter" for firemen—a leather hood and a hose strapped to the leg—the theory being that the best air during a fire would be near the floor [4].

In 1866 Bernoist Rouquayrol [5] patented the demand regulator, which adjusts the flow of air from the tank to meet the breathing and pressure requirements of the diver, as shown in Figure 2. However, as tanks of sufficient strength to contain air at high pressure could not be built at this time, Rouquayrol adapted his regulator to surface-supplied diving equipment.

In 1878 the first commercially practical self-contained breathing apparatus was developed by H. A. Fleuss [5]. He used a closed-circuit type, using 100% oxygen for breathing, and the gas used by the diver was recirculated in the apparatus. The tanks did not have to be high strength because there was a need for only one-fifth as much volume as with compressed air. The tanks were useful on shallow dives, but oxygen poisoning occurred at depths greater than 25 feet.

In the United States, the U.S. Bureau of Mines [1] was formed in 1910 to regulate safety conditions in coal mines for more efficient and safer operations. The development of respirators and breathing apparatus was carried on mostly by European countries for warfare purposes. During World War I, both the Germans and the Allies used various poison gases as a chemical warfare technique. As respirator protection brought about improvements in gas sorbents and better filters, the Germans tried to disperse highly toxic particulates onto the battlefield. The gas mask, as the respirator was referred to, was not effective against these types of particulates. During World War II, German blitzkrieg warfare emphasized the use of airplanes and high-mobility troops. In research conducted in the United States, Leslie Silverman and other pioneers, like Philip Drinker

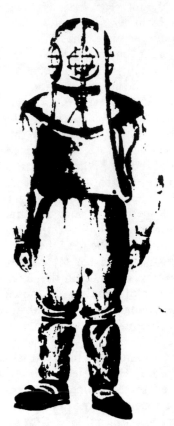

Figure 1.   Siebe's first closed diving dress and helmet, a forerunner of the air-supplied respirator and abrasive blast helmet [5].

[3], studied various German and Japanese respirator techniques. In occupied France, Captain Jacques-Yves Cousteau and Emile Gagnon combined an improved demand regulator and high pressure air tank system to create the first truly efficient and safe open-circuit "self-contained underwater breathing apparatus" (SCUBA).

Perhaps even more important were the U.S. Navy and Harvard School of Public Health Industry Hygiene courses, which recognized the need for trained medical doctors on the wartime industrial scene; the formation of the American Conference of Governmental Industrial Hygienists (ACGIH); and the theory of a threshold limit value (TLV) [6] system of breathing a measurable amount of a toxic material for an eight-hour day was acceptable and would not harm or impair the worker. The creation of the atomic bomb, synthetic gasolines and chemical agents ushered in a

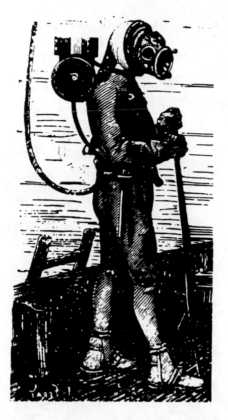

Figure 2. Rouquayrol's demand regulator [5].

whole new era, which industry referred to as the petrochemical complex. The toxic waste handling and disposal problems gave rise to the term "environmental" and to the Environmental Protection Act.

The 1970 Occupational Safety and Health Act [2] contained these requirements: (1) the U.S. Department of Health, Education and Welfare-National Institute of Occupational Safety and Health (NIOSH) should do research on hazardous chemicals and engineering control methods, such as respiratory protection; and (2) the employer should provide a safe workplace for his employees (the general duty clause). The question of worker protection to possible exposure to chemicals seemed endless! As OSHA covered almost all manufacturing functions, the need for better respiratory protection in all phases of industry demanded tremendous response by the employers of America.

In 1981 President Reagan and his Administration outlined the current responsibilities of NIOSH for OSHA and the Federal Mine Safety and

Health Act of 1977: to "conduct research necessary to ensure, insofar as possible, that no worker will suffer diminished health, reduced functional capacity, or decreased life expectancy as a result of his or her work experience" [7]. Thorne Achter, the new head of OSHA, remained firmly committed to improving the safety and health of the nation's workforce, while trying to stay within the budgetary guidelines of Congress.

CHAPTER 2

ANATOMY AND PHYSIOLOGY OF HUMAN RESPIRATION

INTRODUCTION

The most common complaint associated with respirators is the fatigue experienced by the user, which is caused by the added exertion to the lungs and muscular systems of the body when air is drawn through a respirator-filter mechanism. Before a person is assigned a respirator, the company must give the user a thorough physical examination. OSHA Standard 1919.134(b)(10) states "Persons should not be assigned to tasks requiring use of respirators unless it has been determined that they are physically able to perform the work and use the equipment" [8]. OSHA considers "should" as *advisory* in nature and "shall" as *required* or *mandatory*. At present, a company is legally required by two OSHA standards—1919.1001(J) Asbestos and 1910.1043(H) Cotton Dust—to determine pulmonary function. Pulmonary function can be defined as a measurement of the lung's ability to exchange gases or ventilate itself by moving volumes of air in and out during breathing. Tests of lung function vary from simple measurements of vital capacity to the use of gaseous radioisotopes to determine regional ventilation and blood flow. The tests fall into two groups: (1) lung volume and air movement tests; and (2) gas exchange tests. A pulmonary function test, combined with medical history and physical examination, is the only true way to determine whether a person is physically able to wear a respirator.

Opposition to such tests arises from both union and management. Management opposition in some companies includes the cost, previous unstandardized terminology and equipment, lack of trained personnel and, in general, the concept of possible legal situations arising from testing long-time employees and finding respiratory impairment. The union generally feels the testing is justified for the young, but can, or will, be used as a method to remove or retire older or impaired workers. Once found to be impaired, these workers are not able to work or maintain their present standard of living.

The authors feel that these tests must be done so that industry can properly determine the hazards encountered and develop the technology to deal with them. The situation is similar to noise control. The employee exposed to high noise levels loses his or her hearing gradually, the amount of loss being measured by audiometric testing. The loss is established by comparison to nationally established hearing level tables. In pulmonary function testing, the person blows into a spirometer, a device that measures volumes of air relative to time, and either a graph or digital readout is presented by the machine for comparison to standardized medical charts.

ANATOMY [9]

The tracheobronchial system contains two types of airways: the bronchi, which consist of cartilage, and the bronchioles, which are noncartilaginous, or membraneous, airways [9]. The primary function of the airway is to conduct air between the outside environment and the respiratory system. From the trachea downward, the airways divide progressively, similar to the branching of a tree. The branching may be symmetrical or nonsymmetrical. The total cross-sectional area of some 23 generations of airways increases, the significance being that resistance to airflow actually decreases as the air moves down from the larger airways to the bronchioles. The smaller bronchi and bronchioles less than 2 mm in diameter often are referred to as the "small airways." It is in this portion of the tracheobronchial tree that airborne substances are thought to exert their harmful effects. As these small airways contribute only 15% to total airway resistance, considerable disease must be present in them before usual spirometric tests become abnormal.

The bronchioles, or noncartilaginous airways, continue to subdivide in a distinctive fashion (Figure 3) and serve mainly as conductors of air. Once the level of the respiratory bronchioles is reached, gas exchange can occur because there are respiratory tissues in their walls. The conducting airways, therefore, refer only to the trachea, bronchi and nonrespiratory bronchioles. Gas exchange of oxygen and carbon dioxide takes place in the respiratory unit consisting of the respiratory bronchiole, alveolar duct, alveolar sac and individual alveoli. Deoxygenated blood reaches the alveoli via the pulmonary arterial system, the branching bronchi and

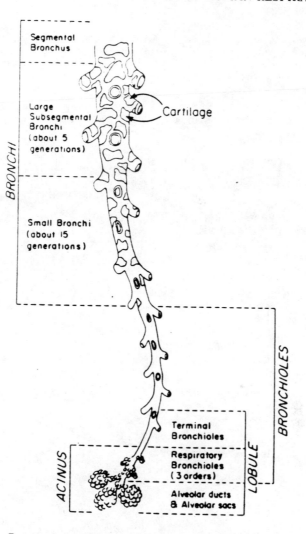

Figure 3. Progressive subdivision of the tracheobronchial tree, illustrating both conducting airways and the respiratory unit.

bronchioles. This capillary plexus is in intimate proximity to the alveolar epithelium, so that red blood cells are separated from the inhaled air only by the thickness of the alveolar-capillary membrane (Figure 4). The alveoli have a surface area of about 70 m^2, providing a contact area for gas exchange equivalent to the size of a tennis court.

The lung has two separate blood supplies: one for the pulmonary circulation and the other for bronchial circulation. The pulmonary circula-

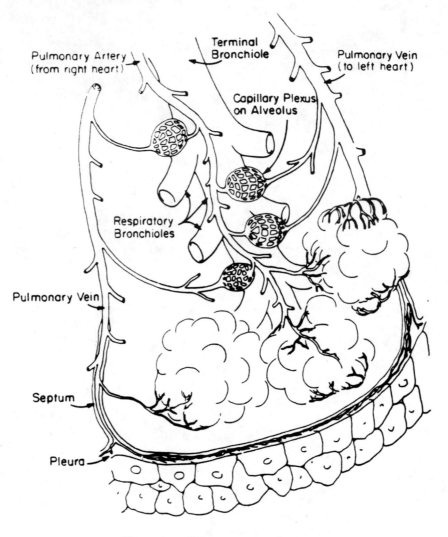

Figure 4. Pulmonary vascular system.

tion handles the cardiac output, its major function being to oxygenate the blood. The bronchial circulation arising from the aorta receives only a small portion of cardiac output and contains only oxygenated blood. These bronchial arteries are the principal source of nutrient blood to the pulmonary tissue itself, including the tracheobronchial tree, pulmonary nerves, lymph tissue and the visceral pleura.

Many hazardous materials are prevented from going down into the alveoli area by the lining of the airway. The lining of the airways (Figure 5) as far as the terminal bronchiole consists of two basic cell types: ciliated columnar epithelial cells and goblet cells. Goblet cells create a mucous layer that rests on top of the cilia and is swept mouthward by coordinated movement of the cilia. This mucous blanket, sometimes referred to as ciliary escalator, is an important defense mechanism for the removal of inhaled particulate matter. Unfortunately, its efficiency may be impaired or destroyed by acids and bases or by cigarette smoke. Excessive mucous secretion, which occurs during chronic bronchitis, may impose an undue burden on cilia and contribute to plugging and narrowing of the airways. The cellular elements of the lung are supported mainly by a framework consisting of reticulin, elastin and collagen fibers. The presence of these fibers helps determine the compliance (stiffness) and the elastic recoil properties of the lung. Figure 6 illustrates the flow of air from the nose and mouth through the trachea into the lungs to the alveoli.

Respiration is the utilization of oxygen and the various exchanges of

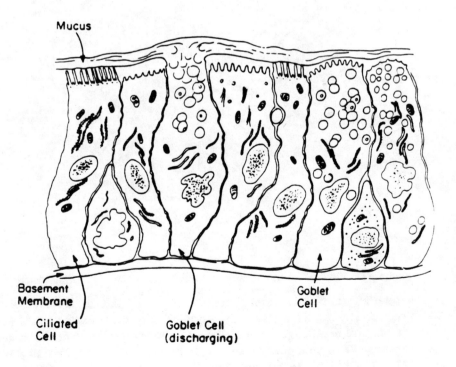

Mucus

Basement
Membrane

Goblet
Cell

Ciliated
Cell

Goblet Cell
(discharging)

Figure 5.   Mucociliary escalator.

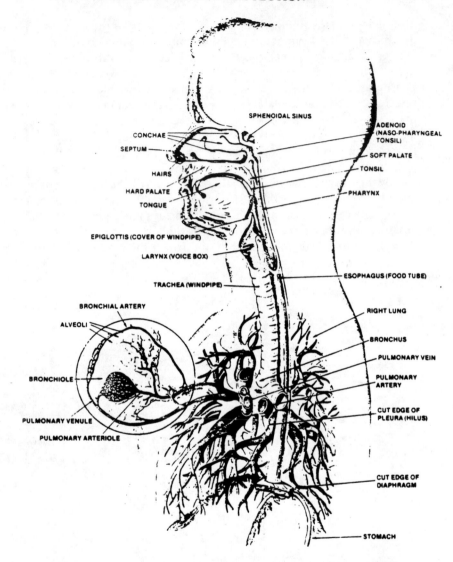

Figure 6.   Flow of air to the lungs (courtesy American Medical Association).

gases that take place throughout the body as part of the metabolic process. The respiratory system is comprised of those parts of the body that involve breathing: the lung, the air passages leading to the lungs and the rib cage, the diaphragm and other other muscles that help produce the movement of air into and out of the lungs. Figure 7 illustrates the movement of the rib cage during the breathing cycle.

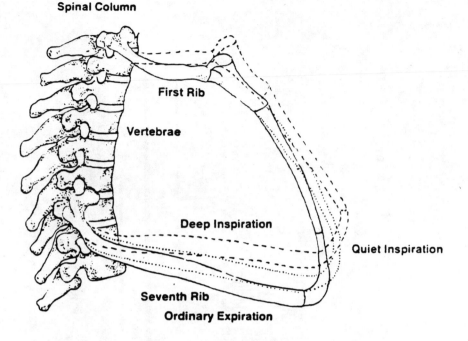

Figure 7.   Rib cage movement during the breathing cycle.

THE PHYSIOLOGY OF BREATHING [5]

Breathing is the result of a combined movement of the rib cage and the diaphragm, which increases or decreases the volume of the chest cavity [10]. For inspiration, the ribs are raised and the diaphragm (which forms the bottom of the chest cavity) is lowered. In accordance with Boyle's law, the pressure in the chest is decreased as the volume is increased, and air from outside the body will move into the lungs because it is at a relatively higher pressure. When the rib cage is lowered and the diaphragm raised, the volume is decreased and air is forced out of the lungs. However, no matter how hard a person might try, he cannot expel all the air from his lungs. A residual volume of 1–1.5 liters will remain always. Figure 8 illustrates the basic terminology of lung function. Later, we will examine specific lung terminology, as modified by the physician, to measure the performance of the lung during the pulmonary function testing.

Tidal volume is the amount of air moved in and out of the lungs during a single breathing cycle. Tidal volume may vary from breath to breath, and usually will range from about 0.5 liters, when a person is at rest and

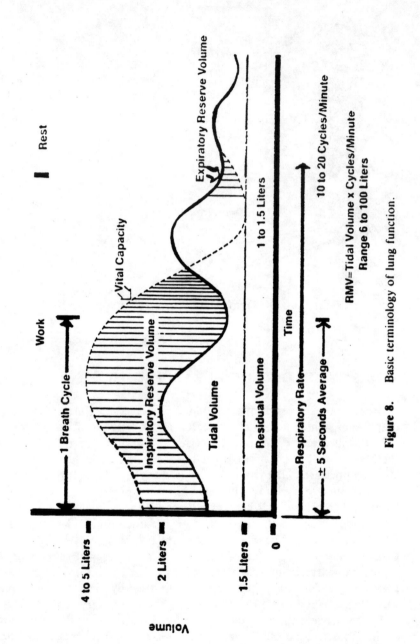

Figure 8. Basic terminology of lung function.

breathing easily, to more than 2 liters, when he is working and breathing heavily.

Vital capacity of the lungs is the greatest amount of air that can be moved in and out of the lungs in a single breath. It is measured starting with the largest possible inspiration and then forcing out as much of the breath as possible, leaving only the residual volume.

Respiratory rate is the number of breathing cycles in one minute. A normal rate would be between 10–20 cpm.

Respiratory minute volume (RMV) is the total volume of air moved in and out of the lungs in one minute. It is computed by multiplying the tidal volume by the respiratory rate. RMV ranges from about 6 l/min to more than 100 l/min.

Inspiratory reserve volume measures the amount of air that can be added to the lungs forcibly after taking a normal breath. Similarly, **expiratory reserve** is the amount of air that can be expelled forcibly after a normal expiration. Vital capacity = inspiratory reserve volume + expiratory reserve.

Respiratory dead space is that fraction of a breath that does not reach the alveoli and, therefore, does not participate in the gas exchanges in the lungs. This would include air remaining in the mouth and the other air passages, which is brought in at the end of a breath and is pushed out ahead of the "used" air. The amount of dead space usually makes up about one third of the tidal volume in normal relaxed breathing.

Compliance generally describes stiffness or distensibility of the lung. It represents the relationship between the change in volume of air within the lung and the accompanying pressure change needed to cause that volume change. When the pressure needed to change the volume is great, the lung is stiff and compliance will be low. This is a situation found in various forms of pulmonary fibrosis, such as asbestosis. In contrast, with emphysema the volume change occurs when less pressure is exerted and compliance is increased or the lung is less stiff. **Dynamic compliance** is measured during tidal breathing; **static compliance** is measured at different lung volumes. Because compliance measures the distensibility of the respiratory system, it reflects the elasticity of the lungs or, more specifically, the elastic recoil properties of the lung and chest wall. Elastic recoil refers to the tendency of the lungs to return to the relaxed state at functional residual capacity. This elastic property is given by the intrinsic qualities of the lung tissue itself, as well as a film of surface-active material that lines the lung. Elastic recoil pressure varies with the type of disease; pulmonary fibrosis demonstrates increased elastic recoil pressure, and emphysematous lungs are more distensible due to loss of supporting tissue and have less elastic recoil.

Spirometry is the measurement of the ventilatory capacity of the lungs.

Forced vital capacity (FVC) is the maximum volume of air that can be exhaled forcefully after a maximum inspiration.

Forced expiratory volume in one second (FEV$_1$) is that volume of air that can be expelled forcibly during the first second of expiration.

Body temperature, ambient pressure, saturated with water vapor (BTPS) occurs when the person tested exhales a volume of gas at body temperature (37°C). When collected in the spirometer, this volume rapidly cools to approach the lower ambient temperature and contracts. This reduced volume must be multiplied by the appropriate BTPS conversion factor to correct it to what it should be at normal body temperature (Table I).

Forced expiratory flow during the middle half of the 25–75% FVC (FEF) is the average rate of flow during the middle two quarters of the forced expiratory effort.

BREATHING CYCLE [9]

Before the air ever reaches the lungs, it is possible for it to be heated, moistened and cleaned of foreign particles and bacteria while being drawn across the moist mucous lining of the nasal passages [10]. Once the air moves into the lungs, it comes into contact with the walls of the alveoli. Here, it is separated from the blood circulating in the lungs only by the membrane walls of the alveoli and the capillaries. The oxygen, driven by its relatively high partial pressure in the lung, is dissolved quickly by the moist lining of the alveoli and diffused through the membranes into the blood. The partial pressure of oxygen in the blood entering the lungs is relatively low because much of the dissolved oxygen has been consumed in the various cells. At the same time, the partial pressure of the carbon dioxide in the blood is relative to that in the lungs, and a quantity of carbon dioxide will diffuse quickly into the area of lower partial pressure in the alveoli.

As an example, at atmospheric conditions the partial pressure of oxygen in the blood entering the lungs is about 40 mm of mercury (Hg), while the partial pressure of the carbon dioxide is about 46 mm Hg. The partial pressures of oxygen and carbon dioxide in the inspired air are about 158 mm Hg and 0.30 mm Hg, respectively. The partial pressure gradients of each gas are high, and diffusion into and out of the blood will proceed almost instantaneously. The partial pressures in alveolar air are almost the same as those for blood leaving the lungs because the exchange of gas takes place so rapidly that the composition of the

Table I.   Factors Used to Convert Gas Volumes from
Ambient Temperature to BTPS

Temperature ($^{\circ}C$)	Conversion Factor
18	1.114
19	1.111
20	1.102
21	1.096
22	1.091
23	1.085
24	1.080
25	1.075
26	1.068
27	1.063
28	1.057
29	1.051
30	1.045
31	1.039
32	1.032
33	1.026
34	1.020
35	1.014
36	1.007
37	1.000

inspired air is changed as it reaches the walls of the alveoli. This alveolar air mixes with used air in the respiratory dead spaces on the way out of the body and then becomes expired air. This has a partial pressure of about 116 mm Hg for oxygen and 28.5 mm Hg for carbon dioxide.

OXYGEN CONSUMPTION

The concentration of oxygen and carbon dioxide in the arterial blood is relatively constant whether the body is at rest or at work. It is determined primarily by the partial pressure of the gases in the alveoli. When a working body requires greater quantities of oxygen, the additional supply is provided by an increase in the cardiac output. A corresponding increase in the RMV provides more fresh air to match the larger flow of blood moving through the lungs. Oxygen consumption indicates the amount of oxygen being taken into the system and used. Oxygen consumption may vary from 0.25 l/min for a man at rest to more than 3 l/min when doing hard work.

ABNORMAL CARDIOPULMONARY PHYSIOLOGY

The American Thoracic Society refers to this as chronic obstructive pulmonary disease (COPD) [10]. Airway obstruction brings about an increase in airway resistance and results in reduced expiratory flowrates and increased work of breathing. Blood pH levels are determined by the ratio of bicarbonate ion concentration to CO_2 concentration, normally 20:1, a ratio physiologically maintained by means of disposal of CO_2 by the lungs and of bicarbonate by the kidney. As impairment of alveolar ventilation increases, CO_2 retention appears. Generally, medical technicians obtain a microsample of blood from an ear puncture for determining the pH and other acid-base values.

The respiratory therapist and physician would be interested in the patient's respiratory acidosis, which is the excess CO_2 resulting from inadequate alveolar ventilation. **Respiratory alkalosis** is a deficit of CO_2 resulting from alveolar hypersensitivity. The area we will examine is the use of the spirometer and the accompanying charts for comparison. The medical terminology of inhalation therapy is more directed to pulmonary disease treatment, which one is attempting to prevent with the use of respirators. It should be noted that once the worker or person impairs his lungs, modern medicine cannot reinstate previous capacity. At best, present technology can only ease the pain.

SPIROMETRY

As spirometry is the measurement of the ventilatory capacity of the lungs, one should be concerned about the validity and reproducibility of this type of test and the factors that affect these considerations.

There are several types of equipment on the market today, whose principal differences are the methods in which the recorded data are presented. Some equipment models produce an accurate graph on which calculations are made to determine values such as FEV_1, FVC, etc., which produce the numbers in tabulated form. In a recent study evaluating commercially available spirometers [11] and the use of room air for testing was completed, the results showed that testing with room air is easier and simpler and, for most devices, just as effective as heated and humidified air. An important conclusion was that most available spirometers can faithfully record forced spirograms; therefore, any spirometer that meets the American Thoracic Society requirements can be used to record the spirogram. OSHA has stipulated in 1910.1043 how the instruments are to be manufactured. The Cotton Dust Standard [8] also requires that the employer must assure that all medical examinations and procedures are performed by, or under the supervision of, a licensed physician and must provide them without cost to the employee. Section (h)(1)(iii) states, "Persons other than licensed physicians, who administer the pulmonary function testing required by the section shall complete an NIOSH-approved training course in spirometry." In January of 1976 [11] the Bureau of Medical Devices of the U.S. Food & Drug Administration (FDA) listed 35 manufacturers of spirometers.

SPIROMETRIC TECHNIQUE [9]

The spirometric technique test measures FVC and FEV_1. The person performing the test must blow as hard and fast as possible into the tube connected to the spirometer. The person doing the testing should advise the person doing the test to relax. Smoking or the use of an aerosolized bronchodilator can alter the accuracy of testing. The individual may sit or stand; nose clips are provided but generally are not worn. The following three graphs (Figures 9a,b,c) are unacceptable for the reasons given. In these situations, some people get nervous and cough; some either cheat or think they are supposed to show improvement with testing; and others do not blow hard enough. The two best FVC must be within 5% (100 ml) of each other. Figure 10 illustrates this mathematically.

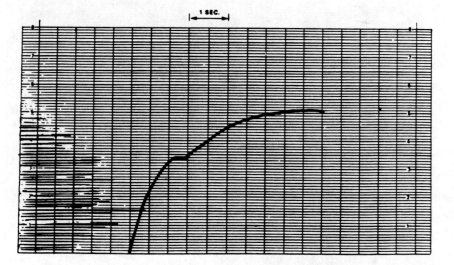

Figure 9a.   Unacceptable tracing—cough [9].

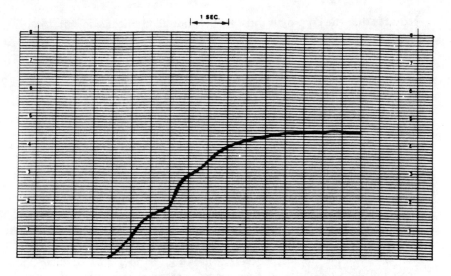

Figure 9b.   Unacceptable tracing—inconsistent effort [9].

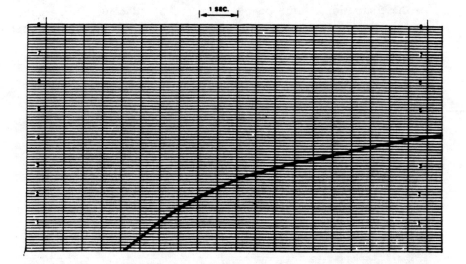

Figure 9c.   Unacceptable tracing—early termination of expiration and failure to "plateau" [9].

NOMOGRAPHS

Figures 11–16 are the nomographs currently used by NIOSH for various calculations, and Table II comprises the spirometry for normal males and females [9]. From the standpoint of testing, as illustrated by Figure

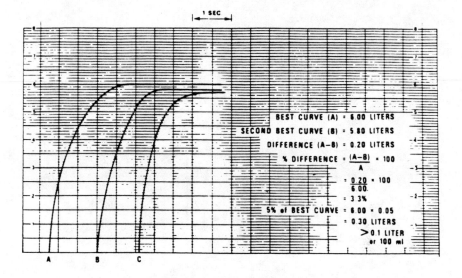

Figure 10.   Valid spirogram—two best curves within 5% [9].

10, the comparison of the curves to the 5% difference and the fact the tracing plateaus are consistent are the important factors.

Because of the budget constraints and the cost of compliance, the OSHA cotton dust standard has met much opposition. Regardless whether the standard is in effect, the important factor is that it will be used as a model for future pulmonary function standards. These standards will specify the characteristics of the apparatus, techniques for measurement, interpretation of spirogram results and who will be qualified to give these tests.

Figure 17 lists the current requirements for OSHA's Cotton Dust Standard, 1910.1043 Appendix D—Pulmonary Function Standard for Cotton Dust [8]. It should be mentioned that the FEF 200 to 1200 test, which is the flow between 200 and 1200 cc of the FVC, formerly known as the maximal expiratory flowrate (MEFR), reflects changes in the large airways but adds little to information already available from the FEV_1 and FVC. The maximum voluntary ventilation (MVV) test is usually unpleasant, exhausting and involving much effort. The Social Security and Black Lung Acts sometimes require this type of test to evaluate pulmonary disability.

EXAMPLES OF WORK AND DISEASE

A problem faced by most young professionals, such as engineers and managers, is how to deal with the relationship of work to disease [14].

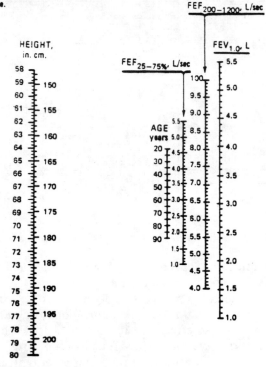

TO USE NOMOGRAM:
Lay a straight edge between the patient's height as read on the HEIGHT scale, and his age as it appears on the AGE scale.

$FEF_{200-1200} = 0.109\ H_{in} - 0.047\ A + 2.010\ [0.44\ 1.66]$

$FEF_{25-75\%} = 0.047\ H_{in} - 0.045\ A + 2.513\ [0.53\ 1.12]$

$FEV_{1.0\ sec} = 0.092\ H_{in} - 0.032\ A - 1.260\ [0.73\ 0.55]$

$FVC = 0.148\ H_{in} - 0.025\ A - 4.241\ [0.65\ 0.74]$

Morris, J. F., et al.: Am. Rev. Respir. Dis., 103:57–67, 1971

Note: The predicted FEV₁ and FVC in non-Caucasians must be multiplied by 0.85.

Figure 11.   Spirometric standards for normal males (BTPS) [9] (derived from Morris et al. [12]).

Until the 1900s, the only way a disabled worker or his family could obtain compensation for job-related injuries was to sue the employer. By 1920 all but six states had passed workmen's compensation statutes that made employers responsible for economic loss due to worker's injuries

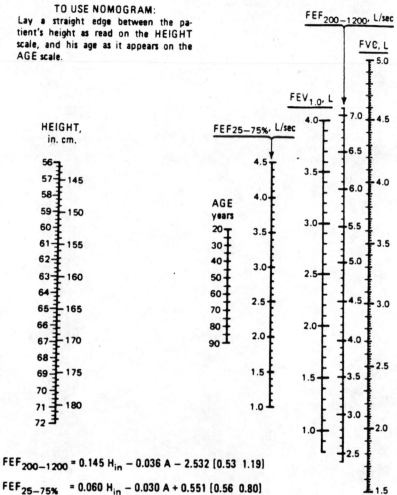

TO USE NOMOGRAM:
Lay a straight edge between the patient's height as read on the HEIGHT scale, and his age as it appears on the AGE scale.

HEIGHT, in. cm.

FEF$_{25-75\%}$, L/sec

AGE years

FEV$_{1.0}$, L

FEF$_{200-1200}$, L/sec

FVC, L

$$FEF_{200-1200} = 0.145\ H_{in} - 0.036\ A - 2.532\ [0.53\ 1.19]$$

$$FEF_{25-75\%} = 0.060\ H_{in} - 0.030\ A + 0.551\ [0.56\ 0.80]$$

$$FEV_{1.0\ sec} = 0.089\ H_{in} - 0.025\ A - 1.932\ [0.73\ 0.47]$$

$$FVC = 0.115\ H_{in} - 0.024\ A - 2.852\ [0.71\ 0.52]$$

Morris, J.F., et al.: Am. Rev. Respir. Dis., 103:57—67, 1971

Note: The predicted FEV$_1$ and FVC in non-Caucasians must be multiplied by 0.85.

Figure 12.   Spirometric standards for normal females (BTPS) [9] (derived from Morris et al. [12]).

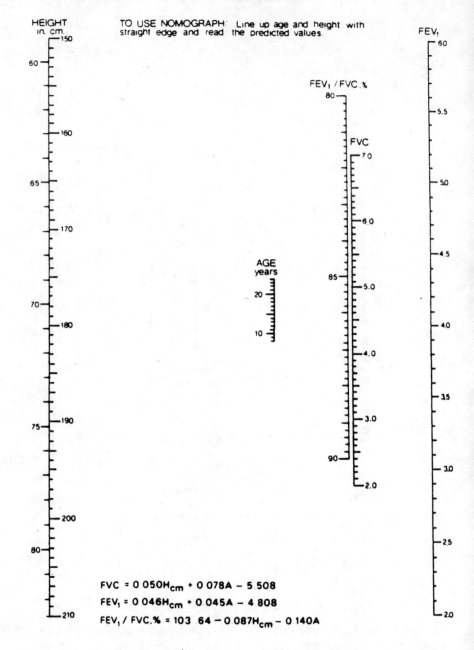

$$FVC = 0.050H_{cm} + 0.078A - 5.508$$
$$FEV_1 = 0.046H_{cm} + 0.045A - 4.808$$
$$FEV_1 / FVC.\% = 103.64 - 0.087H_{cm} - 0.140A$$

Figure 13.   Spirometric standards for normal males under 25 years of age [9].

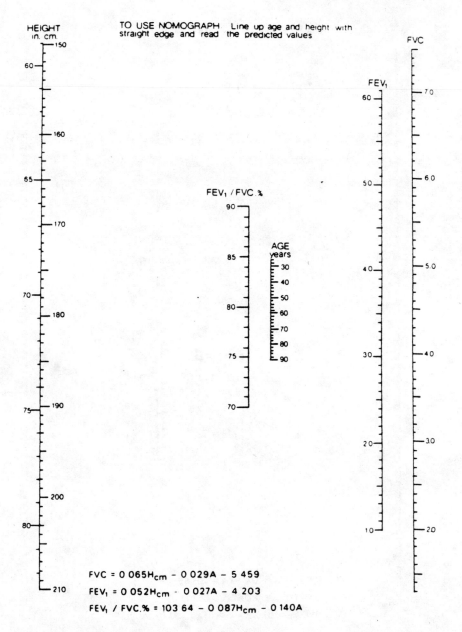

Figure 14.   Spirometric standards for normal males 25 years of age and over [9] (prepared by NIOSH, derived from Knudson [13]).

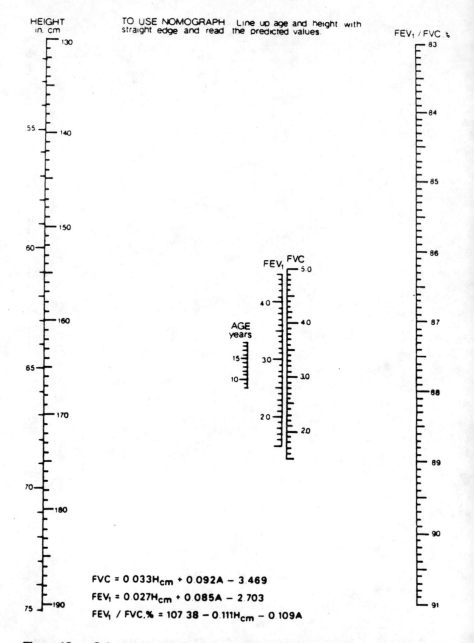

FVC = 0.033H$_{cm}$ + 0.092A − 3.469

FEV$_1$ = 0.027H$_{cm}$ + 0.085A − 2.703

FEV$_1$ / FVC.% = 107.38 − 0.111H$_{cm}$ − 0.109A

Figure 15. Spirometric standards for normal females under 20 years of age [9] (prepared by NIOSH, derived from Knudson et al. [13]).

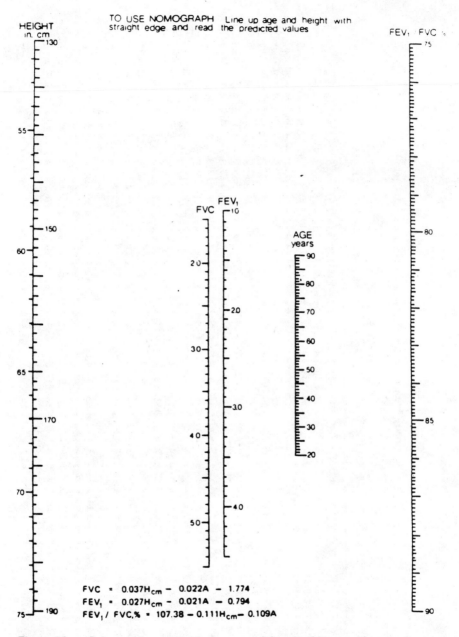

Figure 16. Spirometric standards for normal females 20 years of age and over [9] (prepared by NIOSH, derived from Knudson et al. [13]).

Table II.   Spirometry Prediction Tables for Normal Males and Females [9]

Predicted FVC for Males [13]

Height	Age 17	19	21	23	25	27	29	31	33	35	37	39	41	43	45	47	49	51	53	55	57	59	61	63	65
60.0	3.44	3.59	3.75	3.91	3.72	3.66	3.61	3.55	3.49	3.43	3.37	3.32	3.26	3.20	3.14	3.08	3.03	2.97	2.91	2.85	2.79	2.74	2.68	2.62	2.56
60.5	3.50	3.66	3.81	3.97	3.80	3.75	3.69	3.63	3.57	3.51	3.46	3.40	3.34	3.28	3.22	3.17	3.11	3.05	2.99	2.93	2.88	2.82	2.76	2.70	2.64
61.0	3.56	3.72	3.88	4.03	3.89	3.83	3.77	3.71	3.66	3.60	3.54	3.48	3.42	3.37	3.31	3.25	3.19	3.13	3.08	3.02	2.96	2.90	2.84	2.79	2.73
61.5	3.63	3.78	3.94	4.10	3.97	3.91	3.85	3.80	3.74	3.68	3.62	3.56	3.51	3.45	3.39	3.33	3.27	3.22	3.16	3.10	3.04	2.98	2.93	2.87	2.81
62.0	3.69	3.85	4.00	4.16	4.05	3.99	3.94	3.88	3.82	3.76	3.70	3.65	3.59	3.53	3.47	3.41	3.36	3.30	3.24	3.18	3.12	3.07	3.01	2.95	2.89
62.5	3.76	3.91	4.07	4.22	4.13	4.08	4.02	3.96	3.90	3.84	3.79	3.73	3.67	3.61	3.55	3.50	3.44	3.38	3.32	3.26	3.21	3.15	3.09	3.03	2.97
63.0	3.82	3.97	4.13	4.29	4.22	4.16	4.10	4.04	3.99	3.93	3.87	3.81	3.75	3.70	3.64	3.58	3.52	3.46	3.41	3.35	3.29	3.23	3.17	3.12	3.06
63.5	3.88	4.04	4.19	4.35	4.30	4.24	4.18	4.13	4.07	4.01	3.95	3.89	3.84	3.78	3.72	3.66	3.60	3.55	3.49	3.43	3.37	3.31	3.26	3.20	3.14
64.0	3.95	4.10	4.26	4.41	4.38	4.32	4.27	4.21	4.15	4.09	4.03	3.98	3.92	3.86	3.80	3.74	3.69	3.63	3.57	3.51	3.45	3.40	3.34	3.28	3.22
64.5	4.01	4.17	4.32	4.48	4.46	4.41	4.35	4.29	4.23	4.17	4.12	4.06	4.00	3.94	3.88	3.83	3.77	3.71	3.65	3.59	3.54	3.48	3.42	3.36	3.30
65.0	4.07	4.23	4.39	4.54	4.55	4.49	4.43	4.37	4.32	4.26	4.20	4.14	4.09	4.03	3.97	3.91	3.85	3.79	3.74	3.68	3.62	3.56	3.50	3.45	3.39
65.5	4.14	4.29	4.45	4.60	4.63	4.57	4.51	4.46	4.40	4.34	4.28	4.22	4.17	4.11	4.05	3.99	3.93	3.88	3.82	3.76	3.70	3.64	3.59	3.53	3.47
66.0	4.20	4.36	4.51	4.67	4.71	4.65	4.60	4.54	4.48	4.42	4.36	4.31	4.25	4.19	4.13	4.07	4.02	3.96	3.90	3.84	3.78	3.73	3.67	3.61	3.55
66.5	4.26	4.42	4.58	4.73	4.80	4.74	4.68	4.62	4.56	4.51	4.45	4.39	4.33	4.27	4.22	4.16	4.10	4.04	3.98	3.93	3.87	3.81	3.75	3.69	3.64
67.0	4.33	4.48	4.64	4.80	4.88	4.82	4.76	4.70	4.65	4.59	4.53	4.47	4.41	4.36	4.30	4.24	4.18	4.12	4.07	4.01	3.95	3.89	3.83	3.78	3.72
67.5	4.39	4.55	4.70	4.86	4.96	4.90	4.84	4.79	4.73	4.67	4.61	4.55	4.50	4.44	4.38	4.32	4.26	4.21	4.15	4.09	4.03	3.97	3.92	3.86	3.80
68.0	4.45	4.61	4.77	4.92	5.04	4.98	4.93	4.87	4.81	4.75	4.69	4.64	4.58	4.52	4.45	4.40	4.35	4.29	4.23	4.17	4.11	4.06	4.00	3.94	3.88
68.5	4.52	4.67	4.83	4.99	5.13	5.07	5.01	4.95	4.89	4.84	4.78	4.72	4.66	4.60	4.55	4.49	4.43	4.37	4.31	4.26	4.20	4.14	4.08	4.02	3.97
69.0	4.58	4.74	4.89	5.05	5.21	5.15	5.09	5.03	4.98	4.92	4.86	4.80	4.74	4.69	4.63	4.57	4.51	4.45	4.40	4.34	4.28	4.22	4.16	4.11	4.05
69.5	4.64	4.80	4.96	5.11	5.29	5.23	5.17	5.12	5.06	5.00	4.94	4.88	4.83	4.77	4.71	4.65	4.59	4.54	4.48	4.42	4.36	4.30	4.25	4.19	4.13
70.0	4.71	4.86	5.02	5.18	5.37	5.32	5.26	5.20	5.14	5.08	5.02	4.97	4.91	4.85	4.79	4.74	4.68	4.62	4.56	4.50	4.44	4.39	4.33	4.27	4.21
70.5	4.77	4.93	5.08	5.24	5.46	5.40	5.34	5.28	5.22	5.17	5.11	5.05	4.99	4.93	4.88	4.82	4.76	4.70	4.64	4.59	4.53	4.47	4.41	4.35	4.30
71.0	4.83	4.99	5.15	5.30	5.54	5.48	5.42	5.36	5.31	5.25	5.19	5.13	5.07	5.02	4.96	4.90	4.84	4.78	4.73	4.67	4.61	4.55	4.49	4.44	4.38
71.5	4.90	5.05	5.21	5.37	5.62	5.56	5.50	5.45	5.39	5.33	5.27	5.21	5.16	5.10	5.04	4.98	4.92	4.87	4.81	4.75	4.69	4.64	4.58	4.52	4.46
72.0	4.96	5.12	5.27	5.43	5.70	5.65	5.59	5.53	5.47	5.41	5.36	5.30	5.24	5.18	5.12	5.07	5.01	4.95	4.89	4.83	4.78	4.72	4.66	4.60	4.54
72.5	5.03	5.18	5.34	5.49	5.79	5.73	5.67	5.61	5.55	5.50	5.44	5.38	5.32	5.26	5.21	5.15	5.09	5.03	4.97	4.92	4.86	4.80	4.74	4.68	4.63

73.0	5.09	5.24	5.40	5.56	5.87	5.81	5.75	5.69	5.64	5.58	5.52	5.46	5.40	5.35	5.29	5.23	5.17	5.11	5.06	5.00	4.94	4.88	4.82	4.77	4.71
73.5	5.15	5.31	5.46	5.62	5.95	5.89	5.83	5.78	5.72	5.66	5.60	5.54	5.49	5.43	5.37	5.31	5.25	5.20	5.14	5.08	5.02	4.96	4.91	4.85	4.79
74.0	5.22	5.37	5.53	5.68	6.03	5.98	5.92	5.86	5.80	5.74	5.69	5.63	5.57	5.51	5.45	5.40	5.34	5.28	5.22	5.16	5.11	5.05	4.99	4.93	4.87
74.5	5.28	5.44	5.59	5.75	6.12	6.06	6.00	5.94	5.88	5.83	5.77	5.71	5.65	5.59	5.54	5.48	5.42	5.36	5.30	5.25	5.19	5.13	5.07	5.01	4.96
75.0	5.34	5.50	5.65	5.81	6.20	6.14	6.08	6.02	5.97	5.91	5.85	5.79	5.73	5.68	5.62	5.56	5.50	5.44	5.39	5.33	5.27	5.21	5.15	5.10	5.04
75.5	5.41	5.56	5.72	5.87	6.28	6.22	6.17	6.11	6.05	5.99	5.93	5.88	5.82	5.76	5.70	5.64	5.59	5.53	5.47	5.41	5.35	5.30	5.24	5.18	5.12
76.0	5.47	5.63	5.78	5.94	6.36	6.31	6.25	6.19	6.13	6.07	6.02	5.96	5.90	5.84	5.78	5.73	5.67	5.61	5.55	5.49	5.44	5.38	5.32	5.26	5.20
76.5	5.53	5.69	5.85	6.00	6.45	6.39	6.33	6.27	6.21	6.16	6.10	6.04	5.98	5.92	5.87	5.81	5.75	5.69	5.63	5.58	5.52	5.46	5.40	5.34	5.29
77.0	5.60	5.75	5.91	6.06	6.53	6.47	6.41	6.35	6.30	6.24	6.18	6.12	6.06	6.01	5.95	5.89	5.83	5.77	5.72	5.66	5.60	5.54	5.48	5.43	5.37
77.5	5.66	5.82	5.97	6.13	6.61	6.55	6.50	6.44	6.38	6.32	6.26	6.21	6.15	6.09	6.03	5.97	5.92	5.86	5.80	5.74	5.68	5.63	5.57	5.51	5.45
78.0	5.72	5.88	6.04	6.19	6.69	6.64	6.58	6.52	6.46	6.40	6.35	6.29	6.23	6.17	6.11	6.06	6.00	5.94	5.88	5.82	5.77	5.71	5.65	5.59	5.53
78.5	5.79	5.94	6.10	6.26	6.78	6.72	6.66	6.60	6.54	6.49	6.43	6.37	6.31	6.25	6.20	6.14	6.08	6.02	5.96	5.91	5.85	5.79	5.73	5.67	5.62
79.0	5.85	6.01	6.16	6.32	6.86	6.80	6.74	6.68	6.63	6.57	6.51	6.45	6.39	6.34	6.28	6.22	6.16	6.10	6.05	5.99	5.93	5.87	5.81	5.76	5.70
79.5	5.91	6.07	6.23	6.38	6.94	6.88	6.83	6.77	6.71	6.65	6.59	6.54	6.48	6.42	6.36	6.30	6.25	6.19	6.13	6.07	6.01	5.96	5.90	5.84	5.78
80.0	5.98	6.13	6.29	6.45	7.02	6.97	6.91	6.85	6.79	6.73	6.68	6.62	6.56	6.50	6.44	6.39	6.33	6.27	6.21	6.15	6.10	6.04	5.98	5.92	5.86
80.5	6.04	6.20	6.35	6.51	7.11	7.05	6.99	6.93	6.87	6.82	6.76	6.70	6.64	6.58	6.53	6.47	6.41	6.35	6.29	6.24	6.18	6.12	6.06	6.00	5.95
81.0	6.10	6.26	6.42	6.57	7.19	7.13	7.07	7.02	6.96	6.90	6.84	6.78	6.73	6.67	6.61	6.55	6.49	6.44	6.38	6.32	6.26	6.21	6.15	6.09	6.03
81.5	6.17	6.32	6.48	6.64	7.27	7.21	7.16	7.10	7.04	6.98	6.92	6.87	6.81	6.75	6.69	6.63	6.58	6.52	6.46	6.40	6.34	6.29	6.23	6.17	6.11
82.0	6.23	6.39	6.55	6.70	7.35	7.30	7.24	7.18	7.12	7.06	7.01	6.95	6.89	6.83	6.77	6.72	6.66	6.60	6.54	6.48	6.43	6.37	6.31	6.25	6.19
82.5	6.30	6.45	6.61	6.76	7.44	7.38	7.32	7.26	7.20	7.15	7.09	7.03	6.97	6.91	6.86	6.80	6.74	6.68	6.62	6.57	6.51	6.45	6.39	6.33	6.28
83.0	6.36	6.51	6.67	6.83	7.52	7.46	7.40	7.35	7.29	7.23	7.17	7.11	7.06	7.00	6.94	6.88	6.82	6.77	6.71	6.65	6.59	6.53	6.48	6.42	6.36
83.5	6.42	6.58	6.73	6.89	7.60	7.54	7.49	7.43	7.37	7.31	7.25	7.20	7.14	7.08	7.02	6.96	6.91	6.85	6.79	6.73	6.67	6.62	6.56	6.50	6.44
84.0	6.49	6.64	6.80	6.95	7.68	7.63	7.57	7.51	7.45	7.39	7.34	7.28	7.22	7.16	7.10	7.05	6.99	6.93	6.87	6.81	6.76	6.70	6.64	6.58	6.52
84.5	6.55	6.71	6.86	7.02	7.77	7.71	7.65	7.59	7.53	7.48	7.42	7.36	7.30	7.24	7.19	7.13	7.07	7.01	6.95	6.90	6.84	6.78	6.72	6.66	6.61
85.0	66.1	6.77	6.92	7.08	7.85	7.79	7.73	7.68	7.62	7.56	7.50	7.44	7.39	7.33	7.27	7.21	7.15	7.10	7.04	6.98	6.92	6.86	6.81	6.75	6.69

sustained at the workplace. However, several large corporations sold their manufacturing operations to employees, who now run the plant themselves. For example, General Motors sold the Hyatt Bearing Plant in Linden, New Jersey to the employees. In this situation would employees sue themselves? Perhaps government agencies should be available to consult with companies and groups of this type about this problem on a more frequent basis.

APPENDIX D—PULMONARY FUNCTION STANDARDS FOR COTTON DUST STANDARD

The spirometric measurements of pulmonary function shall conform to the following minimum standards, and these standards are not intended to preclude additional testing or alternate methods which can be determined to be superior.

I. APPARATUS

a. The instrument shall be accurate to within ±50 milliliters or within ±3 percent of reading, whichever is greater.

b. The instrument should be capable of measuring vital capacity from 0 to 7 liters BTPS.

c. The instrument shall have a low inertia and offer low resistance to airflow such that the resistance to airflow at 12 liters per second must be less than 1.5 cm H_2O/(liter/sec).

d. The zero time point for the purpose of timing the FEV_1 shall be determined by extrapolating the steepest portion of the volume time curve back to the maximal inspiration volume (1, 2, 3, 4) or by an equivalent method.

e. Instruments incorporating measurements of airflow to determine volume shall conform to the same volume accuracy stated in (a) of this section when presented with flow rates from at least 0 to 12 liters per second.

f. The instrument or user of the instrument must have a means of correcting volumes to body temperature saturated with water vapor (BTPS) under conditions of varying ambient spirometer temperatures and barometric pressures.

g. The instrument used shall provide a tracing or display of either flow versus volume or volume versus time during the entire forced expiration. A tracing or display is necessary to determine whether the patient has performed the test properly. The tracing must be stored and available for recall and must be of sufficient size that hand measurements may be made within requirement of paragraph (a) of this section. If a paper record is made it must have a paper speed of at least 2 cm/sec and a volume sensitivity of at least 10.0 mm of chart per liter of volume.

h. The instrument shall be capable of accumulating volume for a minimum of 10 seconds and shall not stop accumulating volume before (1) volume change for a 0.5 second interval is less than 25 milliliters or (2) the flow is less than 50 milliliters per second for a 0.5 second interval.

i. The forced vital capacity (FVC) and forced expiratory volume in 1 second (FEV_1) measurements shall comply with the accuracy requirements stated in paragraph (a) of this section. That is, they should be accurately measured to within ±50 ml or within ±3 percent of reading, whichever is greater.

j. The instrument must be capable of being calibrated in the field with respect to the FEV_1 and FVC. This calibration of the FEV_1 and FVC may be either directly or indirectly through volume and time base measurements. The volume calibration source should provide a volume displacement of at least 2 liters and should be accurate to within ±30 milliliters.

II. TECHNIQUE FOR MEASUREMENT OF FORCED VITAL CAPACITY MANEUVER

a. Use of a nose clip is recommended but not required. The procedures shall be explained in simple terms to the patient who shall be instructed to loosen any tight clothing and stand in front of the apparatus. The subject may sit, but care should be taken on repeat testing that the same position be used and, if possible, the same spirometer. Particular attention shall be given to insure that the chin is slightly elevated with the neck slightly extended. The patient shall be instructed to make a full inspiration from a normal breathing pattern and then blow into the apparatus, without interruption, as hard, fast, and completely as possible. At least three forced expirations shall be carried out. During the maneuvers, the patient shall be observed for compliance with instruction. The expirations shall be checked visually for reproducibility from flow-volume or volume-time tracings or displays. The following efforts shall be judged unacceptable when the patient:

1. has not reached full inspiration preceding the forced expiration,

2. has not used maximal effort during the entire forced expiration,

3. has not continued the expiration for at least 5 seconds or until an obvious plateau in the volume time curve has occurred,

4. has coughed or closed his glottis,

5. has an obstructed mouthpiece or a leak around the mouthpiece (obstruction due to tongue being placed in front of mouthpiece, false teeth falling in front of mouthpiece, etc.)

6. has an unsatisfactory start of expiration, one characterized by excessive hesitation (or false starts), and therefore not allowing back extrapolation of time 0 (extrapolated volume on the volume time tracing must be less than 10 percent of the FVC.)

7. has an excessive variability between the three acceptable curves. The variation between the two largest FVC's and FEV_1's of the three satisfactory tracings should not exceed 10 percent or ± 100 milliliters, whichever is greater.

b. Periodic and routine recalibration of the instrument or method for recording FVC and FEV_1 should be performed using a syringe or other volume source of at least 2 liters.

III. INTERPRETATION OF SPIROGRAM

a. The first step in evaluating a spirogram should be to determine whether or not the patient has performed the test properly or as described in II above. From the three satisfactory tracings, the forced vital capacity (FVC) and forced expiratory volume in 1 second (FEV_1) shall be measured and recorded. The largest observed FVC and largest observed FEV_1 shall be used in the analysis regardless of the curve(s) on which they occur.

b. The following guidelines are recommended by NIOSH for the evaluation and management of workers exposed to cotton dust. It is important to note that employees who show reductions in FEV₁/FVC ratio below .75 or drops in Monday FEV₁ of 5 percent or greater on their initial screening exam, should be re-evaluated within a month of the first exam. Those who show consistent decrease in lung function, as shown on the following table, should be managed as recommended.

IV. QUALIFICATIONS OF PERSONNEL
ADMINISTERING THE TEST

Technicians who perform pulmonary function testing should have the basic knowledge required to produce meaningful results. Training consisting of approximately 16 hours of formal instruction should cover the following areas.

a. Basic physiology of the forced vital capacity maneuver and the determinants of airflow limitation with emphasis on

the relation to reproducibility of results.

b. Instrumentation requirements including calibration procedures, sources of error and their correction.

c. Performance of the testing including subject coaching, recognition of improperly performed maneuvers and corrective actions.

d. Data quality with emphasis on reproducibility.

e. Actual use of the equipment under supervised conditions.

f. Measurement of tracings and calculations of results.

[43 F.R. 27394, June 23, 1978.]

[corrected at 43 F.R. 28473, June 30, 1978, and 43 F.R. 35032, August 8, 1978.]

Figure 17.   Standards and interpretations [8].

Decisions concerning respirators also must consider the protection afforded by it and the consequences of not wearing it or wearing it improperly. Most plant managers who deal with OSHA do not realize the potential harm that employees may encounter in the workplace. If they did, respirators would be used.

AUTOMATED BREATHING
METABOLIC SIMULATOR (ABMS)

Scanning the available literature on respirators, one notes the minimal success achieved in developing apparatus to simulate breathing. Using computers and mechanical simulation, IBM Corp. designed and fabricated (for the Bureau of Mines, Dust Control and Life Support Group in Pittsburgh), a mechanical man, which simulates man's respiratory and metabolic functions during a sequence of assorted work tasks [15,16].

For each work task, the breathing rate, breathing depth energy expenditure, functional residual capacity (amount of air remaining in the lungs at the end of expiration) and breathing waveform are simulated. The Bureau of Mines requires breathing apparatus to be used in simulated rescue activities—climbing, running and lifting—for varying time periods. As the various activities require varying levels of oxygen and carbon dioxide, exhalations are produced. Therefore, a researcher can examine at length the performance of the apparatus under a sequence of controlled test conditions. Figure 18 illustrates the ABMS system, whose goal is to produce more extensive and safer evaluations in hazardous environments when human fatigue is the limiting factor.

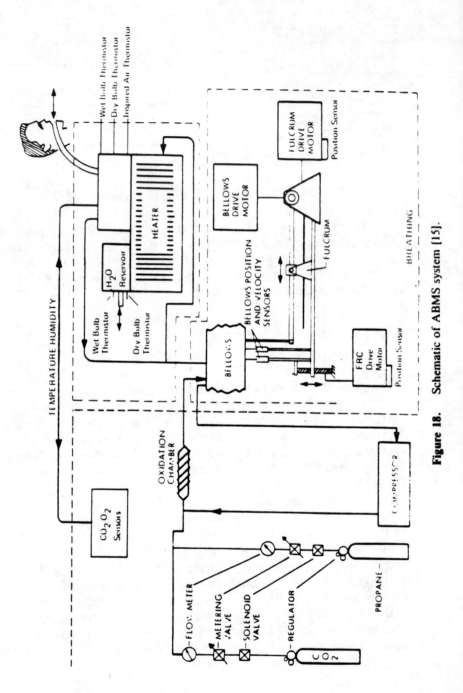

Figure 18. Schematic of ABMS system [15].

All functions can be remotely controlled from either the operational console during manual control, or the computer when in the automatic mode. With computer control, a sequence of test conditions, breathing and metabolic states, can be programmed. Also, the tests can be conducted for several hours with no operator intervention. Figure 19 illustrates the ABMS software program subroutines during simulation of a steady-state work test.

The machine is not only the state-of-the-art of test equipment, but represents the rapid development of respirators and human engineer-biomechanical simulation fields.

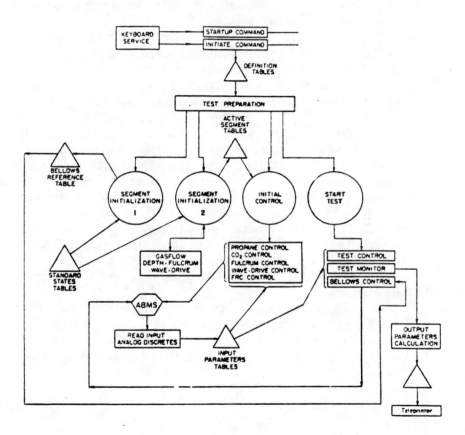

Figure 19.   Schematic of the ABMS software program subroutines during simulation of a steady-state work test [15].

DRUGS AND THE INDIVIDUAL
WEARING A RESPIRATOR

Drugs should be taken only with the direct consent of the physician who is familiar with the person's medical history, medical tests, physical examinations and job description. Persons who take spirogram tests are asked whether they have used a bronchodilator. Drugs can be used to cause bronchodilation, which increases the size of the bronchioles and the alveolar ducts and decreases resistance to airflow, resulting in a more normal, or increased volume, spirogram. Epinephine and isoproternol are two aerosol bronchodilators that were used in the early 1970s. They decrease both congestion in the respiratory tract through vasconstriction and mucous membrane swelling [17].

Most employees in dusty areas generally take some medication through the day, whether it is an alcoholic beverage, medicine that can be purchased over the counter, or medicine prescribed without the physician being aware of the working conditions. Even at low levels, throats become dry and irritable, and an employee looks for simple relief. Many simple, unobtrusive dusts such as flour and similar grains dry out the throat. The body response is a protective reflex to clear the respiratory tract of irritants and accumulated secretions. Frequent and prolonged coughing can be exhausting, painful and taxing to the circulatory system and the elastic tissue of the respiratory system. Cough-suppressant medications include narcotic as well as nonnarcotic antitussives, demulcents, antiseptics, expectorants, etc. Demulcents are the sticky substances that protect the lining of the respiratory tract from the irritation caused by air passing back and forth during inhalation and exhalation. Cough syrups, honey and hard candy are common in this group. Expectorants reduce the viscosity of the mucous in the bronchi and aid in the expulsion of secretions.

As coughing and mucous secretion affect the performance of the respirator, extremely dry areas should be examined and possibly humidified. Coughing generally is a positive indication that the wearer has either experienced problems or that the respirator is not functioning correctly.

CHAPTER 3

INTRODUCTION

To select the proper respirator for use in an environment, the constituents of that environment must be determined as accurately as possible. The different types, concentrations and toxic effects of this environment must be analyzed carefully by a trained industrial hygienist, safety engineer or medical professional. These professionals depend on research data on various substances, and their effects on biological systems and living organisms, whether they be plants, animals or humans. This chapter presents the history, basic terminology, and research methods of the field of toxicology to aid the user in understanding the potential hazard.

HISTORY

Medically speaking, toxicology usually referred to the study of poisons. This stems from early Greek and Roman experiments with various plant poisons and chemical mixtures to be used in warfare. The history of poisons and their use is the basis of retrospective diagnosis [18,19]. Catherine de Medici is considered to have been the first untrained experimental toxicologist. Under the guise of delivering to the sick and the poor, she tested toxic concoctions, carefully noting the rapidity of the toxic response, the effectiveness of the compound (potency), the degree of response of the parts of the body (site of action) and the complaints of the victim (clinical signs and symptoms). Various individuals have been credited with having been the fathers of toxicology; however, today most industrial hygienists, medical and technical people rely on the *Essentials of Toxicology*, by Loomis [20], and *Toxicology, the Basic Science of Poisons*, by Casarett and Doull [21].

Most toxicological research falls into three main categories: environmental, economic and forensic. **Environmental** concerns pollution, residues and industrial hygiene. **Economic** areas involve drugs, food additives, pesticides and insecticides. **Forensic** areas include diagnosis, therapy and medical/legal aspects.

The respirator user is concerned with the work done by groups such as the American Conference of Governmental Industrial Hygienists and the American Industrial Hygiene Association. As early as the 1940s, these groups began to publish lists of commonly encountered chemicals and their tolerable level of worker exposure. For the first time, groups in various segments of industry and government began to correlate these data and seek common grounds in the development of health standards. With the passage of the Occupational Safety & and Health Act of 1970 (OSHA) and the creation of The National Institute of Safety & Health (NIOSH), the mechanism for implementing and enforcing the standards of employee exposure and research finally arrived at the industrial level.

BASIC TERMINOLOGY

Toxicology, as all sciences, has its own terminology. The most basic term is **exposure.** Exposure is the length of time an individual is in contact with a substance. The period of time may be short, usually referred to as being acute, or long, referred to as being chronic.

As in any investigation, the next questions concern how the individual came in contact with the material or what was the route of entry of the material into the body or system. Was it absorbed through the skin, ingested through the gastrointestinal tract or inhaled by breathing? Of the three methods of entry, inhalation is regarded as the most important because it is probably the most frequent point of entry. Substances suspended in the air in the form of fumes, mist or vapors, dusts (particulate) or gases are breathed in easily through the nose and mouth and can be deposited in the lungs. Some of the material passes through the alveoli directly into the blood. Other materials may be acted on by the gastrointestinal tract or the lymphatic system.

As in a chemical reaction, the rate at which the material enters the body depends on the concentration of material, the dose to which the individual is exposed and how fast the material can pass through the body's cell membranes and protective reactions.

In respiratory protection, the objective is to prevent these materials from entering the body system, but the knowledge that the material ultimately will end up in a specific organ is the only proof that a respirator is effective. If that organ is accumulating the material that the respirator is designed to protect against, another type of respirator or additional control methods must be instituted immediately.

Generally, the organs most commonly affected by chemicals in the blood are the liver and kidneys. They have a high capacity to extract many chemicals, and the liver has a high capacity to metabolize them. Two other areas of concern are bone cells and fat cells. Chemicals such as DDT usually are found in the fatty tissues of man, and more than 85% of the lead in the body is found in the skeleton (bone structure). Methods of respiratory protection are designed to protect those exposed to lead and most pesticides, so correlations are possible between deposition of these materials in areas of the body and respiratory effectiveness. Generally, the U.S. Department of Labor (OSHA) refers to blood-lead levels in industrial experiences to determine exposure to lead.

As mentioned earlier, the body has several defense mechanisms that are important and should be examined. In the measurement of the time a substance is retained in the body, the biological half-life [22] (the time in which one-half the compound present in the body is eliminated from the body) is of great importance. For example, caffeine has a biological half-life of four hours. Substances or chemicals that are absorbed into the body's cells sometimes are bound to a protein and removed by excretion by the kidneys. Researchers in the respiratory protection field are concerned with the excretion of carbon dioxide. The physician is concerned that blood pH level remain normal. Blood pH level is determined by the ratio of bicarbonate ion concentration to CO_2 concentration, normally 20:1, a ratio physiologically maintained by means of disposal of CO_2 by the lungs and bicarbonate by the kidneys.

Biotransformation is the ability of a cell to alter normally existing and foreign compounds, which change into more or less toxic levels than the original chemical. Drug-metabolizing enzymes, abundant in liver cells, usually are involved in the biotransformations.

TOXIC RESPONSES

As mentioned in the introduction, death could be the most immediate response to a toxic substance. The problem with toxic substances that cause dysfunction of an organ or system of the body is the time between exposure and onset of the disease or illness. Reuse of the organ may be partial or complete, but of major concern is the attitude of the respirator user. A common problem can be illustrated as follows: an employee is told he will become sick within 20 to 30 years if he does not wear a respirator. The employee is 50 years old and does not expect to live to be 70. At 68 years of age, another individual, who was not required to wear a respirator 18 years earlier, retires from the firm with a pension—and cancer. He sues the company for $12 million, claiming willful disregard for his health and stating that the company knew or suspected that the material he was working with could cause cancer. This type of situation keeps enrollment in law schools almost as high as the legal fees involved in settling the case. Basically, eight typical responses are observed:

Type	Example/Response
1. Behavioral	Oxygen deficiencies/loss of perception Mercury/emotional problems
2. Biochemical	Organophosphorus insecticides/prohibit acetylcholinesterase/result in nerve tremors
3. Carcinogenic	Vinyl chloride/cancer of the liver
4. Mutagenic	DNA and gene changes in infants
5. Pathological	Silica/lung tissue is deformed
6. Physiological	Ammonia gas/decreased pulmonary function
7. Reproductive	Cadmium/affects the reproductive organs and their ability to function properly
8. Teratogenic	Thalidomide/damage to a developing offspring in a pregnant female

The respiratory tract from the nasal cavities and mouth to the lungs is lined by delicate cells covered by a moist mucous layer. Various chemicals and their compounds can attack this lining and the lungs, producing a variety of results. The most common substances are those that are either acidic or alkaline, which irritate this area and cause inflammation. It is very difficult to distinguish a common throat irritation from inflammation caused by toxic substances in the early stages. The solubility of the material is usually a key factor. Materials that dissolve in the blood are removed. Ethyl ether, for example, is absorbed by the alveoli and does not accumulate to cause damage. Nitrogen dioxide does not dissolve, so it tends to pass onto and irritate the lungs. A common problem with MIG welders of aluminum is that the ozone produced tends to make the walls of the alveoli less elastic, so more effort is required to breathe.

The most common of the lung and respiratory diseases is "pneumoceniosis." It generally means dust in the lung, but really describes a tissue response of the lung to inhaled dust or fibers. Dust generally causes the respirator user the greatest problems. In the past, when miners used nonautomatic or pneumatic tools and drilling equipment, they claimed that the particles were larger and more easily removed by the lungs. Black lung, a type of pneumoconiosis, resulted from the use of automatic equipment. The automatic equipment removed more coal but generated more dust, which either was not removed by ventilation or overloaded the filters used in prevailing respirators. The respirators used created too much of a pulmonary strain on lungs that already were reduced in capacity by years of working in the mines. Once clogged, the respirator strained the wearer to the point where he removed it.

The energy shortage and environmental protection legislation of the middle and late 1970s raised the question of what to do with the dust generated by the typical operations. However, pollution control operations were not cost-effective, causing many small organizations to shut down and severely cutting into profits of many others.

Most textbooks on dust generally deal with it in two categories: fibrogenic and nonfibrogenic. OSHA and ACGIH literature define a fiber as a particle whose length is three times its mean diameter. As most of these fibers tend to be like bundles containing several filaments per bundle, extreme caution should be emphasized for this type of exposure. Asbestos is a typical example.

Silicosis is the classic example of pneumoceniosis. The lung's protective system tries to remove the silica particles by phagocytizing or engulfing them. The silica destroys the phagocytes, and other phagocytes form layer-nodules, which usually are detected by X-rays. Foundry workers exposed to silica experienced relief when green olivine, nonsilica sands were used. OSHA's National Emphasis Foundry Program (1976–1978) experienced some very good results after switching to this type of sand.

The most widely publicized lung-induced disease is asbestosis. This disease results from the chronic inhalation of asbestos, a group of chain silicates that occur in natural forms. Asbestosis may not become apparent until 5–20 years after exposure to asbestos. Although there is strong legal evidence that impairment results from asbestos, what of the employees who worked 30 years in asbestos plants and did not get cancer? In the opinion of the authors, two developments probably will take place due to increased research in respiratory diseases. The first will be to develop a class of chelating type agents to remove or dissolve various substances deposited in the lung. Presently, chelating agents are used to remove lead from the body. The second will be better respiratory equipment to protect the worker from hazards.

The most common form of lung problem that produces immediate death is asphyxia—lack of oxygen sufficient to endanger life. Every year, firemen, utility workers, coal miners, bin and silo workers are exposed to air with concentrations of oxygen less than the normal 16–19.5% by volume. As in other places in the literature, however, the values are not consistent. OSHA values vary from 16.0 to 19.5% of the volume of the atmosphere. OSHA Maritime Standard 1915.81 uses 16.0% oxygen, and the General Industry Standard 1910.94 (ventilation) uses 19.5% oxygen. Physiologically, anoxia is the diminished availability of oxygen to the cells of the body, while asphyxia is the condition of the body due to anoxia. The following data record the oxygen level versus physiological effect [23].

Oxygen—Volume Percent at Sea Level	Physiological Effect
16–12	Increased breathing volume, accelerated heartbeat, impaired attention and thinking, impaired coordination.
14–10	Faulty judgment, very poor muscular coordination, rapid fatigue that may cause rapid heart damage.
10–6	Nausea, vomiting, inability to perform vigorous movement or loss of movement—unconsciousness.
Less than 6%	Death in minutes.

Another form of asphyxia, chemical asphyxia, is common in carbon monoxide deaths. When inhaled, carbon monoxide gas reacts with the hemoglobin, the oxygen carrier in the blood, to form carboxyhemoglobin. The individual dies of oxygen deficiency. A common symptom at low levels of exposure is headache. Higher levels of exposure are usually identified by high levels of redness of the skin.

TESTING WITH ANIMALS

Experimentation on animals is the accepted method for determining toxicity. As a note of caution, however, little is known about the effect of the low dose rates on animals that survive. Some state that there are no safe levels of carcinogens, while some agree that "feasible engineering controls" can reduce the current TLV to an acceptable OSHA level. In regard to the number of animals necessary to determine a low level response, "In essence, as the magnitude of the effect (or its incidence) tends toward zero, the number of experimental subjects needed to demonstrate the effect tends toward infinity" [22].

Experimental animals should be physically small, inexpensive, easily handled, easily fed with inexpensive food, not dangerous to man by direct attack, and (if possible) of a standardized strain of the species used. The life span of the animal is important, as well as its ability to breed easily in captivity. For special purposes, monkeys and apes are chosen. Of great importance here is that the animal be physiologically comparable to the human with regard to the site of toxic action. A classic case was the testing of the drug Thalidomide. This supposedly mild sedative produced more than 10,000 malformed children in Germany, Japan and other parts of the world. Subsequent studies revealed that Thalidomide caused malformations only when taken by pregnant women between days 35 and 50. Prior to, or after, that time, there was no effect on the developing child. Animals tested with the drug showed no sign of birth defects.

Another important aspect is the relative size and weight of the test animal. Table III compares the dosage of the substance by weight and surface area to different species. These data indicate the amount of material that must be fed to the animals [21].

In 1959 the U.S. Public Health Service (USPHS) [24] published criteria for design of exposure chambers. They had to meet three basic criteria:

1. They had to be dynamic air systems.
2. They had to remove toxic products to avoid danger to laboratory personnel.
3. They had to provide accurate determination of the contaminants.

The dynamic air systems required a constant flow of clean air that could be metered over a suitable flow range, as well as apparatus for introducing the contaminant uniformly into the chamber. Most multiple cham-

Table III. Comparison of Dosage by Weight and Surface Area (100 mg/kg) [20]

Species	Weight (g)	Surface (cm²)	Dose by Weight (mg)	Dose by Surface (mg)	Ratio
Mouse	20	46	2	2	1.00
Rat	200	325	20	14	1.43
Guinea Pig	400	564	40	24	1.65
Rabbit	1,500	1,272	150	55	2.74
Cat	2,000	1,381	200	60	3.46
Monkey	4,000	2,975	400	128	3.12
Dog	12,000	5,766	1,200	248	4.82
Man	70,000	18,000	7,000	776	9.08

bers required a cooling system to remove heat generated by the animal above a central point. Door seals had to be under negative pressure so material would not escape from the chambers.

Chamber shape and air movement are important design considerations. The inlet and exhaust are designed so concentrations of air contaminants are uniform across a horizontal cross section of the chamber. Large access doors provide for the efficient loading and unloading of the animal cages. It is suggested that toxicity is often markedly greater in animals being exercised than in sedentary animals in the same atmosphere. To simulate this, rats were exercised in revolving cylindrical wire cages 18 inches in diameter and 24 inches long, rotating at 6.5 rpm. A treadmill also was constructed to simulate conditions for dogs. Although exposure chambers varied according to the size and type of material tested, pilot chambers or small test chambers were constructed for the LD_{50} values and short-term tests.

In the areas of operation and performance, injecting a dust uniformly into the chamber was the major problem. The size of the respirable particles tested, 0.01–5.0 μ in diameter, tended to collect on the animals' fur and then on the cages. As the instruments varied that were used to feed the dust into the chamber, an average reading was taken, and 100-day periods of chamber operation were compared using various dusts. The accuracy was sufficient and the results were reproducible.

Liquid aerosols had droplets with diameters that ranged in size from 0.01 to 5.0 μ to ensure penetration past the upper respiratory tree. As the liquids have an appreciable vapor pressure, the spray or mist test agent will be present in the vapor, as well as in the liquid, phase. Here, the chamber temperature controls are important because the droplets could condense on the cages. The diameter of any single droplet is not fixed because materials with a greater vapor pressure are in the process of constant evaporation. Here again, only a trained toxicologist can interpret data on animals with long fur, considering the amount of absorption through the skin and that exposure through fur might have a greater toxic effect than exposure by inhalation.

The use of gas contaminants usually produces greater accuracy. Its known concentrations, chemical analysis and ease of distribution make gas a much easier material with which to work. However, research by analytical gas companies indicates that mixed gases separate under high pressure over time. There has been some controversy as to whether published TLV values are too high or too low. Published data [25,26] listed vinyl chloride as 1000 ppm in 1943 by agreement of the states; in 1950 it was reduced to 500 ppm.

The present work was based on "Acute Response of Guinea Pigs to Vapor of Vinyl Chloride'' [27]. The current OSHA standard (1910.1017C) for the permissible exposure limit of vinyl chloride states that no employee may be exposed to it at concentrations greater than 1 ppm averaged over any eight-hour period [28], which represents quite a large drop during the last 30 years.

Additional areas of importance include the following: (1) well-balanced diet; (2) sleep; (3) ban on smoking; and (4) care that animals not be overworked.

ROUTES OF ENTRY

Percutaneous Route

The various basic concepts of toxicology have been discussed. In applying them to the respirator user, we will try to correlate these basics with actual field problems. As a respirator is designed to protect the lungs and inhalation system, the skin often is neglected or disregarded. Most respirators disregard the skin and concern themselves only with about 10 square inches of skin covering the nose and mouth. Many substances such as alkaloids may pass freely through the skin. Lipid-soluble compounds such as phenol and phenolic derivatives are readily absorbed into the skin. Strychnine and nicotine, common organic compounds, also can be absorbed into the skin, as well as hormones such as estrogen and progesterone. Therefore, the respirator may offer false comfort if protective clothing is not also worn where required.

Oral exposure is also a problem for workers who do not have a lunch room, smoking area and lavatories to wash properly. The common route of exposure to body lead is often cigarettes left in an open shirt pocket and smoked with dirty hands while the respirator rubs on a shirt with lead dust.

Common in laboratory animal testing is the parenteral route of entry, which, by definition, is as follows: introduction of chemicals into the organism by means of injection of the chemical from a syringe through a hollow needle at specific sites in the animal. As animal testing is very common, the typical method of administration of the test chemical is as:

- Skin (intradermal)
- Beneath the skin (subcutaneous)
- In the muscle (intramuscular)
- Into the blood of the veins (intravenous)
- Into the spinal fluid (intrathecal)

- Into the chest fluid (intrapleural)
- Into the abdominal fluid (intraperitoneal)
- Into single cells (intracellular)—by use of micropipettes

Two common examples of workers who experience fluid injected into their skin are: (1) diesel mechanics, who put their fingers on the diesel fuel injector port, causing the fluid to be injected under the skin; and (2) painters, who use the high-pressure (3000 psi) paint systems with solvent when cleaning the spray gun. As a large volume of the data in toxicology is acquired in studies in which animals are injected, the toxicologist should be consulted before any comparison is made to the other methods.

The most important route of entry to respirator users is inhalation. Every day workers are exposed to particulates, vapors, and gases, or combinations of the three. Most normal manufacturing operations produce these when materials are added, mixed, poured, welded, machined, shaped, cleaned or painted to produce a product. Particulates generally are defined further in the following categories [29]:

1. **Mechanical dispersoid**—particulates of solid or liquid matter formed and dispersed into the air by mechanical means, such as grinding, crushing, drilling, blasting and spraying.
2. **Condensation particulates**—solid or liquid matter formed and dispersed into air by reactions such as combustion.
3. **Dust**—a dust dispersed phase is a solid mechanical dispersoid ranging in size from submicroscopic to visible.
4. **Spray and mist**—a liquid splashed onto the surface for coating or cleaning. While droplets the size of sprays are visible, a mist droplet is not.
5. **Fume**—the condensation of a liquid into a solid, typically a welding alloy. The particles are extremely small, generally less than 1 μm in diameter.
6. **Fog**—a mist dense enough to obscure vision.
7. **Smoke**—the products of incomplete combustion of organic substances in the form of solid and liquid particles suspended in air and gaseous products mixed with air. It is visible and generally obscures vision.

Considering that these various physical states are inhaled easily by the operator and people in adjacent areas, the exposure can be significant.

Dose Response

Of major concern is the **safe level** for a particular substance. Historically, the material tested was to be used as a poison, thus pioneering the **lethal dose** concept. Certain species of animals are fed increasingly higher doses of a substance until the response is death. Lethal dose—the amount to kill 100% of a certain species—or LD_{100}, was born. Lethal doses for 5, 20, 30, 50, 70, and 90% also were established. With the high cost of animal testing, the LD_{50} is generally referenced most. Figure 20 shows two hypothetical dose-response curves for two chemical agents— the LD_{50} lines. That one substance is safer than another is illustrated by the two different LD_5's and LD_{50}'s on the graph. Substance D killed more animals at LD_5 than substance C, but substance C killed more animals at LD_{50} than substance D. The hypothetical dose-response curve for different bodily response typically is divided by parallel sections (Figure 21). The first zone is the unit of normal adjustment of the body. This means that the body is using a defense mechanism to remove the material—excretion, for example. The second zone, or limit of compensation without injury, tries to differentiate between health and impairment. The third area of limit of repair when exposure ceases usually refers to the body's ability to heal itself. The limit of survival with permanent disability is self-explanatory. It should be noted that different studies have arranged toxicological data to illustrate the relative safety or hazard of the substance, depending on whether the data were aimed at

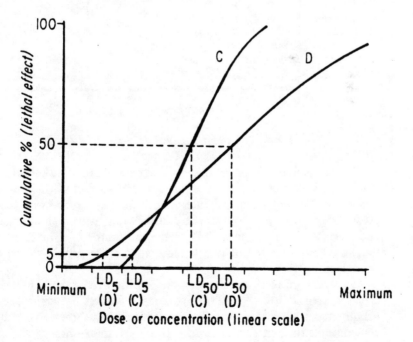

Figure 20. Hypothetical dose-response curves for two chemical agents (C and D) administered to a uniform population of biological specimens [20].

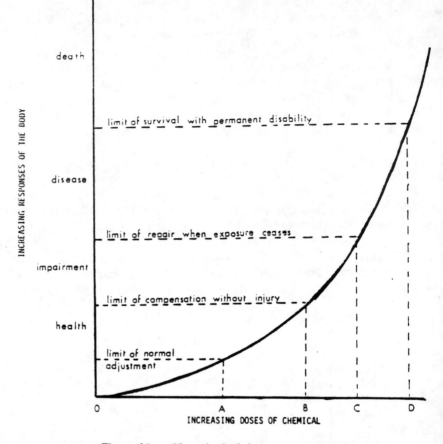

Figure 21.   Hypothetical dose-response curve.

justifying the material or having it removed from the marketplace. Pharmacologists use the relation of lethal dose 50 to effective dose 50 to relate a margin of a drug's safety or therapeutic index. Anyone who has read a prescription drug package recently knows that warnings are numerous and specify a doctor's advice. With the thousands of substances used in the work environment, it is a wonder that more problems are not encountered.

As usually more than one substance is involved in an operation, the term "synergistic" or "combined response" is used. Synergistic responses usually mean additive in nature, but research has shown that substances can combine to form less hazardous responses than when exposed to only one substance at a time. Table IV summarizes classifications categorizing relative toxicities.

Table IV.   Summary of the Classification that Places
Toxicants into Categories Related to their Relative
Toxicities [30]

Toxicity Rating	Commonly Used Term	Probable Human Lethal Dose for a 70-kg (150-lb) Man
6	Supertoxic	<5 mg/kg (a taste), <7 drops
5	Extremely toxic	5–50 mg/kg, 7 drops–1 tsp.
4	Very toxic	50–500 mg/kg, 1 tsp.–1 oz
3	Moderately toxic	5–5 g/kg, 1 oz–1 pint
2	Slightly toxic	5–15 g/kg, 1 pint–1 quart
1	Practically nontoxic	>15 g/kg, >1 quart

Threshold Limit Values

The toxicologist who prepared the data for the LD_{50} did not realize that it would be of little use to an industrial hygienist in determining whether a substance were harmful to workers; therefore, a new concept was born. ACGIH first published a list of the "Maximum Allowable Concentrations to Industrial Atmospheric Contaminants in Industrial Medicine" (MAC) in 1945 [25]. The basic criteria for these MAC limits are protection against impairment of health, reasonable freedom from primary irritation, pharmacological effect and nuisance-induced stress. Later, the term was changed to TLV and, in 1970, OSHA adopted many of these TLVs into federal law. TLVs are expressed in ppm and mg/m^3, and the term "time-weighted average" (TWA) is used to describe the level a worker can be exposed to for an eight-hour day without suffering any ill health. Historically, the early TLVs were important because six states (California, Connecticut, Massachusetts, New York, Oregon, Utah), the USPHS and the American Standards Association, presented comparable data. Currently, OSHA publishes its current levels of concentrations in the *Federal Register,* while ACGIH publishes a pamphlet and a documentation book. The data are published as shown in Table V.

SUMMARY

In the preceding sections, various medical and technical terminology described the field of toxicology in general terms. With the passage of the OSHA Act, a provision was made to determine whether a material could be hazardous to the user. The *OSHA-20 Form* or *Material Safety Data Sheet* (Figure 22) is available from most manufacturers for almost all

Table V.   How TLVs are Published

---

1. OSHA General Industry Standard
   OSHA Publication 2206 Revised June, 1981
   29CFR 1910. 1000   Air Contaminants   Page 632
   Table Z-1

Substance	ppm	mg/m³
Acetic acid	10	25

2. American Conference of Governmental Industrial Hygienists
   Cincinnati, OH
   TLV List   1981   Page 9

Acetic acid	10 ppm	25 mg/m³

3. American Conference of Governmental Industrial Hygienists
   Documentation of TLVs
   Page 4   1981

ACETIC ACID
CH_3COOH
TLV, 10 ppm (≈ 25 mg/m³)
STEL, 15 ppm (≈ 37 mg/m³)

Acetic acid is a clear, colorless liquid with a pungent odor. It has a specific gravity of 1.0492 at 20° C; molecular weight of 60; a boiling point of 188° C, (765 mm) 80° C (202 mm); a melting point of 16.63° C, an open cup flash point of 110° F, refractive index of 1.3716 (20° C) and a vapor pressure of 11 mm Hg at 20° C. It is miscible with water, alcohol, glycerin and ether; insoluble in carbon disulfide.

It is used in the manufacture of acetic anhydride, cellulose acetate and vinyl acetate monomer, acetic esters chloroacetic acid. It is also used in the production of plastics, pharmaceuticals, dyes, insecticides, photographic chemicals, food additives (as vinegar), natural latex coagulant and in textile printing.

Sterner[1] concluded that 10 ppm is relatively nonirritating on the basis of industrial experience. Patty[2] reported that 800–1200 ppm cannot be tolerated for longer than three minutes. Smyth[3] found inhalation of 16,000 ppm by rats killed one of six. Vigliani and Zurlo[4] regard 20 to 30 ppm to be without danger. They reported that workers exposed for 7 to 12 years to concentrations of 60 ppm, plus one hour daily at 100 to 260 ppm, had no injury except slight irritation of the respiratory tract, stomach and skin. However, Parmeggiani and Sassi[5] found conjunctivitis, bronchitis, pharangitis and erosion of exposed teeth, apparently in the same workers. Baldi[6] reported conjunctival irritation from concentrations below 10 ppm. Amdur[7] found minor changes in respiration in guinea pigs inhaling 5 ppm acetic acid, with more pronounced effects at 100 ppm.

A TLV of 10 ppm and a STEL of 15 ppm are recommended to prevent undue irritation.

Other recommendations: Cook (1945) and Elkins (1959) recommended 10 ppm. The Soviet limit (1966) was 2 ppm.

References:

1. **Sterner, J.H.:** *Ind. Med. 12*:518 (1943).

2. **Patty, F.A.:** *Industrial Hygiene & Toxicology*, Vol. II, p. 886, Interscience, NY (1949).

3. **Smyth, H.F. Jr.:** *Am. Ind. Hyg. Assoc. Q. 17*:143 (1956).

Table V, continued

4. **Vigliani, E.C., Zurlo, N.:** *Arch. Gewerbepath. Gewerbehyg. 13:* 528–535 (1955). Abstr. in *Arch. Ind. Health 13*:403 (1956).

5. **Parmeggiani, L., Sassi, C.:** *Med. Iavoro 45*:319 (1954). Cited in **Patty, F.A.,** *Industrial Hygiene & Toxicology,* 2nd ed., p. 1779, Interscience, NY (1963).

6. **Baldi, G.:** *Med Iavoro 44*:403 (1953). Abstr. in *Arch. Ind. Hyg. & Occup. Med. 9:*349 (1954).

7. **Amdur, M.:** *Am. Ind. Hyg. Assoc. J. 22*:1 (1961).

Table VI.   How Acetic Acid is Listed in the 1979 Registry of Toxic Effect of Chemical Substances [28]

AF122500	— Registry number
Acetic Acid	— Prime substance name
UPDT:7911	— Data when substance entry was updated, November 1979
CAS:64-19-7	— *Chemical Abstracts* service registry number
MS:60	— Molecular weight
MOLFM:$C_2H_4O_2$	— Molecular formula
SYN:	Acetic Acid (aqueous solution)—synonyms Essigsäure—German name
MTDS:	— Mutation data, no entry
IRDS:	— Skin-hmn 50 mg/24H MLD—Skin and eye irritation—animal tested MLD—mild; skin reaction was well defined erythema
TXDS:	— Toxicity data
ORL	— Hmn—Administered orally to humans
TDLo	Toxic low dose—lowest dose reported to have a toxic effect on humans
1470µg/kg	— 1470 µg/kg body weight
Ih1-hmn	— Administered by inhalation
816 ppm/3m	— 816 ppm exposed for 3 minutes
Review	— TLV Threshold Limit Value—Air, 10 ppm
Regulations	— OSHA Standard—Air TWA, 10 ppm
	DOT—corrosive material, label corrosive

chemicals. Section two of the OSHA-20 requires hazardous materials to be listed by percentage and current TLV. The sheet provides a rapid and detailed description of most problems generally encountered in industry.

The second method is a NIOSH publication entitled "Registry of Toxic Effects of Chemical Substances" [26]. This publication is probably the single most important source on the toxic effects of materials in the workplace today. To demonstrate the problems in the growth of toxicology and numbers of new chemicals and compounds being used in industry, the 1979 edition had 145,053 listings, with 5300 more new chemical compounds than did the 1978 registry. Acetic acid as it appears in this book is shown in Table VI.

U.S. DEPARTMENT OF LABOR
Occupational Safety and Health Administration

Form Approved
OMB No. 44-R1387

MATERIAL SAFETY DATA SHEET

Required under USDL Safety and Health Regulations for Ship Repairing,
Shipbuilding, and Shipbreaking (29 CFR 1915, 1916, 1917)

SECTION I

MANUFACTURER'S NAME	EMERGENCY TELEPHONE NO.

ADDRESS (Number, Street, City, State, and ZIP Code)

CHEMICAL NAME AND SYNONYMS	TRADE NAME AND SYNONYMS
CHEMICAL FAMILY	FORMULA

SECTION II · HAZARDOUS INGREDIENTS

PAINTS, PRESERVATIVES, & SOLVENTS	%	TLV (Units)	ALLOYS AND METALLIC COATINGS	%	TLV (Units)
PIGMENTS			BASE METAL		
CATALYST			ALLOYS		
VEHICLE			METALLIC COATINGS		
SOLVENTS			FILLER METAL PLUS COATING OR CORE FLUX		
ADDITIVES			OTHERS		
OTHERS					

HAZARDOUS MIXTURES OF OTHER LIQUIDS, SOLIDS, OR GASES	%	TLV (Units)

SECTION III · PHYSICAL DATA

BOILING POINT (°F.)		SPECIFIC GRAVITY (H_2O=1)
VAPOR PRESSURE (mm Hg.)		PERCENT, VOLATILE BY VOLUME (%)
VAPOR DENSITY (AIR=1)		EVAPORATION RATE (_____ =1)
SOLUBILITY IN WATER		
APPEARANCE AND ODOR		

SECTION IV · FIRE AND EXPLOSION HAZARD DATA

FLASH POINT (Method used)	FLAMMABLE LIMITS	Lel	Uel
EXTINGUISHING MEDIA			
SPECIAL FIRE FIGHTING PROCEDURES			
UNUSUAL FIRE AND EXPLOSION HAZARDS			

PAGE (1)   (Continued on reverse side)   Form OSHA-20

SECTION V · HEALTH HAZARD DATA

THRESHOLD LIMIT VALUE

EFFECTS OF OVEREXPOSURE

EMERGENCY AND FIRST AID PROCEDURES

SECTION VI · REACTIVITY DATA

| STABILITY | UNSTABLE | | CONDITIONS TO AVOID | |
| | STABLE | | | |

INCOMPATABILITY *(Materials to avoid)*

HAZARDOUS DECOMPOSITION PRODUCTS

| HAZARDOUS POLYMERIZATION | MAY OCCUR | | CONDITIONS TO AVOID | |
| | WILL NOT OCCUR | | | |

SECTION VII · SPILL OR LEAK PROCEDURES

STEPS TO BE TAKEN IN CASE MATERIAL IS RELEASED OR SPILLED

WASTE DISPOSAL METHOD

SECTION VIII · SPECIAL PROTECTION INFORMATION

RESPIRATORY PROTECTION *(Specify type)*

| VENTILATION | LOCAL EXHAUST | | SPECIAL |
| | MECHANICAL *(General)* | | OTHER |

| PROTECTIVE GLOVES | EYE PROTECTION |

OTHER PROTECTIVE EQUIPMENT

SECTION IX · SPECIAL PRECAUTIONS

PRECAUTIONS TO BE TAKEN IN HANDLING AND STORING

OTHER PRECAUTIONS

Form OSHA-20
Rev. May 72

Figure 22.   Material safety data sheet.

CHAPTER 4

EVALUATING THE HAZARD: SAMPLING AND ANALYSIS

INTRODUCTION

Evaluating the hazard means measuring an individual's level of exposure to a known toxic material relative to a time frame. For a known substance, one can research the toxicological properties from testing data and with analytical instruments measure the concentration present on the day tested. In areas in which the substances cannot be obtained or the levels of contamination present cannot be determined, respirators and proper personal protective equipment must be supplied. Firemen, for example, must assume the worst possible conditions because of the toxic gases generated from combustion of plastics and other material. Our approach is based on the assumption that we know the material and its relative toxicity, but are trying to measure the level of contamination present. Emphasis is placed on the assumption that sufficient time and equipment are available to measure the level of contamination. The reasons for sampling may include startup of a new process, determination of the performance or effectiveness of present engineering control measures, changes in regulatory standards or side-by-side OSHA inspection monitoring.

SAMPLING

Sampling is drawing a discrete quantity of contaminated gas, dust or vapor to represent the atmospheric conditions for an operator or operation at a particular time period. Sampling in the legal sense means measurement of an individual's (an employee) exposure to a gas, dust or vapor for a particular time period.

If the employee is said to have exceeded his TLV for the substance, the company is subject to legal action. If the level is below the TLV, the company is said to be in compliance of the existing standard. Historically, sampling first was initiated on the basis of preventing dust and gas explosions. Use of the canary to determine oxygen and hazardous levels of mine gases was probably the first official method of sampling and testing.

Sampling generally is carried out by direct reading instruments, such as detector tubes, combustible gas indicators and collection methods, in which a known volume of sample is drawn through a filter membrane, cyclone, charcoal tube for absorption or bubble gas in a collecting solution. Direct reading instruments were developed for use in the field as the primary goal, with a direct reading dial or calibrated tubes indicating the quantity measured. Collection-type equipment is generally more accurate but requires offsite laboratory analysis of the sample. Personal monitors, such as a film badge in radiation, measure by color change, absorption or chemical reaction the quantity of contaminant present. However, few such devices are approved for official sampling.

Sampling originally carried out by early industrial hygienists was largely uncorrelated to the physical effects produced and was confined to data taken with a particular instrument. Medical proof is now available that material deposits in the lungs, stomach and intestines have caused disease or impairment. The compartmentalization of electrical systems and power supplies moved the more analytical equipment not only into the field, but onto the individual as well. The ACGIH publication, *Air Sampling Instruments* [31], is a prime source of information on techniques and equipment for air sampling.

The OSHA Act and the creation of NIOSH provided the approved methods of sampling and specified the equipment, analytical procedures and sampling period for a substance (Figure 23) [32]. Note that any sampling equipment must be used as specified by the manufacturer and calibrated as required. Sampling instruments must be calibrated before use and periodically by a certified laboratory to retain their accuracy and acceptability.

Cost generally is considered to be a controlling factor involved in sampling today. As microelectronics has miniaturized many sampling instruments, thus enabling them to be worn by the individual, portability and breathing zone samples are a reality.

Legally, personal sampling is done to correlate actual exposure of an employee to a known contaminant. For the purposes of control or correction of a condition, most industrial hygienists will take an area

Substance:

 Iron oxide

Standard:

 29 CFR 1910.93(a), Table G-1 of October 18, 1972

 8-hour time-weighted average: 10 mg/m

Analytical Procedure:

 Atomic absorption
 Lower working limit: 1.5 μg/filter

Sampling Equipment:

 A personal sampler pump is used to pull air through a 37-mm, 3 piece filter holder. The contaminant is collected on a 0.8-micrometer pore size mixed cellulose ester filter (37 mm in diameter). The filter holder is held together by tape or a shrinking band. If the middle piece of the three-piece holder does not fit snuggly into the bottom piece of the filter holder, the contaminant will leak around the filter. A piece of the flexible tubing is used to connect the filter holder to the pump. Sample at a flow rate of 1.5 liters per minute with face cap on and small plugs removed. After sampling, replace small plugs.

Sample Size:

 A minimum sample size of 30 liters is required. Personal sampler pump betteries should be checked and recharged after four hours.

Blank:

 With each batch of samples, submit one filter labelled as blank. This filter should be subjected to the same handling as the samples, except that no air is drawn through the filters.

Shipping:

 Ship in a container designed to prevent damage in transit.

Figure 23.   Sampling data sheet #25.01, Class E, March 11, 1974.

reading to graphically illustrate the worst areas and formulate control methods. Most plant engineers view sampling as describing the parameters of the material generated, so cost-effective pollution control equipment can be sized properly to remove the contaminant. The dust or material may pollute or infiltrate into the controls of automatic machines and processes, ruining the quality as well as the equipment.

Sampling Strategy

Generally, before any sampling is to be conducted, the company must estimate the cost involved and determine whether the government, a private group or manufacturer of sampling equipment should do the sampling. Most large companies charge costs to a particular "cost center," whether plant engineering, environmental or production. Smaller companies use a general fund or pay out of pocket or a general budget. As sampling can be expensive for even a survey, including actual sampling, laboratory analysis and consulting fees, other alternatives should be explored fully.

Federal groups are subdivided into research and regulatory. Research groups such as the NIOSH Health Hazard Evaluation and Technical Assistance Program (HETA) conduct field investigations of possible health hazards in the workplace. Under Section 20(a)(6) of OSHA, any employer or authorized representative of employees can request in writing that it be determined whether any substance found in the place of employment has potentially toxic effects in such concentrations as used or found. NIOSH also provides, on request, medical, nursing and industrial hygiene technical and consultant assistance to federal, state and local agencies. Figure 24 shows a summary of a HETA survey of the

HETA 80-021-721   NIOSH INVESTIGATOR:
COLGATE-PALMOLIVE COMPANY   Pierre Belanger, I.H.
BERKELEY, CALIFORNIA

SUMMARY

On November 13, 1979, the National Institute for Occupational Safety and Health (NIOSH) received a confidential request from an authorized representative from Local 6 of the International Longshoremen's and Warehousemen's Union to evaluate workers' exposure to 1,4 dioxane, a contaminant of 3EO-Sulfate compound used in liquid detergents at the Colgate-Palmolive Company, Berkeley, California.

Twenty-nine environmental air samples (personal and area) were collected from the storage area, the mixing area, and the finishing line for the measurement of 1,4 dioxane. Also, six bulk samples of liquid detergents and one bulk sample of 3EO-Sulfate were analyzed for 1,4 dioxane concentration. The airborne concentration of dioxane was measured to be below the limit of detection. Furthermore, the concentration of dioxane in the bulk samples was less than 1 percent by weight—the limit recommended in the NIOSH Dioxane Criteria Document for materials where dioxane is present as an unintentional contaminant.

Based on the environmental air results and the analyses of the bulk samples, NIOSH concluded that a health hazard from exposures to 1,4 dioxane did not exist at Colgate-Palmolive, Berkeley, California, during the dates of this survey.

KEYWORDS: SIC 2840 (Soap, Detergents, and Cleaning Preparations), dioxane, 1,4 dioxane, 3EO-Sulfate.

Figure 24.   Summary of HETA survey [34].

Colgate-Palmolive Company, Berkeley, California plant. Figure 25 is an example of the Request for Health Hazard Evaluation form. Regulatory groups such as OSHA routinely conduct inspections on a high hazard basis or as a result of an employee complaint or accident. If a contaminant measured is more than the OSHA TWA or TLV, the company is considered in violation and subject to a possible fine and a correction date (previously referred to as "abatement date") by which the contaminant/employee exposure must be controlled. States such as New Jersey have partially funded programs of Compliance Assistance, in which at the request of an employer, a state inspector will conduct OSHA sampling and provide consulting services at no cost. With the concern about asbestos contamination in schools and public meeting places, many cities, counties and municipalities also are carrying out sampling programs.

Private groups comprise insurance carriers, consultants and research test centers. Consultants are licensed professional engineers, certified industrial hygienists (who have been granted certification to do industrial hygiene work by the American Industrial Hygiene Association) or individuals working in the field [33]. Although having a license issued by a state or group has been in demand, there is no guarantee that a general license will provide the same amount of knowledge as attained from someone working in that field for 20 years.

Equipment or instrument suppliers have worked with companies to field-test their products. As equipment will be used in the field, this type of research can be invaluable to the equipment manufacturer and user. In conjunction with instrument manufacturers, committees such as the Air Sampling Committee of the ACGIH also should be consulted to help find a solution to particular sampling needs. The authors and most experts feel that the best sampling strategy is to have a person or group define the problem areas at little or no cost to the company, and then the company need purchase only the essential equipment. Once aware of the problem areas, if they require constant monitoring for borderline cases, or if OSHA has printed a change of regulation notice specifying a decrease in the TLV, one should use the NIOSH publication *Occupational Exposure Sampling Strategy Manual* [35]. This manual is the statistical reference used by NIOSH and OSHA for determining overexposure or compliance. The problem with it is that it requires a sophisticated knowledge of statistics to use it.

Second, any test for contamination of an area for any substance is subject to variation. Thus, even if the company is in compliance, medical examinations and tests must be conducted on a periodic basis to verify sampling results.

U.S. DEPARTMENT OF HEALTH, EDUCATION, AND WELFARE
NATIONAL INSTITUTE FOR OCCUPATIONAL SAFETY AND HEALTH

REQUEST FOR HEALTH HAZARD EVALUATION

This form is provided to assist in registering a request for a health hazard evaluation with the U.S. Department of Health, Education, and Welfare as provided in Section 20(a)(6) of the Occupational Safety and Health Act of 1970 and 42 CFR Part 85. (See Statement of Authority on Reverse Side.) *The provisions of this section provide for evaluation of health hazards resulting from exposure to chemical substances only: Physical agents (noise, heat, etc.) and safety are not covered by this section.*

Name of Establishment Where Substance(s) Exists _____

Company Address { Street _____ Telephone _____

City _____ State _____ Zip Code _____

1. What Product or Service does the Establishment Produce? _____

_____

2. Specify the particular building or worksite where the substance(s) is located, including address.

_____   _____

3. Specify the name, title, and phone number of the employer's agent(s) in charge. _____·_____

_____

4. Describe briefly the substance(s) which exists by completing the following:

   Identification of Toxic Substance(s) _____

   Trade Name(s) (If Applicable) _____   Chemical Name(s) _____

   _____   _____

   _____   _____

   Manufacturer(s) _____

   Does the material have a warning label? _____Yes _____No. If yes; attach copy of label or a copy of the information contained on the label.

   Physical Form of Substance(s): ☐ Dust ☐ Gas ☐ Liquid ☐ Mist ☐ Other

   How are you exposed? ☐ Breathing   ☐ Swallowing   ☐ Skin Contact

   Number of People Exposed _____ Length of Exposure (Hours Day) _____

   Occupations of Exposed Employees _____

   _____

5. Using the space below describe further the nature of the conditions or circumstances which prompted this request and other relevant aspects which you may consider important, such as the nature of the illness or symptoms of exposure, the concern for the potentially toxic effects of a new chemical substance introduced into the workplace, etc. _____ ___

   _____

   _____

   _____

CDC/NIOSH 2 86
Rev. 2/80

6. (a) To your knowledge has this substance been considered previously by any Government

    agency? _____ (b) If so, give the name and address of each. _____

_____

_____

    (c) and, the approximate date it was so considered. _____

7. (a) Is a similar request currently being filed with or under investigation by any other Govern-

    ment (State or Federal) agency? _____ (b) If so, give the name and address of each ____

_____

8. Requester — (*Employees of State, Local or Federal Agencies are not eligible.*)
    The undersigned Requester believes that a substance (or substances) normally found in the
    place of employment may have potentially toxic effects in the concentrations used or found.

    Signature _____ Date _____

    Typed or Printed Name _____ Phone: Home—_____

    Address { Street _____ Business—_____

             { City _____ State _____ Zip Code _____

Check One:
    ☐ I am an Employer Representative
    ☐ I am an Authorized Representative of, or an officer of the organization representing the
      employees for purposes of collective bargaining. State the name and address of your

      organization. _____

_____

    ☐ I am an employee of the employer and an Authorized Representative of two or more
      employees in the workplace where the substance is normally found. Add signatures of
      authorizing employees below:
      Name _____ Phone _____

      Name _____ Phone _____
    ☐ I am one of three or less employees in the workplace where the substance is normally
      found.

Please indicate your desire: ☐ I do not want my name revealed to the employer.

                       ☐ My name may be revealed to the employer.

Authority:
Section 20(a)(6) of the Occupational Safety and Health Act, (29 U. S. C. 669(a)(6)) provides as
follows: The Secretary of Health, Education, and Welfare shall . . . determine following a written
request by any employer or authorized representative of employees, specifying with reasonable
particularity the grounds on which the request is made, whether any substance normally found
in the place of employment has potentially toxic effects in such concentrations as used or found;
and shall submit such determination both to employers and affected employees as soon as possible. If the Secretary of Health, Education, and Welfare determines that any substance is potentially toxic at the concentrations in which it is used or found in a place of employment, and such
substance is not covered by an occupational safety or health standard promulgated under section
6, the Secretary of Health, Education, and Welfare shall immediately submit such determination to
the Secretary of Labor, together with all pertinent criteria.

For further information
Telephone AC 513-684-2176
Send the completed form to:
    National Institute for Occupational Safety and Health
    Hazard Evaluation and Technical Assistance Branch
    4676 Columbia Parkway
    Cincinnati, Ohio 45226

Figure 25.   OSHA request for health hazard evaluation.

Detector Tubes

Direct reading colorimetric indicators comprise three basis groups: liquid reagents, chemically treated papers, and detector or glass-indicating tubes, containing solid chemicals. Sometimes the tubes are referred to as Kitagawa tubes after the Japanese inventor who first introduced them to the marketplace. The equipment required includes the detector tube and pump. The detector tube is a small glass tube, fire-sealed at both ends and usually containing a granular silica gel packing. The small grains of silica gel are coated with a reactive chemical such as lead acetate, which, when contacting hydrogen sulfide, produces a brown stain from the reaction between the hydrogen sulfide and lead acetate, producing lead sulfide. The length of the brown stain is proportional to the level of hydrogen sulfide in the atmosphere sampled. The concentration of the airborne contaminant is read directly on the calibrated tube in ppm vol %. Some of the tubes require the manufacturer's scale in the tube package to be compared to the length of the stain. The pump draws a calibrated volume of air to be sampled through the detector tube at a constant rate for a short period of time (Figure 26). Table VII shows the available range of indicator tubes and sensitivity.

The general method of operation is simple to learn and use. The pump is pressure-tested to check for leakage. The ends of the tube are broken off in the hole at the head or tube end of the pump, and then the tube is inserted, with the sampling arrow head pointing in the direction of the contaminant source in the rubber collar. The number and length of strokes—full, half or quarter—are specified by the manufacturer and

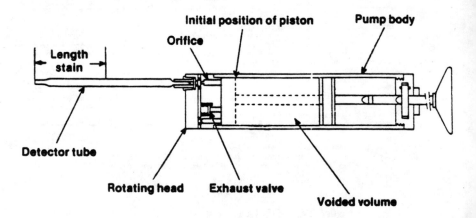

Figure 26.   MSA universal sampling pump.

Table VII.   Indicator Detector Tubes Available and
Sensitivity Ranges

Contaminant Parameter to be Measured	Reaction Principle (reagent system)	Measuring Range
Acetone	Dinitrophenylhydrazine	100–12,000 ppm
Acrylonitrile	Via hydrogen cyanide	5–30 ppm
Alcohol	Chromic acid	100–3000 ppm
Ammonia	Bromophenol blue	5–700 ppm
Ammonia	Mercury (1)-nitrate	25–700 ppm
Aniline	Furfurol + acid	1–20 ppm
Arsine	Gold salt	0.05–60 ppm
Benzene	Formaldehyde + sulfuric acid	15–420 ppm
Carbon Dioxide	Hydrazine + redox indicator	0.1–60 vol %
Carbon Disulfide	Copper thiocarbomate	13–3200 ppm
Carbon Monoxide	Iodine pentoxide + selenium dioxide + fuming sulfuric acid	8–7000 ppm
Carbon Tetrachloride	Via phosgene	10–100 ppm
Chlorine	0-Tolidine	0.2–500 ppm
Cyanogen Chloride	Pyridine + barbituric acid	2–40 ppm
Ethyl Acetate	Chromic acid	200–3000 ppm
Formaldehyde	Xylene + sulfuric acid	2–40 ppm
Hydrazine	Bromophenol blue	0.25–3 ppm
Hydrocarbons	Iodine pentoxide + fuming sulfuric	0.1–1 vol %
	Selenium dioxide + fuming sulfuric	2–25 mg/l
Hydrochloric Acid	Bromophenol blue	1–2 ppm
Hydrogen	Via water vapor	0.5–3 vol %
Hydrogen Cyanide	Mercury (2) chloride + methyl red	2–150 ppm
Hydrogen Fluoride	Zirconium-alizarin lac	0.5–15 ppm
Hydrogen Sulfide	Lead salt	5–2000 ppm
	Copper (2) salt	0.02–7 vol %
	Iodine	0.02–7 vol %
Mercaptan	Copper salt	2–100 ppm
Mercury vapor	Mercury chloride + gold chloride	0.1–2 mg/m^3
Methyl Bromide	Via bromine	5–50 ppm
Monostyrene	Resinification (sulfuric acid)	50–400 ppm
Nickel Carbonyl	Iodine + dioxime	0.1–1 ppm
Nitrogen Dioxide	Diphenylbenzidine	0.5–10 ppm
Nitrous Fumes	Diphenylbenzidine	0.5–100 ppm
	Dianisidine	100–5000 ppm
Olefins	Permanganate	1–55 mg/l
Oxygen	Via carbon monoxide	5–21 vol %
Ozone	Indigo bleaching	0.5–300 ppm
Perchlorethylene	Via chlorine	10–400 ppm
Phenol	Indophenol	5 ppm
Phosgene	(Dimethylanaline-Dimethylaminobenzaldehyde)	0.05–75 ppm
Phosphine	Gold salt	0.1–3000 ppm
Sulfur Dioxide	Iodine	20–2000 ppm

Table VII, continued

Contaminant Parameter to be Measured	Reaction Principle (reagent system)	Measuring Range
Suptox	Gold chloride + N-chloramide	0.5 mg/m^3
Toluene	Sulfuric acid + iodine pentoxide	5–400 ppm
	Fuming sulfuric + selenium dioxide	25–2000 ppm
Trichlorethylene	Via chlorine	10–400 ppm
Vinyl Chloride	Potassium permanganate	100–3000 ppm
Water Vapor	Selenium dioxide + sulfuric acid	0.1–40 mg/l

relate to the level of contamination and the TLVs. Ozone with 0.1-ppm detector tubes requires more full strokes than a high volume or tube used to measure carbon monoxide levels. Generally, it should be noted that tubes are available to measure sometimes three levels of contamination by varying the types of tube and number of strokes.

Advantages include the following: (1) it is inexpensive to operate; (2) it is easy to train the user; (3) it requires little calibration and stands up well to handling and abuse; (4) a large variety of gases can be sampled (more than 120); and (5) readings are available immediately.

Disadvantages include inaccuracies of measurement, temperature, altitude, humidity channeling and nonspecificity. NIOSH-certified detector tubes specifically should be within ±25% error range at one, two and five times the TLV of a contaminant. There is also a quality assurance requirement of ±35% accuracy at half the TLV of the substance. Increased temperature tends to produce a longer stain because the chemical reaction will be more complete and decreased temperature produces correspondingly less stain. Increased humidity sometimes interferes with the reaction, so some manufacturers provide a small desiccant tube to absorb moisture before the contaminated air enters into the samping tube. Channeling is the result of vibrations, induced by falling or storing the tubes in a car trunk, which may alter the array of silica gel, producing blotches of stain.

Nonspecificity is a typical problem of not being able to measure the level of one solvent, when several solvent vapors are present. A typical coating operation could have methyl isobutyl ketone (MIBK), toluene and methol ethyl ketone (MEK) in use at any one time. The detector tube would have difficulty discerning the concentration of one from another.

Combustible Gas Indicator

The most common gas detection instrument used in manufacturing, shipyards, utility workrooms and coal mines probably was the combustible gas indicator. A combustible gas or vapor mixture is passed over a filament heated above the ignition temperature of the substance of interest. If the filament is part of a bridge circuit, the resulting heat of combustion changes the resistance of the filament, and measurement of the imbalance is related to the concentration of the gas or vapor in the sample mixture (Figure 27). The method is nonspecific but may be made more selective by choosing appropriate filament temperatures for individual gases or vapors or by using an oxidation catalyst for a desired reaction.

These instruments are portable and stand up well to abuse, but several limitations should be considered. They are electrically rated instruments for Class I, Groups C & D, and should not be turned on in explosive atmospheres or used in acetylene and hydrogen atmospheres (Class I Group A atmospheres). One isolated case was reported in New Jersey, in which an employee who turned on such a meter in an explosive atmosphere was injured. There are usually two scales: (1) the high, with readings of 0–100% explosibility, and the low—0–10% explosibility. Most manufacturers supply a chart to convert percentage reading to ppm of the gas being tested (Table VIII). If a mixture such as toluene or methyl ethyl ketone is present, the reading does not consider the gases separately. Testing leaded gasoline will destroy the filaments that are routinely supplied by most manufacturers. Cold weather affects the batteries, so the readings are much lower than actual concentrations present.

Sampling Collection Methods

Collection of a gas or material in a special container followed by laboratory analysis is the method most industrial hygienists use for accuracy when time is not a critical factor. Many collecting schemes were devised and developed to count fibers and measure particulate levels of contamination, hoping they would be correlated at a later time to a person's physical condition and to demonstrate human resistance to adverse environments and the cause of disease in individuals. In the 1930s, Drinker and Hatch [3] discussed the subjects of "dusty trades" and described measurement techniques such as sedimentation cells, thimble

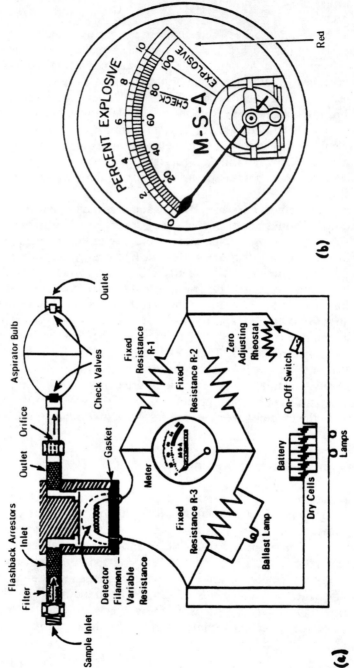

Figure 27. (a) Schematic flow system and wiring diagram; (b) indicator dial gauge/meter (courtesy MSA).

Table VIII. A Typical Calibration Chart (MSA)

LEL = % by volume (US Bom Bulletin #503)
TLV = threshold limit values (ACGIH 196-4) (ppm)

O.S. = OFF SCALE

No.	Name	LEL	TLV	Meter Reading 1	2	3	Parts per Million (in squares) 10% LEL Switch Setting 4	5	6	7	8	9	10	2X TLV	3X TLV	5X TLV	Meter Reading (in squares) % LEL Switch Setting 5% LEL	10% LEL	20% LEL	50% LEL	75% LEL	Formula	No.
1	Acetone	2.6	1000	338	676	1026	1378	1716	2055	2418	2756	3133	3432	7	11	18	5	9	19	48	72	CH_3COCH_3	1
2	Acetaldehyde	4.1	200	328	697	1025	1394	1722	2091	2419	2788	3116	3414		2.5	4.5	5	15	30	75	OS	CH_3CHO	2
3	Acrylonitrile	3.0	20	240	480	720	960	1200	1410	1650	1860	2070	2280				8	16	32	78	OS	C_2H_3CN	3
4	Allyl Alcohol	2.5	2	225	450	650	875	1100	1325	1525	1750	1975	2175			4	8	15	28	61	83	C_3H_6OH	4
5	Amyl Alcohol	1.2	100	180	216	504	660	804	948	1092	1224	1344	1452				5	10	18	37	50	$C_5H_{11}OH$	5
6	Benzene	1.4	25	140	294	434	574	728	868	1008	1162	1302	1442				6	12	24	58	83	C_6H_6	6
7	Butyl Acetate	1.7	200	170	340	527	697	884	1071	1275	1420	1720	1955		1.5	4	2.5	5	11	28	42	$CH_3COOC_4H_9$	7
8	Butyl Alcohol	1.4	100	210	406	602	798	980	1148	1316	1456	1568	1666	1	2	3	4	8	15	33	46	C_4H_9OH	8
9	Carbon Disulfide	1.25	20	275	625	1000	1375	1750								2.5	2.5	5	10	24	35	CS_2	9
10	Carbon Monoxide	12.5	100	750	1500	2250	3000	3750	4500	5250	6000	6750	7500	7	10	18	10	22	42	100	OS	CO	10
11	Cyclohexane	1.3	400	143	286	429	572	715	845	988	1118	1261	1404				6	11	23	57	83	C_6H_{12}	11
12	Dimazine (UDMH)	2.5	0.5	200	450	725	1000	1325	1675	2025	2375	2750	3100			18	5.5	11	21	53	77	$(CH_3)_2N_2H_2$	12
13	Ethyl Acetate	2.5	400	325	675	1025	1400	1775	2175	2625	3050	3450	4000	3	5	8	5	10	20	50	75	$CH_3COOC_2H_5$	13
14	Ethyl Alcohol	4.3	1000	215	473	774	1075	1419	1763	2107	2494	2871	3311	8.5	12	18	9	17	31	70	101	C_2H_5OH	14
15	Ethyl Ether	1.9	400	114	247	399	570	741	931	1021	1311	1520	1729	5	7.5	12.5	6	12	23	56	82	$C_2H_5OC_2H_5$	15
16	Ethylene Chloride	6.2	50	496	1054	1590	2140	2666	3224	3720	4250	4774	5270				7	14	28	68	98	CH_3ClCH_2Cl	16
17	Ethylene Oxide	3.0	50	405	780	1155	1530	1890	2265	2640	3000	3345	3705			5.5	5.5	11	21	54.5	90	C_2H_4O	17
18	Gasoline (leaded—with inhibitor)	1.4	500	140	294	448	608	770	924	1085	1246	1400	1580	8	12	20	6	11	22	55	82	C_7H_{16}	18
19	Heptane	1.2	500	132	270	402	540	672	804	936	1068	1200	1332	9	13.5	21	6	11	21	50	73	C_7H_{16}	19
20	Hexane	1.2	500	144	288	444	600	750	900	1056	1212	1368	1512	8	11.5	19.5	6	9.5	18.5	47	69.5	C_6H_{14}	20
21	Hydrogen Sulfide	4.3	10	516	1011	1485	1935	2387	2838	3290	3741	4171	4622				12	12	24	56	79	H_2S	21
22	Isopropyl Acetate	1.8	200	252	504	738	990	1224	1476	1728	1962	2214	2468	1.5	2.5	4.5	4.5	9.5	18.5	47	70.5	$(CH_3)_2CHOOCCH_3$	22
23	Isopropyl Alcohol	2.0	400	280	550	810	1100	1380	1660	1950	2230	2510	2790	3.5	5	8.5	4.5	8.5	17.5	45	67	$(CH_3)_2CHOH$	23
24	Isobutyl Methyl Ketone (MIBK)	1.4	100	182	350	512	665	826	980	1141	1288	1442	1596	1.4	2.1	3.6	5	10	22	50	73	$CH_3COC_4H_9$	24
25	Methyl Acetate	3.1	200	465	930	1395	1891	2372	2853	3317	3813	4278	4743				4.5	8.5	17	43	65	CH_3COOCH_3	25
26	Methyl Alcohol	6.7	200	402	838	1273	1740	2210	2700	3200	3680	4180	4690				9	18.5	36.5	88	OS	CH_3OH	26
27	Methyl Ethyl Ketone (MEK)	1.8	200	180	378	585	837	1080	1350	1620	1908	2180	2448	2	2	3	9	10.5	21	47.5	71	$CH_3COC_2H_5$	27
28	Octane	1.0	500	130	255	380	510	640	770	915	1060	1210	1365	9.5	14	23	6	9.5	18.5	44	64	C_8H_{18}	28
29	Pentane	1.4	1000	140	294	448	608	770	924	1085	1246	1400	1580	16	24	39	5	11	22	55	82	C_5H_{12}	29
30	Styrene	1.1	100	66	143	242	341	457	583	715	847	990	1133	2	4	4.5	6	10.5	21	52.5	75	$C_6H_5CHCH_2$	30
31	Tetrahydrofuran	2.0	200	200	400	630	860	1050	1260	1480	1700	1930	2160	2	4	6	6	12	25	60	88	C_4H_8O	31
32	Toluene	1.4	200	112	231	350	476	602	728	846	973	1099	1218	3.5	5.5	9	6.5	13	25	60	87.5	$C_6H_5CH_3$	32
33	Xylene	1.0	200	110	220	330	450	560	680	800	920	1055	1200	5	7.5	12.5	6	12	23	42	52	$C_6H_5(CH_3)_2$	33
53	Chlorobenzene	1.3	75	130	267	409	546	682	822	962	1105	1248	1391	2	3	4.5	4.5	8.5	16.5	39	55.5	C_6H_5Cl	53
55	1, 4 Dioxane	2.0	100	280	560	830	1100	1370	1640	1910	2180	2450	2720	1	1.5	2.5	5	10	20	50	75	$C_2H_4OC_2H_4O$	55

filters and Konimeters. Since the 1930s, the field of equipment used to measure contaminants has expanded greatly. We will consider four areas of which a respirator user must be aware: total dust, respirable dust, solvent vapors and metal fumes. With the vast changes in government agencies since 1980, data from NIOSH and OSHA will be used. Table IX lists common gases and vapors with significant properties for plant safety.

Table IX.   Common Gases and Vapors—Some Significant Properties for Plant Safety

Vapor or Gas	Threshold Limit Value (ppm)	Threshold of Smell (ppm)	Lower Ignition Limit (vol %)	Upper Ignition Limit (vol %)	Flash Point (°C)	Boiling Point (°C)
Acetone	1000	—	2.5	13	< −20	56.2
Acetylene	—	—	1.5	32	—	−83.6
Acrylonitrile	20	—	2.8	28	−5	78.5
Ammonia	5	5	15.0	28	—	−33.5
Aniline	5	0.5	1.2	11	76	184.4
Arsine	0.05	—	—	—	—	−62.5
Benzene	25	< 100	1.2	8.0	−11	80.1
Benzylbromide	—	—	—	—	—	198
Bromine	0.1	< 0.01	—	—	—	58.8
Bromoform	—	—	—	—	—	149.6
(1,3) Butadiene	1000	—	1.1	12.5	—	−4
n-Butane	1000	—	1.5	8.5	—	−1
n-Butanol	100	—	1.4	11.3	35	117.8
2-Butanol	150	—	—	—	24	99.5
Carbon Dioxide	5000	Odorless	—	—	—	−78.5
Carbon Disulfide	20	1-2	1.0	60	< −20	46.2
Carbon Monoxide	50	Odorless	12.5	74	—	−191.5
Carbontetrachloride	10	70	—	—	—	76.7
Chloral Hydrate	—	—	—	—	—	98
Chlorine	1	0.02	—	—	—	−34.1
(Chlorobromo-methane)	200	—	—	—	—	68
Chloroform	50	200	—	—	—	61.2
Ethyl Acetate	400	—	2.1	11.5	−4	77
Ethyl Alcohol	1000	350	3.5	15	12	78.4
Ethylene	—	—	2.7	34	—	−103.7
Ethylene Oxide	50	700	2.6	100	—	10.7
Formaldehyde	5	—	7.0	73	—	−19
Hydrazine	1	3	4.7	100	—	113.5
Hydrocyanic Acid	10	2	5.4	46.6	< −20	26
Hydrogen	—	Odorless	4.0	75.6	—	−253
Hydrogen Chloride	5	—	—	—	—	−85.0

Table IX, continued

Hydrogen Fluoride	3	—	—	—	—	19.5
Hydrogen Sulfide	10	0.1	4.3	45.5	—	-60.4
Kerosene	—	—	0.6	12.0	—	82.4
Mercury Vapor	0.1 mg/m^3	Odorless	—	—	—	357
Methane	—	—	5	15	—	-161
Methyl Alcohol	200	2000	5.5	44	11	64.6
Methyl Bromide	20	Odorless	8.6	20	—	3.5
Methyl Ethyl Ketone	200	<25	1.8	11.5	-1	79.6
Methyl Mercaptan	10	—	4.1	21.0	—	6
Monostyrene	100	25	1.1	8	32	145
Nickel-Carbonyl	0.001	—	2.0	—	< -20	43.2
Nitrogen Dioxide	5	1.3	—	—	—	—
Nitrogen Monoxide	—	Odorless	—	—	—	151.8
Ozone	0.1	0.015	—	—	—	—
Perchlor-Ethylene	100	50	—	—	—	121.2
Phenol	5	0.5	—	—	79	182
Phosgene	0.1	0.5	—	—	—	7.6
Phosphine	0.3	2.7	—	—	—	-88
Propane	1000	—	2.1	9.5	—	-42
Sulfur Dioxide	5	3	—	—	—	-10
Toluene	200	50	1.2	7.0	6	110.6
Trichlorethylene	100	50	1.2	7.0	6	110.6
Vinyl Chloride	500	—	3.8	29.3	—	-14

TOTAL DUST SAMPLING

Process and workroom atmospheres must be sampled for the following reasons:

1. to determine the nature and quantity of contaminants and to ensure that levels are within acceptable and legal standards;
2. to evaluate efficiencies of ventilation systems and/or environmental control equipment;
3. for the selection and design of equipment;
4. to project any potential problems in additions of new equipment; and
5. as evidence for regulatory compliance and for maintenance of safe working conditions for employees.

The theory involved in single particle settling is straightforward. For most practical applications of settling in work areas, settling velocities are low enough to make use of Stokes' law, which implies that

$$C_D = \frac{24}{Re_s} = \frac{24\mu}{D_p\rho_g U_y}$$

where Re_s is the particle's settling Reynolds number, and μ is the viscosity of the gas stream. Stokes' law provides a convenient means of estimating the settling velocity of particles. Stokes' law for settling velocity of a particle can be expressed as

$$U_y = \frac{(\rho_p - \rho_g)D_p^2 g}{18\mu}$$

where
U_y = settling velocity of the particle (cm/sec)
ρ_p = density of the particle (g/cm)
ρ_g = density of the gas stream (g/cm)
g = gravitational force constant (980.6 cm/sec^2)
D_p = equivalent diameter of a spherical particle (cm)
C_p = drag coefficient of the particle (dimensionless)

The settling velocity (U_y) therefore is directly proportional to the density difference and the square of the particle's equivalent diameter.

A convenient measure of the relative rates of travel of the particle in each diameter is the gravitational separation number, N_{sg}. This is defined as the ratio of the settling velocity to the linear velocity and is expressed as

$$N_{sg} = \frac{U_y}{U_x} = \frac{(\rho_p - \rho_g)}{18\mu U_x}$$

where U_x is the horizontal velocity of the particle.

Total dust sampling is the collection of all dust to which the individual would be exposed from operations such as crushing, grinding, cutting, sanding and packaging. The geometric shape of the particulate is generally assumed to be spherical, and Stoke's equation can be modified so that the falling rate is proportional to the specific gravity of the particle diameter times the square of its diameter, d.

The diameter size expressed in microns, the terminal velocity of a particle falling freely in air, is approximately 0.003 d^2 × density, or cm/sec. A 1-μ particle with a density of 5 would travel $(0.003)(1)^2 \times (5) =$ 0.015 cm/sec or, in 10 minutes, (60 sec/1 min) × 1 min × 0.015 cm/sec = 9.0 cm, provided the fall were straight down with no air currents.

To compare particle size to travel distance, we will consider a common grinding operation. A metal particle flies off a grinding wheel with the peripheral wheel speed at 5000 cm/sec and a 1-mm diameter particle that is readily visible can travel 70 ft through the air. Comparing a respirable particle of 10 μ in diameter, the particle will travel only about 4 cm through the air before air friction stops it. Flake-sized particles, which are long and narrow particles defined as the length and width, must be much greater than five time the thickness or depth. They also follow Stoke's law but tend to float in the air. These shaped particles are used in metallic-type car paints and, because of the surface area to volume size, can produce violent explosions when oxidized. Early studies of dusts were concerned with the explosibility, and devices such as the Hartman apparatus developed by the Bureau of Mines reported on the explosive index of dusts. The National Electrical Code recognized this and requires special electrical installation in section 500 of its code for Class II Division 1 and Division 2 atmospheres. Therefore, hazardous dusts such as those from sugar, aspirin, coffee and grain-cereals, have produced explosions when in very fine particle size. Sampling equipment must be approved for the atmosphere being tested as well as the method of test.

Second, the amount of material referred to here is relatively small. The OSHA nuisance dust level is 15 mg/m^3 of air. Considering that the average worker can inhale 10 m^3 of air in 8 hours, this person would inhale a total of approximately 150 mg/day, disregarding losses due to such respiratory cleaning actions as mucus and ciliar responses. This is not a large amount of material but if one spreads this out in a layer one-particle thick, it would cover a tremendous surface area due to the fine nature of the dust. The human lung averages 70 m^2 of surface—the area of a tennis court—but the constant exposure to such levels would reduce the lung's efficiency greatly and would put them under strain at such conditions.

The method of sampling in current use is to place a battery-owned pump onto the individual being sampled and, with the use of a flexible plastic tube, to draw the contaminated air into a porous filter medium.

FILTERS

Although the filter medium would be specified by the NIOSH or OSHA sampling method as an example, we will examine two typical filters in use: the Millipore® brand AA and the Mine Safety MSA FWS-B.

For metal fume sampling, the Millipore brand AA filter 0.8-μ pore size is used for the sampling. The AA designation refers to the filter type, which consists of mixed esters of cellulose. The 0.8-μ pore refers to the size of the pores in the filter and indicates their average diameter. The actual thickness of the filter is about 150 μ (37 mm in diameter). The filter has a very high collection efficiency and is not attacked by dilute acids or alkalis. It also is very effective for collecting particulates without too much regard to the flowrate. It should be noted that standard filters such as the Whatman 41 paper filters, commonly used in chemistry labs, have efficiencies directly proportional to flow rates. With a pore diameter of only 0.8 μ in size, any particle larger than that usually is captured on the surface of the filter. Particles smaller than 0.8 μ are the result of two major factors:

1. The particle usually has an electrical charge based on static, and the filter captures the particle by electrostatic attraction, although not necessarily on the surface.
2. As the pores do not pass on a straight line through the filter, particles will impact the surface as well. Efficiency of the filter also increases after a few minutes of sampling as a layer of particulate is built up on the surface and tends to act as an additional filtering medium.

The FWS-B filter has an average pore size of 5 μ and is made of polyvinyl chloride. The larger pore diameter is used because the size of the dust particles varies greatly and the filter could become plugged, reducing the flowrate. This filter does not absorb moisture from the air readily and is more suitable for weighing. These filters have efficiency rates that are the ratio of the weight of total particulates passing through the filter to that of total particulates applied to the filter. Usually, selected aerosol particle sizes of 5 μ or less are used as testing materials. The ratio is expressed as percentage efficiency and it varies with flowrates through the filter and size of the particles.

A final consideration is the level of dust loading to which the operator is exposed. As OSHA and NIOSH methods use time-weighted averages, the number of samples can correspond to the best and worst conditions. This should be done to help determine whether a ventilation or respiratory protection system should be used.

Hypothetical Example

An employee packages various-sized parcels of titanium dioxide, a white pigment inhouse paint, with TLV of 15 mg/m³ for an 8-hour day. Was he exposed to a hazardous amount?

The Data			Time (min)
Small Bags	7:10–9:10	Sample #1	120
	—break		
Small Bags	9:20–11:20	#2	120
	11:20–12:00—lunch		

Large Bags	12:00–2:00	#3	120
	2:00–2:10 —break		
Large Bags	2:10–3:20	#4	70
			430

Sampling Results

After sampling, cassettes were weighed and results were shown in mg/m^3:

	Time (min)	Collected Amount (mg/m^3)		
Sample #1	120	10	=	1200 mg-min/m^3
#2	120	12	=	1440 mg-min/m^3
#3	120	31.6	=	3792 mg-min/m^3
#4	70	33.0	=	2310 mg-min/m^3
Total time = 430 min			=	8742 mg-min/m^3

$$\text{Time-Weighted Average} = \frac{8742 \text{ mg-min/m}^3}{430 \text{ min}} = 20.33 \text{ mg/m}^3$$

This exceeds the 8-hour TWA of 15 mg/m^3; however, our data give us the following information. Filling the large bags produces three times the dust. If we were to fill small bags all day we would be within the legal standard of 15 mg/m^3. We might want a special ventilation system for large bags or a special control system for wearing respirator on the few days or times in a year the operation is carried out. Many employees suffer from discomfort at levels even below the allowable threshold limits or standards.

The company would be well advised to provide a better method because most union-management groups make this job a "punishment"-type task, so the employee who is disliked may get the job. Many a grievance or OSHA complaint has been filed because of apprehension about the nonexistence dangers of such a job. Plant engineers know that the more the dust, the more the waste, and the greater the cost of cleanup, the operator's salary and total profit loss.

RESPIRABLE DUST SAMPLING

The intent of this technique is to collect only that portion of dust in the air that is respirable, or would enter the worker's lower lungs and be retained. The method of testing is to secure a pump drawing a known constant volume of air sample into a cyclone separator (Figure 28) worn by the individual in the work environment. The device works in much the same way as the large industrial-type units. Air is drawn into the unit through an orifice (0.7 mm) set tangentially to the center line, at which time the entering air is accelerated and at a high velocity inside the cyclone. The heavier particles are thrown out to the side of the airstream and dropped down into a grit pot at the bottom of the cyclone, while the small particles (the respirable dust particles) that remain in the center of the airstream are pulled up and collected on the filter.

The cyclone separates particulates with an aerodynamic diameter of 10 μ or larger, and the filter collects the particulates in the 1- to 10-μ range. Because the separation of particles depends on air velocity and particle acceleration inside the cyclone, maintaining flowrate in the sampling system is critical.

PARTICLE FRACTIONATING SAMPLER

This instrument collects and sizes airborne particles for subsequent gravimetric and/or chemical analyses. Its features include the following:

1. Particles $\geq$10.0 μm to 0.4 μm are sized aerodynamically in eight stages.
2. It is used universally by federal and state regulatory agencies, universities, research facilities and industry.
3. Its flowrate is 1 cfm, ideal for in-plant particulate levels.
4. A high-capacity preimpactor eliminates bouncing and reentrainment.
5. It has a constant pressure drop for accurate flow measurement.
6. Its patented concept includes a multiorifice, multistage impactor.
7. It uses 115/230-V ac or 12-V dc vacuum pumps with 1.4-cfm flow capacity.
8. It has corrosion-resistant aluminum impactor components.

Designed to meet the industrial hygienist's requirements for in-plant sampling, the Andersen 1-cfm ambient sampler collects and aerodynamically sizes all airborne particulate matter (solid or liquid) in the working environment. In this manner, an assessment can be made of the potential health hazards from workroom air contaminants. The 8-stage, multijet, multistage cascade impactor automatically separates the particles into 8 fractions from $\geq$10.0 μm to 0.4 μm in diameter. A backup filter gives absolute collection of the submicrometer particles.

The design concept of the Andersen sampler evolved from the follow-

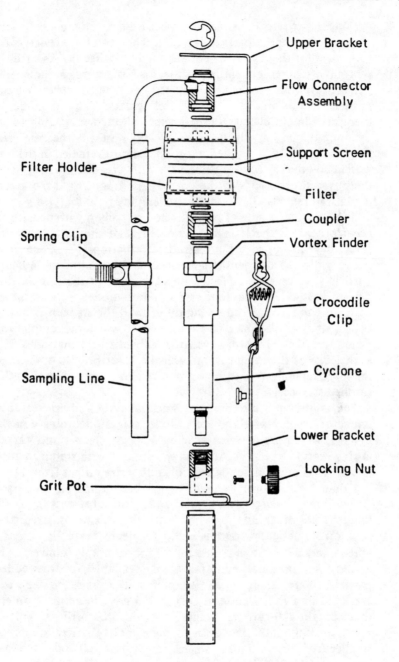

Figure 28. Cyclone/filter holder assembly.

ing facts: The human respiratory tract is an aerodynamically classifying system for airborne particles [36,37]. The sampling device is used as a substitute for the respiratory tract as a dust collector. As such, it should reproduce to a reasonable degree the dust-collecting characteristics of the human respiratory system [37,38] so that lung penetration by airborne particles can be predicted from sampling data. The sampling instrument therefore should classify the particles collected according to the aerodynamic dimension which, as Wells [39] states, is the true measure of lung penetrability. The fraction of inhaled dust retained in the respiratory system and the site of deposition vary with size, shape and density and all the physical properties of the particles that constitute the aerodynamic dimension [36,40–42]. Methods that employ light scattering or filtration and microscopic sizing of particles do not reckon with density and some other properties that affect the movement of the particle in air. Therefore, they do not give the desired information [37]. Because the lung penetrability of unit density spherical particles is known [40,43] and the particle sizes that are collected on each stage of the sampler have been determined [44], then as long as a standard model of this sampler is used according to standard operating procedure, the stage distribution of the collected material will indicate the extent to which the sample would have penetrated the respiratory system. With this information and with the knowledge of the chemical, biological and/or radiological properties of the material collected, the exact nature and extent of the health hazards can be assessed [45].

The Andersen 1-cfm ambient sampler design comprises an optional impactor preseparator and 9 aluminum stages (including a backup filter holder), which are held together by 3 spring clamps and gasketed with O-ring seals (Figure 29). An 8-stage impactor with standard absolute filter classifies particulates or aerosols into 9 size ranges from 11 μ down to less than 0.4 μ. Normally used for in-plant sampling, it operates at 1.0 cfm and may be used with special collection substrates (glass fiber, aluminum foil, membranes, etc.). It features Andersen's patented multicircular orifice design, permitting highly efficient size fractionations. It meets OSHA and EPA design requirements for respirable/nonrespirable segregation. An optional preimpactor is available for the collection of particles larger than 10 μ. Stages 0 and 1 have 96 tapered orifices arranged in a radial pattern. Stages 2–6 have integral air inlet sections that contain 400 orifices. Stage 7 contains 201 orifices. This section is approximately 3.125 inches in diameter. The orifices are progressively smaller from top to bottom stages, ranging from 0.1004 inch in diameter in stage 0 to 0.0100 inch in diameter in stage 7. Each stage has a removal stainless steel or glass (3.25-inch diameter) collection plate. The exhaust

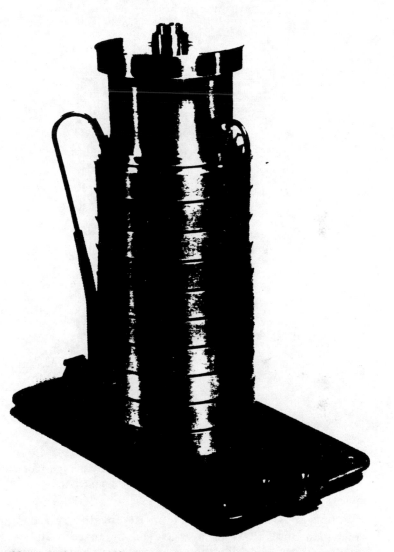

Figure 29.   Andersen 1-cfm ambient sampler with preseparator (courtesy Andersen Air Samplers Inc.).

section of each stage is approximately 0.75 inch larger in diameter than the collection plate, allowing unimpacted particles to flow around the plate and into the next stage (Figure 30). Progressively smaller orifices increase the orifice velocity in 8 successive stages, causing impaction of smaller particles onto the collection discs of each succeeding stage. A

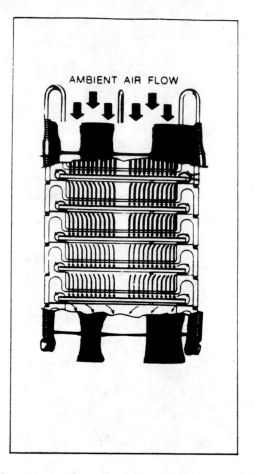

Figure 30.   Schematic cross section of the nonviable impaction stages of the Andersen Sampler (courtesy Andersen Air Samplers Inc.).

constant air sample flow of 1 cfm is provided by a continuous-duty vacuum pump. Flowrate is controlled by an adjustable valve on the pump and periodic calibration is recommended. Requirements for flowrate adjustments can be found in the Andersen 1-cfm *Ambient Sampler Operating Manual.* The sampler is supplied with a built-in backup filter holder that will accommodate an 81-mm filter disc. Normally, Type A glass fiber filter media are used because of their high collection efficiency for submicrometer particles.

To collect sized particles, the preweighed collection plates are placed on each stage. (The stainless steel plates should be placed with the curved lip down so that a raised, smooth surface is exposed for particle impingement). If the impactor preseparator is used, it should be mounted directly on top of stage 0 in place of the inlet cone. When the vacuum source is turned on, particulates entrained in the air stream are impacted inertially onto the collection plates or preseparator. The particle size range collected at the preseparator and each of the eight stages depends on the orifice velocity of the specific stage, the distance between the orifices and the collection surface and the collection characteristics of the preceding stage. The combination of a constant flowrate and successively smaller diameter orifices increases the velocity of sample air as it cascades through the impactor, resulting in the impaction of progressively smaller particles in succeeding stages. At 1 cfm, the particle fractionation ranges from 10.0 to 0.4 μm in diameter (Figure 30). Particles too small to be impacted on the last collection plate are collected in the backup filter, which is an integral part of the sampler. Many people use specific collection substrates other than glass or stainless steel plates because of lighter tare weight and/or specific analytical requirements. These collection materials consist of glass fiber, cellulose, aluminum foil, Gelman Spectro Grade and other materials that can be placed into an inverted stainless steel collection plate. The substrate surface must be level with the top of the curved SS lip to maintain jet to collection surface spacing. In this position, the sampler should be used in an upright position at all times. As airborne particulates have hygroscopic characteristics, all collection media used in the impactor should be desiccated both before and after a sampling cycle. Filter weighing should be made to an accuracy of $\pm$0.02 mg and a precision of $\pm$0.01 mg.

Normally, the sampler is disassembled, loaded with preweighed collection discs and a backup filter, and reassembled before being carried to the sampling site. When ready to sample, the vacuum source is turned on and a sample stream of 1 cfm will flow through the sampler. Normally, there is no variation in flowrate throughout the sampling period because a constant pressure drop is maintained. (No filtration occurs except at the backup filter, resulting in minimal pressure changes).

Normal sampling periods vary from a few minutes to several hours, depending on the workroom contamination levels and the sensitivity of the analytical procedure. An amount of 10 mg of particulate matter on any one stage represents an approximate upper limit because of reentrainment problems. Overloading the sampler can be detected easily by visual inspection and is rarely encountered in industrial hygiene applications. The preseparator is designed to capture several grams of particulate matter without overloading.

After the sampling has been completed, the sampler is disassembled. The collection plates and backup filter are removed and replaced with fresh, preconditioned, preweighed collection media. After conditioning, the collection media can be weighed for net particulate accumulations, or the particulate matter can be analyzed chemically for the various components of interest. The particulate matter in the preseparator should be brushed out carefully and weighed or analyzed separately; however, for data presentation purposes, the weight in the preseparator should be grouped with that for stage 0.

One should keep in mind that whenever a sample has been collected, the particle sizing has been completed. To determine the nature of the size distribution, simply perform the required gravimetric and/or chemical analyses.

FUMES AND VAPORS

A fume is created from a material that is solid at room temperature and is heated until it vaporizes. It condenses to form small particles that can grow with time but generally remain smaller than 10 μ in diameter. Molten metals are a common source of fume generation. The cellulose ester (AA) filter with an 0.8-μ pore size is used and field notes made by industrial hygienists in the laboratory analysis for the conditions sampled. The analysis may be for iron, if it is an iron welding rod, for fluoride, if the process uses a flux coating on the rod, or for copper in wire welding machines that use continuous lengths of wire instead of welding rods.

Vapors are collected in a medium that will absorb them and later, in the laboratory, they will be desorbed and tested. The sampling pump, calibrated flow method is used only in the case of a substance such as toluene. A charcoal tube is used for adsorption of the organic. The charcoal tube consists of two sections containing different mesh-activated charcoal types. The front section contains more charcoal than the second and they are separated by a urethane foam. Figure 31 illustrates a typical MSA sampling setup and calibration kit.

Figure 32 shows an instrument used for personal monitoring of respiratory dust. For personal monitoring of respirable dust in coal mines and other industrial atmospheres, the MSA gravimetric dust sampler kit is a rugged, compact monitor designed to meet the new concept in measuring airborne dust and the requirements of the Federal Coal Mine Health and Safety Act of 1969. MSA's gravimetric dust sampling kit consists of three basic components: (1) a battery-powered, diaphragm-type pump with three precalibrated flowrates; (2) a dual-rate battery charger; and (3) a cyclone assembly and a preweighed cassette or filter holder designed for personal monitoring.

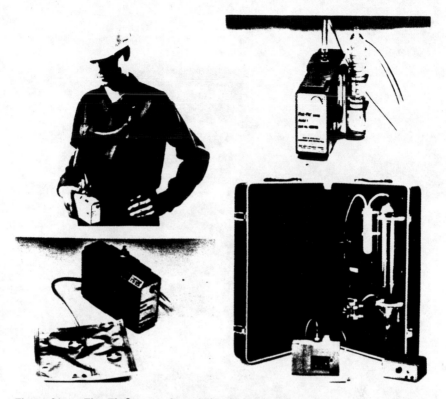

Figure 31.   Fixt-Flo® pump from Mine Safety Appliance Company, Pittsburgh, Pennsylvania, shown with charcoal sampling tube (upper left), impinger flask assembly (upper right), bag sampler for storing samples (lower left), and calibration kit (lower right).

In operation, the sampler is quite simple: the pump draws dust-laden air through the cyclone assembly and filter at a preselected flowrate. The cyclone stage of the assembly discards the larger nonrespirable (above 10 μ in size) particles. The smaller particles are trapped by a preweighed filter on a sensitive balance prior to sampling. At the end of the appropriate sampling period, the total weight of dust is established on the filter medium and the dust concentration of the air determined in mg/m^3. Figure 33 is sampling data sheet No. S343 from NIOSH for toluene.

GENERAL SAMPLING NOTES

1. As all sampling results will be compared to a time-weighted average, the times of exposure sampling must be recorded accurately.

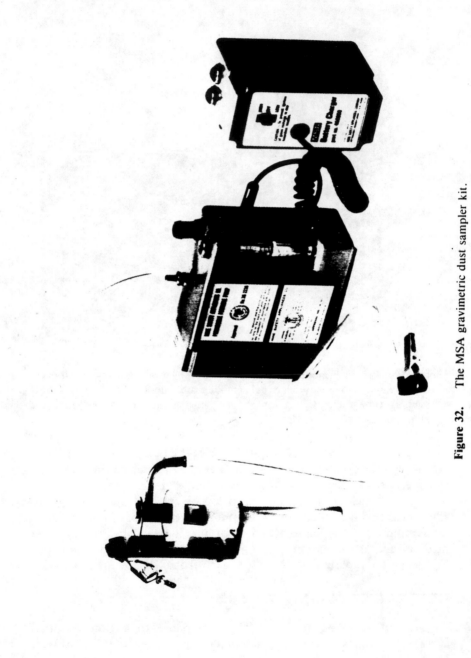

Figure 32.   The MSA gravimetric dust sampler kit.

Substance:

Toluene

Standard:

Ceiling - 300 ppm
Peak - 500 ppm
8-hr. TWA - 200 ppm

Reference: 29 CFR 1910.93

Method:

A known volume of air is drawn through a charcoal tube to trap the toluene vapors present. The analyte is desorbed from the charcoal tube with carbon disulfide, and the sample is separated and analyzed using a gas chromatograph with a flame ionization detector. The method has been validated over the range of 145.5 to 582 ppm for a 2-liter sample at 22°C and 766 mm Hg atmospheric temperature and pressure.

Sampling Equipment:

A calibrated personal sampling pump whose flow can be determined accurately, ±5%, over the range of 0.05 to 0.2 l/min, plus a charcoal tube containing two sections of 20/40 mesh-activated charcoal separated by a 2-mm portion of urethane foam. The charcoal tube is 7 cm long with a 4-mm i.d. The front section of the tube contains 100 mg of charcoal and the backup section contains 50 mg.

Sample Size:

At the ceiling concentration, a sample size of 2 liters is recommended. Sample for 10 minutes at a flowrate of 0.20 l/min.

At the 8-hour TWA concentration, a sample size of 12 liters is recommended. Sample at a flowrate of 0.20 l/min.

Sampling Procedure:

1. Immediately before sampling, the ends of the tube should be broken to provide an opening at least one-half the internal diameter of the tube.

2. The smaller section of charcoal is used as a backup and should be positioned nearest the sampling pump. The charcoal tube should be placed in a vertical position during sampling to avoid channeling and subsequent premature breakthrough of toluene.

3. Air being sampled should not be passed through any hose or tubing before covering the charcoal tube.

4. Set the flowrate as accurately as possible using the manufacturer's directions. Record the temperature and pressure of the atmosphere being sampled. If the pressure reading is not available, record the elevation. If the pump is a low flowrate pump, set the approximate flowrate and record the initial and final counter reading. The sample volume is obtained by multiplying the number of counter strokes times the cc/stroke factor.

5. The charcoal tubes should be capped with the supplied plastic caps immediately after sampling. Masking tape is the only suitable substitute for sealing the tubes. Under no circumstances should rubber caps be used.

6. With each batch of ten samples, submit one tube from the same lot of tubes that was used for sample collection and that is subjected to exactly the same handling as the samples, except that no air is drawn through it. Label this as a blank.

Special Considerations:

1. When interfering compounds are known or suspected to be present in the air, such information, including their suspected identities, should be transmitted with the sample.

2. Due to the high resistance of the charcoal tube, this sampling method places a heavy load on the sampling pump. Therefore, no more than eight hours of sampling should be done without fully recharging the battery.

3. If high humidity or water mist is present, breakthrough volume can be reduced severely. If condensation of water occurs in the tube, the substance will not be trapped quantitatively.

4. The desorption efficiency of charcoal varies from batch to batch. Therefore, all tubes used to collect a set of samples should contain charcoal from the same batch. Several unused charcoal tubes should accompany the samples. Information on the batch number of the charcoal must be supplied.

Bulk Samples:

A bulk sample of the suspected compound should be submitted to the laboratory in a glass container with a Teflon®*-lined cap. Label of the bulk sample should match air samples for identification purposes.

Shipping Instructions:

Capped charcoal tubes should be packed tightly and padded before they are shipped to minimize tube breakage during shipping. Never transport, mail or ship the bulk sample in the same container as the sample or blank tube.

Reference:

Toluene, NIOSH Method No. S343.

---

* Registered trademark of E. I. du Pont de Nemours and Company, Inc., Wilmington, Delaware.

Figure 33.   Sampling data sheet for toluene [32].

The time for lunch, breaks and normal operation must be noted and made part of the record.

2. Review the sampling procedure carefully.

3. Sampling Equipment:

Must be fully charged or have power source available.
Equipment must be approved for atmosphere being tested.
Must be calibrated periodically by NIOSH or approved laboratory.
Personal equipment should be attachable to individual and/or spare belt, and filter cassette holder should be provided (Figure 34).
Flowrate and calibration limits must be prepared for the specific sampling.

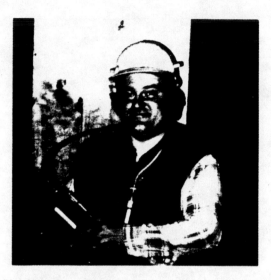

Figure 34.   Checking for respirable dust in the work area with a portable instrument.

4. Sample Size:

- What volume of sample atmosphere must be drawn through filter or medium?
- Bulk sampling of material may be requested.
- A number of samples of the same operation should be obtained to determine variation and consistency.

5. Blank Sample:
This method is comparable to radiation testing background counts to determine whether the filter medium was dirty or soiled or whether quality control was good.

6. Shipping and packaging should be adequate to ensure that the sample arrives at the laboratory undamaged.

7. A preconference with employees should be held to gain confidence and trust of the program. Many employees are afraid of job loss if they are exposed to a hazardous amount. Some employees tamper with the equipment; some managers schedule the least dangerous jobs for the sampling date; and both tend to distort actual conditions and results.

CHAPTER 5

INDUSTRIAL VENTILATION

IS THERE A NEED FOR RESPIRATORS?

It is hard to pinpoint when mankind decided to use respirators, but economics seemed a prime force. We will examine three principal areas of interest: *manufacturing, uncontrolled situations* and *confined spaces.*

Manufacturing historically began outdoors, but weather, atmospheric conditions and seasonal temperature variations accompanied the industrial revolution, which took place in the colder climates of Europe. Therefore, man's primary concern was to build weather- and waterproof shelters and provide heating and cooling for the seasonal changes. As solar energy and light were cheaper than fossil fuels, and, especially, safer than open flames and exhausts, windows were utilized in building design for light, air circulation and to keep out water. Although this explanation is simplistic, the United States built its buildings with this in mind until World War II. Typically, the roofs of many factory buildings were sawtoothed in nature, with parallel or alternating rows of windows or skylights, for light, and ventilation and room for power transmission shafting (Figure 35). Factories were large sets of buildings in which a relatively specific set of products (e.g., textiles, steel mills, foundries, etc.) were manufactured on a large scale. Dusty or dirty operations were usually confined to one area or building where cross-ventilation could be an aid to removing particulates. The soil and geography or neighborhood usually identified the type of manufacturing carried on in nearby factories; Gary, Indiana and its steel mills, as well as New England and its textile mills are examples.

With the technology of World War II and the use of high-speed, higher-temperature, multiple-head or automatic machines, more dust and small particulates were generated than the building's natural ventila-

Windows or Skylights

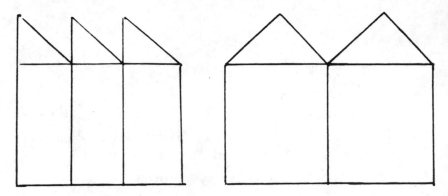

Sawtooth Roofs Typical Mill Construction

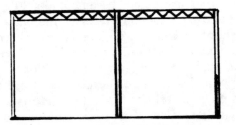

Modern-Flat Roof with Steel Joists
Separated with a Fire Wall

Figure 35.   Sawtoothed roofs—typical mill construction.

tion generally was able to handle. The development of industrial and plant engineering dictated that buildings must be large, one-story segmented structures designed to have raw material fed to the process on a programmed flow basis. Problems immediately arose because some employees had trouble breathing. Usually they were handed a dust mask but then had difficulty seeing the work, resulting in poor tolerances and defective parts. As a turbine moved steam pressure in pipes and the boiler used metal exhaust ducts to remove gas and particulates, plant engineers developed the turbine fans and sheet metal duct systems we know today.

Two main groups researched these problems: (1) *The American Conference of Governmental Industrial Hygienists* (ACGIH), and (2) the *American Society of Heating, Refrigeration, and Air Conditioning Engineers* (ASHRAE) [46]. Because of the lack of existing equipment to collect these materials from the plant before being dispersed into the local atmosphere and in response to the increased documentation on the rise of respiratory diseases, the U.S. Environmental Protection Agency (EPA) eventually developed regulatory policies in the 1970s. The EPA would regulate emissions outside the workplace, while OSHA would monitor and regulate emissions within. Figure 36 shows the legislative authorities affecting the life cycle of a chemical.

Many people may be exposed to a material liberated due to uncontrolled situations, such as pipe breaks, tank ruptures, spills, fires and relief valve venting. Concentrations of released materials may range from detectable odors of nuisance value to hazardous or even life-threatening levels. Many gases are shipped/stored under pressure in cylinders. Once converted into gases, they will occupy the confines of atmospheric pressure. If the only ventilation present consists of natural air currents, these will be transported and diffused into the atmospheric environment to dilute levels and eventually may achieve satisfactory levels. Respirators must be used in these instances in the plant until it can be determined whether the concentration is at safe levels. Civil defense units, firemen, state and local police, the hazardous spill units of the state, or the EPA usually provide this information. Figure 37 shows a sequence of probable response for a hazardous materials or spill accident under existing federal regulations. Instances like this may require self-contained breathing apparatus (SCBA), which will be discussed later in the book.

The third case, or confined space entry, means an area such as a sewer, tank, bin, culvert or reaction vessel, in which either a lack of sufficient oxygen exists to support human life and/or a toxic gas such as hydrogen sulfide may be present in sufficient concentration to kill or produce unconsciousness.

In general practice, an examination of the atmospheric conditions is made by a competent expert wearing an atmosphere-supplied respirator or using sufficiently long sampling probes. The explosibility of the atmosphere and oxygen content must be determined. Many applications require the wearing of an atmosphere-supplied respirator because the volumes of air required to be introduced are too large, too expensive, or too time-consuming to bring the contaminants to a safe level. (**Confined space entry** will be covered in detail in Chapter 12.)

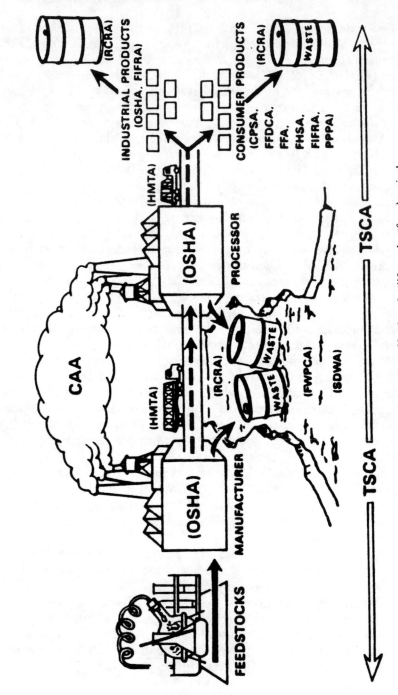

Figure 36.   Legislative authorities affecting the life cycle of a chemical.

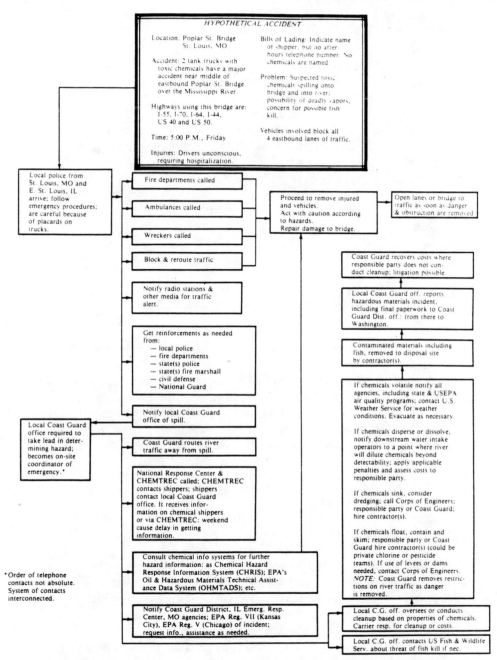

Figure 37. Response to a hazardous materials accident under existing federal regulations.

OCCUPATIONAL HEALTH AND
ENVIRONMENTAL CONTROLS

An explanation of the effects of certain environmental hazards and the rationale used in reducing their effects to acceptable levels is presented here to assist the reader in applying the standards to his workplace. These hazards are air contaminants, noise and radiation.

Two controllable factors that determine the effect of the hazard on employees are concentration of intensity and time of exposure. The product of these two factors is the dose.

The effect (response) on the body of a given dose is dependent on the employee's health status, which, in turn, is affected by many factors that mainly are beyond the employer's control.

Shown below are four degrees of response dependent on the dose (Figure 38):

- No response
- Minimal response
- Reversible response
- Irreversible response

Irreversible response means that permanent or incurable damage has been done.

The allowable dosage prescribed by the standard is called the TLV and is the concentration of hazard that will be within the response area with a safety factor of 2 to 10. The safety factor takes into account uncontrollable factors, e.g., variables in employee health status and others.

To control the dose, one should follow these instructions:

1. Reduce the time that the employee is exposed to the hazard.
2. Through engineering controls/redesign, reduce the concentration or intensity of the hazard by adequate ventilation, exhaust.
3. Provide personal protection equipment. This method is considered to be a last resort.

Keeping the concentration within the TLV is the best method for controlling air contaminants. Figures 39 and 40 illustrate relationships between exposure time and contaminant concentration. In Figure 39, the TLV is 6 mg/m^3 and the excursion factor is 2. The excursion factor has not been exceeded. For the TWA exposure to be less than the TLV, the area of the curve above the TLV must be less than the area below it. Contaminants and their sources include dust from abrasive blasting, dust

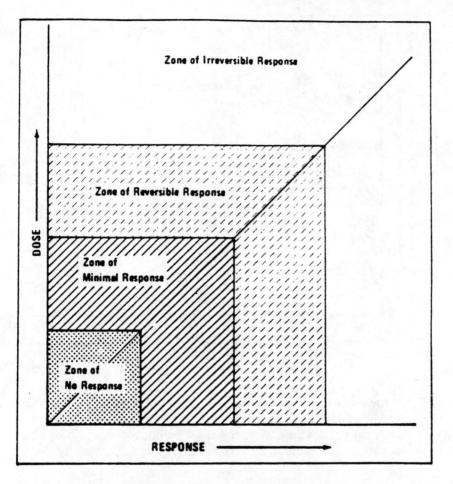

Figure 38.   Dose relation to response.

from dry bulk cargo, mists for pickling or plating tanks, vapors and gases from liquid cargo residue or cleaning solvents and fume gases, vapors, dusts and mists from any operations in places of employment. Employee exposures to contaminants must not exceed the TLV. In emergency situations, or when exposure exceeds the TWA or ceiling limits, protective equipment must be provided and used.

Ventilation is the basic method of reducing the concentration of air contaminants. Contaminated air may be discharged outside the building and replaced with fresh air or reused after being forced through dust collectors, traps or filters in the ventilation system, which remove the

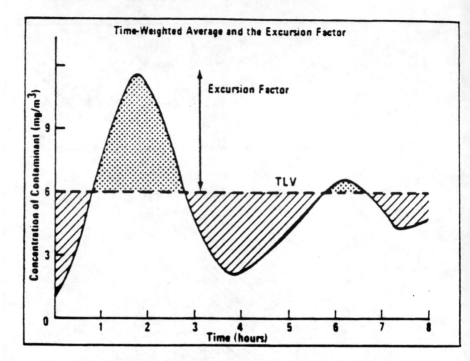

Figure 39.   TWA and the excursion factor.

contaminants. Air that contained toxic heavy metals (lead, cadmium, etc.) must not be reused. If contaminants are from an explosive mixture, electrical equipment and wiring must be nonsparking; no open flames, sparks or other ignition sources are permitted in the vicinity.

ABRASIVE BLASTING

Abrasive blasting operators must have protective devices when blasting is done in the open. Exhaust ventilation and protective devices are required when blasting is done indoors. Air must be filtered through dust collectors. A ventilator should be of sufficient volume to clear the air in the space as soon as the blasting stops. Static pressure drop across the filters must be monitored and not allowed to drop below the designed pressure. Personnel required inside the blasting enclosure must be provided heavy canvas or leather gloves and an apron to protect hands and bodies from the blast. They also must be given goggles, face shields,

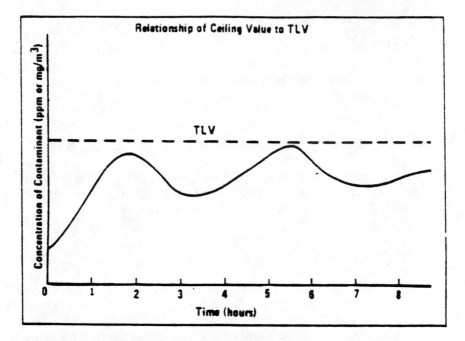

Figure 40. For chemical agents x with a ceiling value, the TLV should not be exceeded.

safety shoes (if heavy materials are being handled) and heavy clothing. Air for abrasive blasting hoods must meet ANSI standards for purity.

GRINDING, BUFFING, POLISHING

Hoods are required on polishing wheels and belts. Hoods must be connected to exhaust ventilation and designed so dirt particles are projected into the hoods in the direction of airflow.

SPRAY-FINISHING OPERATIONS

Spray-finishing operations must be conducted in spray rooms or enclosed booths. Booths and exhaust ducts must be of noncombustible material. Ductwork must not be connected to vent ducts for other processes. There must be an adequate collector system, and no sources of ignition shall be permitted.

OPEN SURFACE TANKS

Fumes, mists or vapors given off by the tanks must not exceed the threshold limit values. Further concentration must not create an explosive atmosphere. Airflow requirements and tank dimensions will determine airflow requirements.

COMPRESSED GASES, GENERAL REQUIREMENTS

Compressed gas cylinders under an employer's control must be in as safe a condition as can be determined by visual inspection. Adequate safety relief devices must be provided on containers.

Acetylene

Acetylene is a highly flammable gas with a flammable range of 2.5–82%, the widest known flammable range. It is classified as an asphyxiant and, under certain conditions, can form compounds with silver, mercury or copper that can explode spontaneously. Piping, generation and filling systems must be adequate.

Hydrogen

The presence of hydrogen cannot be detected by any of the senses. It is flammable in oxygen or air—a mixture of 10–65% hydrogen by volume in air will explode if ignited. Proper delivery, storage and discharge of hydrogen are required by the standards. For gaseous systems, appropriate marked containers, proper safety relief or vent piping and adequate equipment assembly or piping must be provided. The location must be above ground, away from power lines and flammables. Adequate ventilation must be provided, and heating, if provided, must be by an indirect means. Each system must be inspected properly and maintained by a qualified representative of the hydrogen supplier. For liquefied hydrogen systems, containers must be properly marked and well supported. Proper safety relief or vent piping must be provided. Adequate pipe insulation (when warranted), shutoff valve, vaporizer or low-temperature shutoff must be provided. All systems must be bonded and grounded properly. The location must be away from power lines and flammables. System must be ventilated properly. Instructions for operation of equipment must be kept at operating locations and systems must be inspected and maintained properly.

Oxygen

Oxygen must be considered as a potentially hazardous element from the fire hazard standpoint because the ignition temperature of all combustible material is lower in an oxygen-enriched atmosphere. Materials burn much faster in oxygen—the flammable range increases with an increase of oxygen content. When oxygen comes in contact with oil, grease or fuel oils, it may ignite violently. Every possible precaution should be taken to prevent this combination.

Bulk oxygen storage systems must be located aboveground out of doors or installed in a building of noncombustible construction, adequately vented and used for that purpose exclusively.

Proper containers for bulk oxygen storage must be provided. Design, support and construction must be in accordance with DOT or ASME specifications.

Piping or tubing must be suitable for the pressures and temperatures involved and containers must be equipped with adequate safety relief devices.

Liquid oxygen vaporizers must be connected and supported with fittings and devices that can stand the temperature changes. Vaporizers must have proper safety relief devices, heating and grounding.

Each system must be inspected and maintained by a qualified representative of the oxygen supplier.

FLAMMABLE AND COMBUSTIBLE LIQUIDS

The following requirements deal with the storage, handling and use of flammable and combustible liquids. Flammable liquids (Class I and II) and combustible liquids (Class III) are further subdivided as indicated below:

Class	Flash Point (°F)	Boiling Point (°F)
I	100	—
IA	73	100
IB	73	100
IC	73	100

II	Between 100 and 140	—
III	140	—
IIIA	Between 140 and 200	—
IIIB	200	—

TANK STORAGE

Design and Construction

Tanks must be of the proper material and design for their use. Tanks must be located outside, above ground and the proper distance from property lines and public way. Distance between any two flammable or combustible liquid storage tanks must be adequate. Proper venting or emergency relief vents must be provided. The area surrounding the tanks must have adequate drainage. Connections for all tank openings must be vaportight and liquidtight.

Underground Tanks

Tanks must be located the proper distance from buildings. They must have adequate earth cover when stored underground and corrosion protection for the tank and its piping must be provided. Proper venting must be provided, and connections for all tank openings must be vapor- or liquidtight.

Tanks Inside Buildings

Proper venting and an overflow prevention device must be provided. Filling and discharge connections must be closed, liquidtight and properly identified when not in use. Connections for all tank openings must be vapor- or liquidtight.

Supports, Foundations and Anchorage for All Tank Locations

Supports must be installed on firm foundations and constructed of concrete, masonry or protected steel. Supports must be fire-resistant and have adequate flood protection. Sources of ignition must be controlled or eliminated.

PIPING, VALVES AND FITTINGS

The design, materials, assembly and inspection of piping systems containing flammable or combustible liquids must be suitable for the expected working pressures and structural stresses. Adequate joints, supports and corrosion protection must be provided.

CONTAINER AND PORTABLE TANK STORAGE

Each portable tank must have sufficient emergency venting. Containers and portable tanks must meet size specifications.

STORAGE CABINETS AND ROOMS

Cabinets must not exceed gallon capacity (60 for flammable, 120 for combustible liquids) and must be designed and constructed to pass the fire test (internal temperature limited to 325°F if subject to 10-minute fire test). Storage rooms must be constructed to meet the required fire-resistive rating for their use. Electrical wiring and equipment located inside storage rooms must meet specifications. Storage rooms must be provided with either a gravity or a mechanical exhaust ventilation system. Storage in inside storage rooms (storage of flammable or combustible liquids) must be away from exits and containers of proper materials, and be properly stacked. Aisles must not be blocked. Storage outside buildings must not exceed maximum concentration, must be an adequate distance from buildings, must be graded in a manner to divert possible spills away from buildings or other exposures, and must be protected against tampering or trespassers. Adequate fire control devices must be provided.

INDUSTRIAL PLANTS

Where the use and handling of flammable or combustible liquids is only incidental to the principal business, liquids must be stored in adequate tanks or closed containers. The quantity of liquid permitted in a building, except in an authorized storage facility, must not exceed the maximum concentrations of 25 gallons for Class IA and 120 gallons for Classes 1B, 1C, II or III in containers of 660-gallon tanks; transfer methods must be adequate. Where flammable or combustible liquids are handled or used in unit physical operations not involving chemical change, access to firefighting equipment must be provided. Adequate fire separation of area from the rest of plant must be provided, as must proper drainage and ventilation. Tank vehicle and tank car loading and unloading facilities must be separated adequately from other facilities (i.e., aboveground tanks, warehouses, other plant buildings, property lines, etc.). Adequate fire control devices must be provided. Adequate precautions must be taken to prevent the ignition of flammable vapors (i.e., bonding, grounding, etc.). Electrical equipment must meet the standard for prescribed area. Good general housekeeping practices must be maintained.

BULK PLANTS AND TANK STORAGE

Tank storage must be appropriate for the class of liquid. Buildings must have adequate exits and heating units that are not a source of ignition and proper ventilation. Loading and unloading facilities must be separated from other facilities and protected against static sparks during tank loading. Wharves must be an adequate distance from a bridge or tunnel, have proper tanks, pumps, hoses and fittings, and have adequate fire protection. Electrical equipment must be of the proper type for that location. Class I liquids must not be handled, drawn or dispensed where flammable vapors may reach a source of ignition. Adequate fire control devices must be provided.

PROCESSING PLANTS

Processing plants must be an adequate distance from other facilities or the public way. Buildings must be of fire-resistant or noncombustible construction. Proper drainage system, ventilation and explosion relief must be provided. Liquid handling storage (tanks, pipes, etc.) must be adequate. Adequate portable extinguishers and an approved extinguishing system must be provided. Electrical equipment must be designed for the appropriate class of hazardous location.

Refineries, chemical plants and distilleries require that storage tanks meet the standards. Proper pressure vessels and adequate drainage from process units must be provided, and fire control devices installed.

Fires in spray booths and spray booth operations most frequently result from spontaneous ignition of spray deposits. Employers must ensure that spray finishing operations in their plants are safe. Booths must be constructed of noncombustibles and designed to sweep air currents toward the exhaust outlet. Adequate lighting must be available.

ELECTRICAL AND OTHER IGNITION SOURCES

All electrical equipment, open flames and other sources of ignition must meet the requirements of the standard. Wiring must be approved for the location, and equipment must be grounded.

VENTILATION

All spraying areas must have mechanical ventilation adequate to remove flammable vapors, mists or powders to a safe location and to confine and control combustible residues so that life or property are not endangered. Each spray booth must have an independent exhaust duct system discharging to the exterior of the building. Booths must have adequate fans and ductwork. Rotating elements must be nonferrous or nonsparking. Electrical motors and exhaust fans must not be placed inside booths or ducts.

The quantity of liquids kept in the vicinity of spray operations must be the minimum required for operations and should not exceed a supply for one day or one shift. Open or glass containers must not be used for bringing liquids into spray finishing rooms. Hoses must have shutoff valves and heaters must not be located in spray booths or other locations subject to the accumulation of deposits or combustible residue.

Sprinklers protecting spraying areas must be kept as free from deposits as practical by daily cleaning. An adequate supply of suitable portable fire extinguishers must be installed near all spraying areas.

OPERATION AND MAINTENANCE (O&M)

Spraying areas must be kept as free as possible from the accumulation of deposits and combustible residues. Cleaning solvents shall have a flashpoint of more than 100°F. "No smoking" signs must be posted conspicuously at all spraying areas. Booths must not be used for different types of coating materials because the combination of the materials may be conducive to spontaneous ignition.

Fixed Electrostatic Apparatus

Proper electrical equipment must be used in spray areas. Electrostatic apparatus must be equipped with failsafe controls. Adequate guarding, ventilation and fire protection must be provided.

Electrostatic Hand Spraying Equipment

Equipment in the spraying area must not exceed specified maximum surface temperature. The spray gun handle must be grounded. Electrical equipment must be so interlocked with the ventilation of the spraying area that the equipment cannot be operated unless the ventilation fans are in operation.

DRYING, CURING OR FUSION APPARATUS

Booths must not be used alternately for drying purposes in any arrangement that will cause a material increase in the surface temperature of the spray booth, room or enclosure. Adequate ventilation and ventilation interlock with heat must be provided. Powder coating temperature must not be above 150° in electrostatic fluidized beds.

Dip tanks containing flammable liquids subject to ignition at ordinary temperatures and giving off flammable vapors present a severe fire and explosion hazard. Employers must ensure safe dipping operations in the workplace.

An adequate ventilation system must be provided, and tanks must have a properly trapped overflow pipe or bottom drain, when warranted. Large tanks must have an automatic extinguishing device. When dip tank liquids are heated artificially, provision must be made to prevent excessive heating of liquids. The vapor area must be free of sources of ignition.

THRESHOLD LIMIT VALUE AND VENTILATION

The TLV specifies the allowable concentration of a material in the work atmosphere for a legal exposure period (usually eight hours). Under the OSHA Act of 1970, if the concentration of material is greater than the TLV, the plant is in violation and must provide respirators and engineering controls such as ventilation, to lower the concentration below the TLV. If engineering controls are not feasible, then respirators must be used to protect the individual. Respirators generally are considered only as an alternative to general ventilation or engineering and administrative controls. This process is generally termed "dilution ventilation" because it adds more air and, with the exhaust, the concentration of the contaminant is reduced or diluted. In plant engineering practice, the ventilation of a production area can be a complicated and expensive problem. Typically, there are five problem areas that must be considered before the system is said to be balanced environmentally:

- Volume of air
- Temperature changes
- Insulation
- Structure
- Pollution control

The volume of air, or how much ventilation must be introduced into an area to dilute or remove the contaminant, is expressed in cubic feet per minute or air changes per hour. The volume of air depends on the amount of air produced in the contamination process. Makeup air or the air introduced to make up the mass flow balance of the air leaving the room by exhaust is seldom considered. Areas in which toxic substances are handled should be kept under negative pressure to prevent the airborne particle from floating to other areas of the plant and settling out. Negative pressure is understood to mean that the room is under a slight vacuum—more air leaves than enters. As contaminants in the air vary from day to day, several readings should be taken and variable volume systems installed where necessary. Seasonal changes must be noted because the summer weather causes the windows to remain open, producing large amounts of natural ventilation.

Temperature is probably the most misunderstood of all problems. Each type of production machine has its own range of efficient operating temperatures and automatic controls to shut it down or stop it if these ranges are not observed. The radiant heat of the machines is never considered and usually, during the winter, the cold air introduced by ventilation can cause rust or corrosion from condensation. The cost of heating plants in winter and the added cost of additional tempered or heated ventilation air has caused operations to be shut down.

Insulation is seldom, if ever, used on heat-producing equipment, like dyeing vats, vulcanizers or autoclaves used to cure products. During the summer, the "sauna" atmosphere they produce is extreme, and in the winter they act like giant radiators. Ventilation instead of insulation is used to cool the area; however, like a dog chasing its tail, the more evaporative the cooling loss, the more heat that is pumped into the system to maintain process temperature by the automatic controls.

Structural problems usually are encountered in any makeup or ventilation system for two reasons. As mentioned earlier, buildings usually are designed for roof, snow and rain loads, not heavy, high-speed rotary equipment. The riggers who place the fan on the roof (unless it is done by helicopter), generally damage the sealed layers, and leaks spring up after the first few heavy rains.

The area of pollution control is very general, but the following example is typical of most systems. The exhaust duct of factory A blows into the clean air intake of factory B. The noise and vibration cause neighbors to sign a petition complaining to regulatory authorities. The exhaust material turns Wednesday laundry into a pink polkadot contest.

We will confine our examination of ventilation to the determination of the hazard and whether ventilation is required because the concentration is above the TLV. For convenience, we will use the terminology of OSHA and examine typical data of a hypothetical inspection. OSHA determines exposure by sampling an employee for a period of time with a sampling instrument. Although sampling is explained more fully in another chapter, a typical inspector would measure the concentration of the harmful atmosphere by a direct reading instrument or a collecting device.

The direct reading instrument draws a known volume of material through a known medium of a collector material, which produces a color change (a detector tube). Alternatively, a volume of a gas over a Wheatstone Bridge comparing the electrical difference provides a direct reading. The sampler draws the contaminated atmosphere into a collector employing a filter, solution or absorption process, much like a vacuum cleaner. Whatever the method, a concentration of contaminant is read off the equipment and compared to the OSHA 1910.1000 Tables Z1, Z2 or Z3 [47] regulations to determine whether the concentration is above or below the OSHA legal limits. It should be noted in comparing the three tables that Table Z2 also considers the "Acceptable maximum Peak" above the acceptable ceiling concentrations for an eight-hour shift. The concentration of the material and the maximum duration also are noted.

In OSHA, those doing the sampling are *industrial hygienists*. They usually do exposure profiles, which are graphic representations of the degree of air contamination in a process plotted against a time frame, or spot-sampling. For legal purposes, when spot-sampling is done, if the exposure reading is within the statistical error of the sampling device for the TLV, no further sampling is required. If not, a sampling pump would be worn by an employee for a full shift, measuring his or her exposure for that period of time to that particular substance. Such a device also is known as a dosimeter.

Figure 41 illustrates a typical example of a hypothetical metal operation:

1. At 8:00 a.m., before the operation starts up, the level of contaminants present is not zero, due to either a long settling time (following Stoke's law) for the "fine" particles or the dust generated by the third shift.

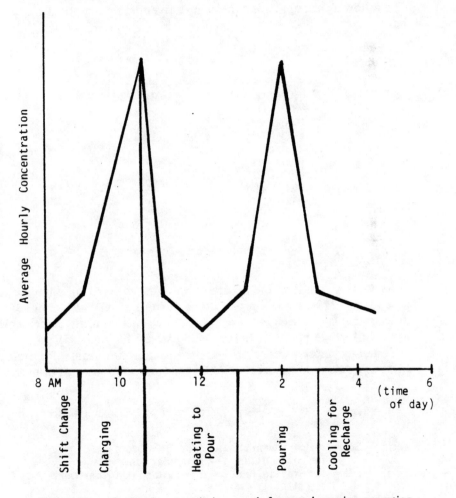

Figure 41.   Contaminant emission graph for metal pouring operation.

2. As production starts up, the furnace is charged and the emission rate rises due to aeration and mechanical mixing employed.

3. The melt is checked for metallurgical purity and the pour operation is ready.

4. While the metal is poured into the mold, the concentration climbs rapidly again.

5. The concentration drops during cooling.

As in this case, most production operations are cyclic in nature. With the high cost of sampling equipment and related calibration and laboratory fees, some hygienists use detector tubes and average out the reading. The following example was done using a five-minute sample each quarter hour.

Time	Average Concentration (ppm)
0800–0900	34
0900–1000	40
1000–1100	20
1100–1200	15
Lunch	
1300–1400	15
1400–1500	20
1500–1600	15
1600–1700	25
	184

$$\frac{184}{8} = 23 \text{ ppm for an 8-hour day.}$$

As OSHA considers the accuracy or statistical error of the detector tube to be ±35%, the reading could be 31 (plus 35%) or 15 (minus 35%) or even the value measured. For a substance such as nitric oxide, which has a TLV of 25 ppm, further sampling would be required.

Generally, most workers are exposed to concentrations of chemicals from more than one source. OSHA specifies the following formula:

$$Em = \left(\frac{C_1}{L_1} + \frac{C_2}{L_2} + \cdots \frac{C_n}{L_n} \right) \quad \text{The value of Em shall not exceed unity.}$$

where Em = the equivalent exposure for the mixture
   C = the concentration of a particular contaminant
   L = the exposure limit for that contaminant from Tables Z-1, Z-2, Z-3 [47].

Example: An employee was exposed to three solvents during an 8-hour time period, given the following information. Was the exposure too much?

Material (Table Z-1) from OSHA STD 1910.1000	Actual Concentration Measured for 8-hour Exposure (ppm)	8-hour Time-Weighted Average Exposure Limit (ppm)
Acetone	600	1000
2-Butanone	45	200
Toluene	40	200

$$\text{Substituting in formula } Em = \frac{600}{1000} + \frac{45}{200} + \frac{40}{200}$$

$$= 0.600 + 0.225 + 0.200 = 1.025$$

As Em is greater than 1, the employee was overexposed.

Table Z-2 in OSHA Standard 1910.1000 [47] gives the acceptable ceiling concentrations (and maximum peaks above them) and their corresponding time durations for 22 assorted compounds. The survey for exposure should take these substances into account by a graphic method also. Figure 42 illustrates a hypothetical operation in which an employee, who operates a multicolor rotary screen printing machine, is exposed to too much toluene. The legal maximum peak level for toluene (Table Z-2) is 500 ppm at 10 minutes, yet the operator is within the 200-ppm 8-hour TWA. Most operators of this type equipment are required to clean their own screens, usually in a tub of toluene with a scrub brush. To comply with local and state permits, ventilation of this operation generally is costly and time consuming, so the operator generally is provided with an organic filter respirator.

PHYSICAL PROPERTIES OF AIR

Of primary importance in the selection of respirator or the design of a ventilating system is proper consideration of the physical properties of air. Factors such as compression, expansion, temperature difference, moisture and concentration of impurities are common to both systems but seldom considered in respirator protection. Air is a composition of gases, that have properties of molecular weight, density, relative and

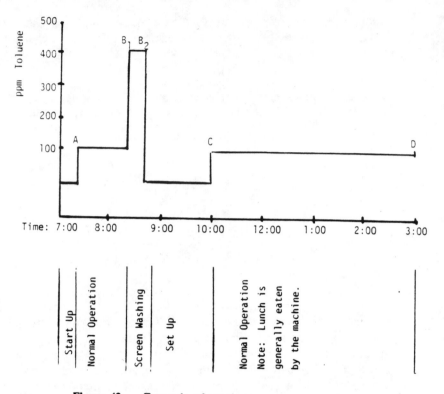

Figure 42. Example of employee exposure to toluene.

absolute humidity, volume and thermodynamic properties. From our first breath we do not question the composition of air—we merely accept it. As the materials being handled in industry become more toxic by legal definition or by physiological testing, or the atmosphere being inhabited becomes less life supporting, respirator design has moved from the simple facepiece to the space suit or environment-atmosphere type design. Man's own body becomes the source of toxic gases or pollution, which must be controlled to survive. The reader is reminded that whether one is ventilating a process, a human set of lungs or a space suit, the basic principles apply. As the thermodynamic and physical properties of air handling systems are book-length subjects, a quick review is provided for reader convenience.

Evangelista Toricelli, an Italian mathematician, summarized that we all live at the bottom of an ocean of air and that we must be under some pressure. Toricelli created the first crude barometer by inverting a tube of mercury over a bowl of mercury. He determined that the weight of air pressing on the mercury in the bowl was equal to about 30 inches of water, or 760 mm of mercury (Hg). It also follows that if 1 inch of mercury (Hg) equals 13.6 inches of water pressure, 30 inches of mercury equals 407 inches of water. To correlate the information, we must consider the physical state of the air with regard to pressure. In ventilation, a fan flows air with slight pressure, a blower compresses the air more and a compressor pressurizes the air in a receiver and pipe system. Duct systems are usually low pressure and are measured with a water-filled U-tube manometer for pressure drops across the system. Air line respirators use air compressed from a compressor whose pressure is measured in pounds per square inch (psi). Scuba tanks developed by divers use atmospheres absolute (ata) or kilograms per centimeter squared (kg/cm^2) to express their required pressures. A practical example would be Figure 43, which shows what the relative values would be if a U-tube manometer filled with mercury were placed on an air compressor receiver tank.

Air is composed of oxygen (21%), nitorgen (78%), argon (0.9%) and various rare gases (neon, helium, hydrogen), 0.1% which Boyle's and Charles' gas laws apply and the perfect gas equation, PV = nRT. In ventilation problems, an easy method of dealing with the equation is presented by James May in the *Physics of Air* [48]:

$$PQ = WRT$$

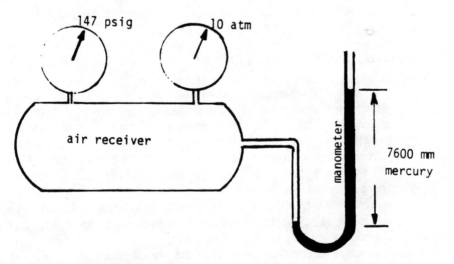

Figure 43.   Comparison of pressure terminology: 1 atm = 14.7/psig = 760 mm Hg/30 in. Hg = 407 in. water.

where   P = the absolute pressure (psf)
         Q = the total volume of the gas (ft³)
         W = the total weight of the gas (lb)
         R = the gas constant = 53.34
         T = the absolute temperature = $(460 + t)°F$

R is derived by dividing 1545.4 by the molecular weight (28.941) of the air mixture, which equals 53.34. Typical errors in calculation include temperatures that often are expressed in degrees farenheit rather than in degrees absolute. Concentrations of oxygen, nitrogen and argon always should be monitored or certified.

In diving, if a man breathes pure oxygen under pressure he can experience oxygen poisoning. If a diver ascends too fast, he can suffer the "bends" from the nitrogen. A fire fighter could become engulfed in a ball of flames if he brought a tank of oxygen instead of compressed air into a fire situation. Typically, the part water vapor plays in breathing systems is often forgotten. Air must contain a small percentage of water vapor or an individual's sinus tissues will dry out or dehydrate. In cold climates, too much water vapor will produce fogged faceplates and frozen valves in air line respirators. Engineers refer to the properties as psychrometric and use a chart to aid in these calculations. The individual who specifies atmosphere-supplied suits must be familiar with this approach because once in the suit the individual cannot replace water loss. He also may faint due to heat and/or water loss. We will next examine the psychrometric chart as it applies to air pollution control.

THE PSYCHROMETRIC CHART

Most pollution engineers eventually will be exposed to a project that requires a knowledge of terms and calculations common to industrial air pollution control. With the exception of a pencil and slide rule, the handiest tool for simplifying these calculations is a psychrometric chart. Psychrometrics, in the modern sense, means the evaluation of air properties and the processes that alter them. Psychrometrics has a special vocabulary often used in air pollution control work.

Absolute humidity or humidity ratio is the mass of water vapor per unit mass of dry air in a mixture of air and water vapor. This mixture is commonly called *gas*.

Relative humidity is the ratio of the partial pressure of the water vapor in a mixture to the saturation pressure of pure water at the same temperature.

Dry (DA) is the mixture of all the normal components of atmospheric air except water vapor.

Saturated air is a mixture of dry air and saturated water vapor or, alternatively, a mixture having relative humidity equal to 1.00.

Dewpoint temperature is the temperature at which the mixture, or gas, becomes saturated (or condensation begins) when a mixture of air and water vapor is cooled at constant pressure from an unsaturated state.

Dry bulb temperature (DB) is the actual temperature of the gas.

Wet bulb temperature is the temperature indicated by a thermometer having its bulb covered by a film of water when the thermometer is exposed to an air-vapor mixture in turbulent flow.

Adiabatic saturation temperature is that reached by an airstream after it has been saturated with water vapor with no sensible heat transfer. The wet bulb temperature and the adiabatic saturation temperature are numerically very close for air-vapor mixtures only. It is largely this fact that makes the wet bulb temperature useful. Adiabatic saturation occurs at constant enthalpy.

Humid volume is the volume occupied by one pound of dry air, with its water vapor, in a mixture.

A psychrometric chart graphically displays the above properties over a range of temperatures and humidities. Its great usefulness is that processes can be traced easily and computations are simplified greatly. A typical high-temperature psychrometric chart is shown in Figure 44 [49]. The following examples explain use of the psychrometric chart.

Example One

Convert 33,000 acfm at 300°F dry bulb and 0.10 lb H_2O/lb dry air to standard conditions (70°F and dry).

Solution. This problem asks to determine the volume flow at standard conditions that will yield the same mass flow as the given conditions. This can be done by multiplying 33,000 acfm by the ratio of standard density to actual density. The density of air at standard conditions is 0.075 lb/ft³. By referring to the psychrometric chart and schematic chart (Figure 45), it may be seen that at 300°F dry bulb and 0.10 lb H_2O/lb dry air the humid volume is about 21.5 ft³/lb DA, therefore, the actual gas density is

$$\frac{1 \text{ lb DA} + 0.10 \text{ lb } H_2O}{2.15 \text{ ft}^3/\text{lb DA}} = 0.0512 \text{ lb/ft}^3$$

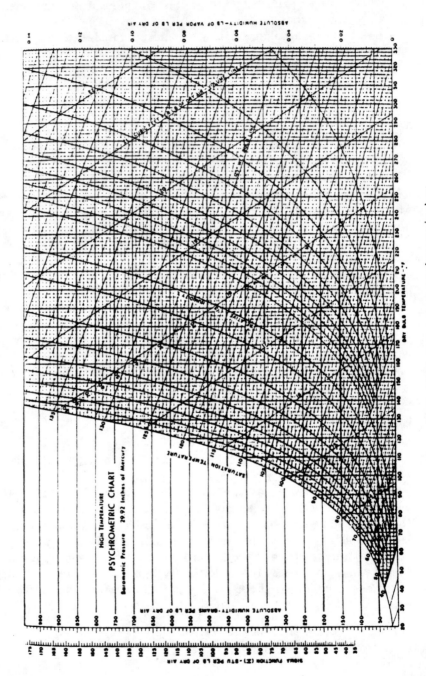

Figure 44.   Typical high-temperature psychrometric chart.

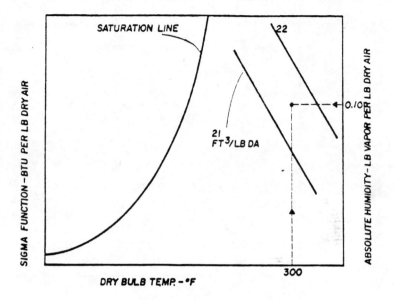

Figure 45.

$$\text{Standard flowrate} = 33,000 \times \frac{0.0512}{0.075} = 22,528 \text{ acfm}$$

Example Two

Suppose the gas in Example One is cooled to 200°F DB. What is the new volume?

Solution. As the gas is cooled without adding or condensing moisture, it must occur along a constant absolute humidity line (Figure 46). The new volume will be the initial volume multiplied by the ratio of final to initial humid volume:

$$\text{New volume} = 33,000 \text{ acfm} \times \frac{19 \text{ ft}^3/\text{lb DA}}{21.5 \text{ ft}^3/\text{lb DA}} = 29,163 \text{ acfm}$$

Example Three

How much water is required to cool the gas in Example One by adiabatic saturation, and what is the resultant gas volume?

Solution. For purposes of calculation, adiabatic saturation can be

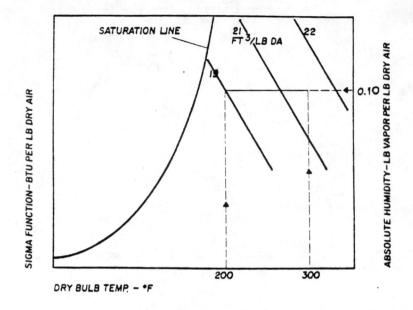

Figure 46.

assumed to take place along a constant wet bulb line (Figure 47). The gas initially contains 0.10 lb H_2O/lb DA and, after cooling, contains 0.126 lb H_2O/lb DA. Therefore, the added water is

0.126 lb H_2O/lb DA − 0.10 lb H_2O/lb DA = 0.026 lb H_2O/lb DA

The mass flowrate is

$$\frac{33,000 \text{ acfm}}{21.5 \text{ ft}^3/\text{lb DA}} = 1535 \text{ lb DA/min}$$

$$\text{Water requirement} = \frac{1535 \text{ lb DA}}{\text{min}} \times \frac{0.026 \text{ lb } H_2O}{\text{lb DA}} \times \frac{\text{gal}}{8.3 \text{ lb } H_2O}$$

$$= 4.8 \text{ gpm}$$

$$\text{New volume} = \frac{33,000 \text{ acfm} \times 19.7 \text{ ft}^3/\text{lb DA}}{21.5 \text{ ft}^3/\text{lb DA}} = 30,237 \text{ acfm}$$

Example Four

What is the mass and volume flowrate of the water component of the gas mixture in Example One?

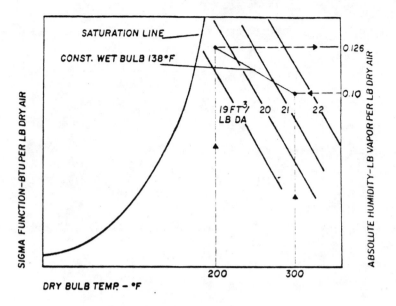

Figure 47.

Solution. By referring to Example One, each pound of dry contains 0.10 lb of water vapor. From Example Three, the mass flowrate of dry air was 1540 lb DA/min. Therefore:

$$\text{Mass flow of vapor} = \frac{1535 \text{ lb DA}}{\min} \times \frac{0.10 \text{ lb } H_2O}{\text{lb DA}} = 154 \text{ lb } H_2O/\min$$

As all components in a gas mixture occupy the same volume, the volume flowrate of water vapor is 33,000 acfm.

Example Five

How much heat energy must be added to 150,000 acfm of gas at 150 F DB and 0.02 lb H_2O/lb DA to raise the temperature to 300°F DB?

Solution. If the products of combustion are assumed to contribute little to the total mass, then the initial state can be represented by point A on Figure 48 and the final state is point B. Point B is determined by the intersection of the required dry bulb temperature and a constant absolute humidity line. By referring to 44, one can see that the heat energy content of the various combinations of gas mixtures is given by sigma function expressed in Btu/lb DA. The sigma function is analogous to enthalpy

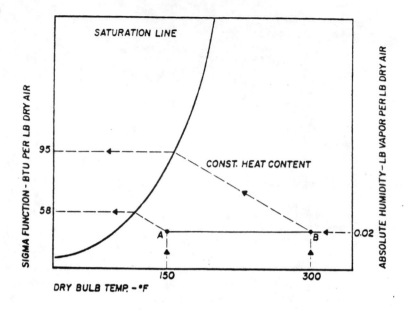

Figure 48.

and differs from enthalpy by an amount equal to the enthalpy of liquid water at the adiabatic saturation temperature. In practice, either sigma function or enthalpy can be used for computation. Constant heat energy lines are approximately parallel to wet bulb lines.

- heat energy at A = 58 Btu/lb DA
- heat energy at B = 95 Btu/lb DA
- heat energy added = (95 – 58) Btu/lb DA = 37 Btu/lb DA

$$\text{lb DA} = \frac{150,000 \text{ acfm}}{19.7 \text{ ft}^3/\text{lb DA}} = 7614 \text{ lb DA/min}$$

Total heat added = 7614 lb DA/min × 37 Btu lb DA = 282,000 Btu/min

The above examples are only a sample of the many calculations needed by a pollution engineer. It should be apparent, however, that use of the psychrometric chart greatly facilitates these and many more calculations.

FANS AND BLOWERS [50,51]

The most common method for moving gases under moderate pressures is by some type of fan. The fan is significant and important in all industrial plants. It is the heart of any system that demands that air be supplied, circulated and removed in a way that provides a safe and comfortable environment. For industrial plants, the needs of heating, ventilating, air conditioning and pollution control are fulfilled by this equipment.

There are two general classes of fans: **axial and centrifugal.** Axial fans employ propellers and are classed into three subtypes—**propeller, tube-axial** and **vane-axial.** Centrifugal fan flow is principally radial rather than axial. Centrifugal fans also are divided into three groups: **forward, backward** and **radial.** A distinction is made in engineering practice between fans for low pressure and centrifugal compressors for high pressure. A boundary separating the two classes of equipment is set at 7% increase in density of air from the inlet to the outlet. Fan action is below this density increase, and the incompressibility of gas moved is assumed.

The choice of fan depends on flow volume required, static pressure, condition of air handled, available space, noise, operating temperature, efficiency and cost. Consideration also should be given to the drive system, whether direct or belt-driven.

Axial Fans

The axial flow fan is used in systems that have low resistance levels. This type fan moves the air or gases parallel to the fan's axis of rotation. Axial flow fans use the screw-like action of their propellers to move the air in a straight-through parallel path. This screw-like action of the propeller causes a helical-type flow pattern. **Propeller-type** axial flow fans move air at pressures from 0 to 1 inch of water. Additional variations of the axial flow fan can move air at somewhat higher pressures.

A variation of the axial flow fan is the **tube-axial fan**—the basic axial flow fan encased in a cylinder. The fan's propeller in the cylinder helps to collect and direct the air flow. The tube-axial fan can move air or gas at pressures between 0.25 and 2.5 inches of water.

A second variation of the axial fan is known as the **vane-axial** fan, which is an adaptation of the tube-axial fan using air guide vanes mounted in the cylinder either on the entry or discharge side of the propeller. These vanes further increase the fan's efficiency and working pressures from 0.5 to 10 inches of water by straightening out the air or discharge flow.

Principal advantages of axial fans are their economy, installation simplicity and small space requirements. The principal disadvantage, aside from operating pressure limitations, is noise. This latter problem is usually apparent at maximum pressure levels. These fans are seldom used in duct systems because of the relatively low pressures developed. They are well adapted for moving large quantities of air against low pressures with free exhaust, as from a room to the outside.

Centrifugal Fans

Centrifugal fans or blowers move the air or gas perpendicular to the fan's axis of rotation (Figure 49). Air is drawn into the center of the revolving wheel, which is on a shaft containing the fan's blades. The gas stream then enters the spaces between the wheel's blades and is thrown out peripherally at high velocity and static pressure. As this occurs, additional air is drawn into the eye of the wheel. This type blower is used where the frictional resistance of the system is relatively high.

There are various adaptations of the centrifugal fan, which are distinguished by the type of blade used. Blade types depend on space limitations, efficiency demanded by the system for particular load conditions and allowable noise levels. There are three general types of blades that are used in blowers: forward-curved, backward-curved and straight or radial type (Table X).

In the **forward-curved centrifugal fan**, the blade is inclined at the tip toward the direction of rotation. This is the most widely used centrifugal

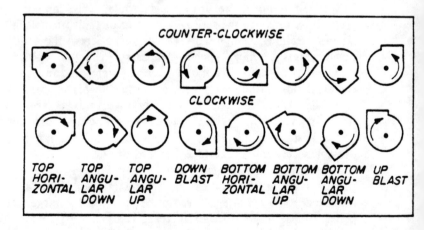

Figure 49. Centrifugal fan rotation and discharge. Two directions of discharge and sixteen discharge positions are possible with centrifugal fans. Rotation direction will be determined by the fan function and is specified according to the view from drive side.

Table X. Relative Characteristics of Centrifugal Fans

	Forward-Curved Blade	Backward-Curved Blade	Radial Blade
First Cost	Low	High	Medium
Efficiency	Low	High	Medium
Operational Stability	Poor	Medium	Medium
Tip Speed	Low	High	Medium
Abrasion Resistance	Poor	Medium	Good
Sticky Material Handling	Poor	Medium	Good

fan for general ventilation purposes. It operates at relatively low speeds and generally is used for producing high-volume airflow and low static pressure. This type of fan is quiet, economical, space-efficient and lightweight. Because of the inherent design of its blade configuration and low operating speeds, the forward-curved fan cannot develop high static pressures.

Backward-curved fans are more suitable for higher static pressure operation. They operate at about twice the speed of forward-curved centrifugal fans and have higher efficiency and a nonoverloading horsepower curve. The higher operating speeds, however, require larger shaft and bearing size. Therefore, greater care must be taken in system balance.

The **radial fan** has a blade curvature tangent to the radius at its outer tip. The radial-type centrifugal fan generally is designed for handling low air volumes at relatively high static pressures. It also is suitable for handling high dust concentration air because of its wheel design.

Fan Selection

When selecting a fan, one must consider which fan will fit the purpose, while being the most economical to operate. Cost considerations before purchase include O&M and equipment costs. It is not necessary to design a new fan for each new application. Choice of a fan that fits the needs usually consists of selecting one commercially available from suppliers.

A fan's capacity is measured in cubic feet per minute. This is equivalent to the number of pounds of air or gas flowing divided by the number of pounds of gas or air per cubic foot at the system's inlet. To meet the fan's capacity, the right horsepower motor must be used to drive the fan. Belt-driven fans are used for motor requirements generally between 1 and 200 hp. Fans of this type are available in a larger number of standard sizes. Economical motor selection can be made, even when its speed is different from that of the fan, by selecting the proper belt-drive ratio. For fans requiring drive motors larger than 200 hp, direct-drive motors generally are used. Direct-drive fans are limited to the fan's motor speed. Principal advantages of this latter type drive are less required maintenance and less power transmission loss than from belt-driven fans.

When ordering a fan, the following data are required:

1. **Flow volume**—the volume of air the fan will handle at the actual temperature conditions that will prevail.
2. **Composition of the gas handled**—moisture, dust load, corrosives present, etc.
3. **Static pressure**—the resistance the fan will have to overcome to deliver the required volume of air, including the resistance or pressure drop in the total system the air flows through from process intake to exhaust stack exit.
4. **Operating temperature**—important not only from the standpoint of affecting the volume of air handled, but because it will determine the materials of construction in many cases.
5. **Efficiency**—the ability of the fan to handle the required volume and pressure with a minimum horsepower motor and expenditure of electrical energy. This parameter will determine the operating costs of the unit.
6. **Noise**—the best guide to the selection of a suitably quiet fan is successful previous performance.
7. **Space requirements and equipment layout**—will include orientation of fan inlet and outlet as many options are available.
8. **Initial cost** of the equipment.

Space requirements and initial cost are usually secondary considerations. Two important factors in fan selection for ventilation, for example, are efficiency, which affects operating costs, and noise.

When ordering a fan, the customer must include information concerning the applicable size of ductwork and the system for which the fan is to be used. From this information, the supplier can make sure the fan will meet pressure requirements. To fulfill the requirements, the fan must be able to accelerate the air or gas from the velocity at the system's entrance to that of its exit. It also must be able to overcome any pressure differences within the system. Finally, it must be able to overcome frictional and shock losses encountered in the system. Additionally, fans achieving their final exhaust through stacks must maintain a minimum exit velocity (usually 60 fps minimum) to ensure that the exhaust stack gas will escape the turbulent wake of the stack. In many cases, it is desirable to have the gas exit velocity on the order of 90 or 100 fps. Another piece of information that the supplier should have is whether the fan will be subject to any unusual conditions. This is particularly important for fans and blowers used with air pollution control devices.

When the system requirements are known, the main points to be considered in fan selection are efficiency, reliability of operation, size and weight, speed, noise and cost.

To assist customers in choosing a fan, manufacturers supply tables or curves that show the following factors for each fan size, operating against a wide range of static pressures:

- Air volume handled, in cfm at standard conditions (68°F, 50% R.H., weighing 0.07496 lb/ft^3)
- Air velocity at the outlet
- Fan speed (rpm)
- Brake horsepower
- Peripheral speed, or blade tip speed (fpm)
- Static pressure (in. H$_2$O)

Tables listing fan capacities indicate the most efficient operating point by printing values in in bold face, italics or in some other way.

Corrosion Resistance

Two major problems that fan and blower designs must overcome are excessive temperatures and corrosive atmospheres. Mild steel is good for fan construction in dry applications up to temperatures of 900°F. Temperatures exceeding this cause scaling. In such cases, steel may be coated with a protective alloy.

Structural and corrosive problems arise at excessive high gas stream temperatures and/or corrosive atmospheres. High temperatures cause many materials to lose their strength and promote chemical reaction in the metal itself, such as scaling. Some methods used to solve these problems include lowering the gas temperature and controlling the concentration of corrosives in the exhaust gas. With lower temperatures, the fan can be coated with a layer of lead, vulcanized rubber or plastic for corrosion protection. Fans fabricated of higher-resistance metals, such as stainless steel and monel, can be used with excellent results if it is impractical to lower the temperature of a corrosive atmosphere. These latter systems, however, are substantially more expensive.

Fans fabricated from fiberglass-reinforced plastics (FRP) also are used under corrosive conditions. Fiberglass plastics are strong, lightweight and economical, as well as corrosion-resistant. Fans also can be coated with fiberglass plastics for protection. The maximum temperature at which fiberglass can be used is 200°F. Aluminum and aluminum alloys also have corrosion-resistant properties and can be used for applications with a maximum operating temperature of 300°F.

Fan Noise

Fan noise is a complex mixture of sounds of various frequencies and intensities. The total pressure rise produced by a fan and the air volume delivered can be measured exactly. These quantities can be rated under pressure and volume of the fan. Sound energy for an absolute noise rating cannot be measured and is limited to comparative intensities of noise produced at some given point. Noise rating of a fan must specify the measurement positions or points. Size of the room, the form and material of the bounding surfaces also will have an effect on the noise intensity at a given point. It is important, therefore, that measurements be compared on a common basis such as the same room, at the same location, with a satisfactory noise level measuring instrument. These limitations should be recognized and noise level values from manufacturers used as guides. The best guide to the selection of a suitably quiet fan is successful previous performance on a similar job. For the reasons indicated, there is no such quantity as an absolute decibel rating of a fan.

Noise may be caused by factors other than the fan itself. For example, too high velocity of air in the ductwork and improper construction of ducts and air passages, as well as unstable housings, walls, floors and foundations, can cause noise. The importance of selecting a fan to suit the characteristics of the duct system accurately cannot be overemphasized.

Where noise responsibility can be attributed to the fan itself, the cause may be improper selection of type or excessive speed for the size. The tip speed required for a specific capacity and pressure varies with the type of blade. An excessive tip speed for forward-curved blades may not be required for a backward-curved type. A fan operating considerably above its maximum efficiency is usually noisy.

Fan Laws

When a given fan is used for a specific system, the following fan laws apply:

1. The air capacity (cfm) varies directly as the fan speed.
2. The pressure (static, velocity or total) varies as the square of the fan speed.
3. The horsepower required varies as the cube of either the fan speed or capacity.
4. At constant speed and capacity, the pressure and horsepower vary directly as the density of the air.
5. At constant pressure, the speed, capacity and horsepower vary inversely as the square root of the density.
6. At constant weight delivered, the capacity, speed and pressure vary inversely as the density, and the horsepower varies inversely as the square of the density.

For conditions of constant static pressure at the fan outlet or fans of different sizes but same blade tip speed, $\pi DR = $ constant:

7. The capacity and horsepower vary as the square of the wheel diameter ratio.
8. The speed varies inversely as the wheel diameter.
9. With constant static pressure, the speed, capacity and power vary inversely as the square root of the air density.
10. At constant capacity and speed, the horsepower and static pressure vary directly as the air density ratio.

At constant weight delivered:

11. The capacity, speed and pressure are inversely proportional to the density. Horsepower is inversely proportional to the square of the density.

These laws can be expressed mathematically, singly or in combination, as follows:

$$Q = A R D^3 \qquad H = B R^2 D^2 d \qquad P = C R^3 D^5 d$$

where
- Q = capacity (cfm)
- D = wheel diameter (ft)
- H = static pressure head, ft fluid flowing
- P = horsepower (hp)
- R = speed (rpm)
- d = density or specific weight of air or gas (lb/ft^3)
- A, B, C = constants

If, when considering two fans, $A = A_1$, then $B = B_1$ and $C = C_1$. The fans are said to be operating at the same equivalent orifice, ratio of opening, point of operation, corresponding points or point of rating. This means the two fans are proportional and the above three equations are applicable, and the fans have identical efficiencies.

Example

A fan is rated to deliver 20,500 cfm at a static pressure of 2 in. of water when running at 356 rpm and requiring 5.4 hp. If the fan speed is changed to 400 rpm, what are the resulting cfm, static pressure and hp required at standard air conditions?

Solution

By fan laws 1, 2 and 3,

$$\text{Capacity} = 20,500\left(\frac{400}{356}\right) = 23,042 \text{ cfm}$$

$$\text{Static pressure} = 2\left(\frac{400}{356}\right)^2 = 2.53 \text{ in. } H_2O$$

$$hp = 5.4\left(\frac{400}{356}\right)^3 = 7.67 \text{ hp}$$

Note: Standard air in fan tabulations usually is taken as air at 68°F, at 29.92 in. Hg and 50% relative humidity, weighing 0.07496 lb/ft³ (0.075 is used most often for approximate calculations).

Example

In the previous example, if, in addition to speed change, the air handled were at 150°F instead of the standard 68 F, what capacity, static pressure and horsepower would be required?

Solution

Air density at 68°F and 29.52 in. Hg is 0.075 lb/ft³:

$$0.075\left(\frac{460 + 68}{460 + 150}\right)\left(\frac{29.92}{29.92}\right) = 0.065 \text{ lb/ft}^3$$

Density at 150°F and the same barometric pressure are obtained by multiplying by absolute temperature and pressure ratio.

By fan law 4,

$$\text{Capacity} = 23,042 \text{ cfm at } 150°F$$

$$\text{Static pressure} = 2.53 \left(\frac{0.065}{0.075} \right) = 2.19 \text{ in. H}_2\text{O}$$

$$\text{hp} = 7.67 \left(\frac{0.065}{0.075} \right) = 6.65 \text{ hp}$$

Fundamental Formulas

Pressure in fan engineering is called **static pressure.** The pressure resulting from velocity impingement is called **velocity pressure.** The sum of static pressure and velocity pressure is the **total pressure.** Fan pressures are determined from duct pressure readings. The total pressure of a fan is the increase in total pressure through the fan, as indicated by a differential reading between the fan inlet and outlet of two impact tubes facing the air current.

Static pressure, p_s, is the total pressure rise, p, less the velocity pressure in the fan inlet.

Velocity pressure, p_v, is the velocity pressure in the fan outlet, expressed in inches of water.

Velocity can be expressed in terms of velocity pressure as follows:

$$V = 18.3\sqrt{p_v/d} \text{ fps} = 1,906\sqrt{p_v/d} \text{ fpm}$$

where d = density of gas in lb/ft^3

Air horsepower, or power-output of the fan,

$$\text{Air hp} = \frac{62.3 \text{ pQ}}{12(33,000)} = 0.0001575 \text{ pQ}$$

where   Q = volume of air (cfm)
         p = pressure rise (in. H$_2$O)

Efficiency of a fan is the ratio between output horsepower (air hp) and the input horsepower (bhp):

$$\text{efficiency} = \text{air hp/bhp}$$

Static efficiency of a fan is the ratio of static pressure power and the input horsepower.

Standard air density is 0.075 lb/ft³. Fan pressures and horsepowers vary directly as air density.

Fan Characteristics

Fan performance should be presented graphically. A chart usually plots volumes against pressures, horsepower inputs and efficiencies. The forms of the pressure and horsepower curves depend on blade type. Figure 50 shows a typical plot of fan performance, volume cfm, against total pressure, static pressure, horsepower and efficiencies. It is drawn for a given size fan at a given speed. Plots of more general application also are used as fans function closely to dimensional theory. Dimensionless plotting of fan curves is accepted practice. A dimensionless plot, Figure 51, shows the percentage of wide-open volume vs percentage pressure, horsepower and efficiencies. These typical performance curves show how efficiency, pressure and power input vary with changing flow volume. Plots are based on fans operating at constant speed and standard air density.

Air Pollution Control with Fans and Blowers

Fans and blowers can be used alone as air pollution control devices or in conjunction with control equipment such as wet scrubbers, baghouses,

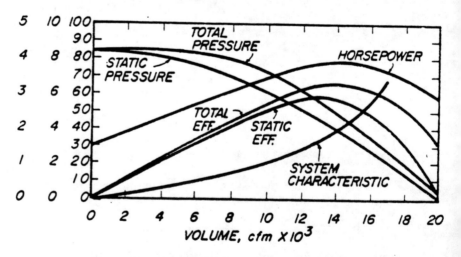

Figure 50.   Typical characteristic curves of a fan.

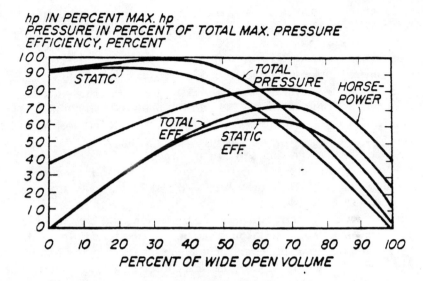

Figure 51.   Typical plot of dimensionless fan characteristics.

electrostatic precipitators and combustion units. In any case, the fan is the heart of the system.

Ventilation fans are used in heat control, for removing heat from rooms or closed areas. Size of the fan depends on the work being done in the area as well as the equipment, such as furnaces, milling machines, etc. In industrial heat relief, insulation and shielding from high heat sources are used as well as spot cooling by fans and fan exhaust systems employing hoods.

Roof ventilators provide positive effective control of the in-plant environment. These compact units remove heat and contamination efficiently at modest cost from work areas. Additionally, the equipment can incorporate split or combined heating control and room air can be recirculated. Mechanical ventilators have other advantages. Unit efficiency can be maintained regardless of weather conditions, and often equipment can be located in otherwise wasted space.

Fans and blowers have innumerable applications as ventilating devices, aside from their industrial use. Systems of fans and blowers are used in large traffic tunnels to reduce carbon monoxide concentrations from automative exhaust to 2½ parts per 10,000 of air. Clean air is fed by blowers into the tunnel through a system of ducts located under the roadway. Exhaust air is removed by fans through ducts in the ceiling of the tunnel. Most traffic tunnels have two large fan rooms located at either end of the tunnel. Large garages also use ventilation systems of fans and blowers to remove carbon monoxide. Fan size units depend on the total number of moving and idling cars in the garage. Most ventilating systems of this type remove between 2800 and 5600 cfm per car to reduce the level of carbon monoxide below 1 part per 10,000.

Underground mining operations also rely on fans and blowers for ventilation. Mine ventilation is a complex problem, requiring units that must supply a continuous flow of fresh air to mine shafts and tunnels, as well as remove dusts and fumes caused by the mining operation. Ventilators used in mines usually are capable of reversing their flow to prevent spread of dusts and fumes in case of fire.

Ventilation is important in the removal of odor and moisture in barns and animal shelters. In most barns exhaust fans usually are located 18 inches above the floor.

In-plant odor control involves the use of fans and blowers to force or induce contaminated air through various control devices. Industrial toxicants and odiferous materials include substances such as ammonia, carbon tetrachloride, phenol, ozone and hydrogen sulfide. Manufacturing processes generate contaminants including irritants, toxic dusts, fibrosis-producing and inert allergy-producing dusts, asphyxiants, inorganic and organic gases.

Activated carbon filters are used in conjunction with fans to control odors and contaminants consisting of organic substances. Fans are used to draw the contaminated air through a bed of activated carbon, which absorbs the odors. All the air may be passed through the carbon bed (a continuous bed system), or some may be diverted around the bed, making it a discontinuous bed. Continuous carbon beds are made of porous tubes filled with charcoal, or that have flat strips with charcoal granules glued to them. Most applications use continuous beds made of pleated or flat cells of charcoal or hollow cylinder canisters filled with charcoal. These absorb most odors in a single pass at air velocities between 50 to 120 fpm. Maximum recommended velocity for continuous bed absorbers is 250 fpm. Continuous bed absorbers are 95% efficient, using 5–50 lb of charcoal/1000 cfm capacity, depending on the required application.

Air washers are used to remove water-soluble vapors, dusts, gases and fumes resulting from plant processes. Air washers exhibit good efficiency on particles larger than 5 μ. The polluted air is drawn into the washer by the fan, and water is sprayed into the air perpendicular to the flow. Water and particulates land on a filter. The water trickles through, and the particulate remains on the filter. Units such as these also can be adapted as humidifiers and dehumidifiers. Air velocity of such units ranges between 200 and 500 fpm, the efficiency increasing with lower velocities. Between 2 and 5 gpm of water/1000 cfm are used for washing, depending on the application.

Dry filters also are employed widely. They consist of a bed or mat of fiberglass or fine synthetic fibers. This type filter actually increases in efficiency as a dust layer builds up, acting as an additional filter surface. Low air velocities of 300-500 fpm also increase efficiency. When filters become dirty they can be washed and reused, disposable filters may be thrown away and replaced.

DUCTING DESIGN [50,52,53]

The time to avert airflow problems in a plant's heating, ventilating and air conditioning ductwork is when the system is being designed. Once the ducts are in place, revisions can be extremely expensive, not only from the standpoint of modification costs, but also because of the disruption created.

There are two occasions in which the engineer is presented with an opportunity to forestall ductwork problems. One occurs when a new plant is being designed, the other when an existing facility is being revised. In both instances, an understanding of the basic principles of practical duct design is essential.

General Principles

Pressure losses in ducting systems are caused by skin friction, flow separation and changes in flow direction produced by bends, splits and takeoffs. Good duct design requires that such pressure losses be minimized so that the required pumping power can be kept as low as possible. Except for laminar or low-velocity streamline flow, most pressure losses can be considered approximately proportional to the dynamic velocity head, which is a function of the square of the duct velocity. Accordingly, the first basic principle of duct design is as follows:

1. Maintain airflow at the lowest practical velocity by using adequately sized ducts.

When flow in a duct separates from the wall, as in a sudden expansion, localized flow reversals and high turbulence occur in the separated region. This condition causes high duct pressure losses. Consequently, the second general design principle is as follows:

2. Maintain gradual deceleration of the airflow through good diffuser design. (A seven-degree diffuser half angle usually is a good compromise.)

Rapid changes in flow direction, such as those created by sharp bends, also can result in flow separation and, consequently, large duct pressure drops. Therefore:

3. Use a generous turning radius wherever possible. A good rule of thumb to follow here is that turning radius should be 1.5 times the duct diameter.

Another contributing factor in pressure losses is duct surface roughness, which creates flow disturbance. Such disturbances, which are the result of protrusions into the fluid stream, cause form drag, local flow separation and increased pressure drop. Thus:

4. Keep the surface of the duct as smooth as possible. Preferably, one should keep the ratio of roughness protrusion height to duct diameter at less than 0.0001.

In some instances, duct resistances can be used to advantage. Screens, grills and other resistance elements in a duct can act to stabilize and strengthen air flow, reducing the possibility of flow separation.

Definitions and Terminology

Basic equations governing fluid flow through a ducting system are developed on the premises that mass and energy are conserved and that Newton's second law of motion is followed.

A segment of a ducting system in which the cross-sectional area changes as the flow moves from one section to another is shown in Figure 52. The continuity equation requires that the mass of fluid per unit time entering section 1 must equal the mass of fluid per unit time leaving section 2. For a compressible fluid, then,

$$\rho_1 A_1 V_1 = \rho_2 A_2 V_2$$

where symbols are defined in the Nomenclature, p. 132. For an incompressible fluid, where mass density, ρ, is constant, this equation becomes

$$A_1 V_1 = A_2 V_2$$

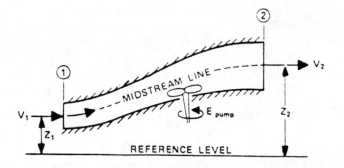

Figure 52.   Typical duct segment with varying cross-sectional area.

This expression of constant volume flow per unit time is valid for liquids or gases in motion where only small variations in density occur. In most ducting systems, air pressure and, hence, density, do not vary substantially from atmospheric conditions. Therefore, assumption of incompressibility is acceptable for purposes of calculation. For example, a relatively high duct pressure level of 10 in. w.g. (referred to atmospheric pressure) is only 2.46% of standard atmospheric pressure (407 in. of water).

Bernoulli's classic equation for steady frictionless flow of an incompressible fluid along a streamline is

$$Z + \frac{P_s}{\rho} + \frac{V^2}{2g_c} = \text{Constant}$$

where each of the terms may be interpreted as a form of energy:

Z = potential energy per pound of fluid based on an arbitrary reference level

P_s/ρ = measure of the work the fluid can do by virtue of its sustained pressure (sometimes called the pressure energy)

$V^2/2g_c$ = kinetic energy per pound of fluid

Application of this equation to the duct situation of figure 52 gives

$$Z_1 - Z_2 + \frac{P_{s1} - P_{s2}}{\rho} + \frac{V_1^2 - V_2^2}{2g_c} = 0$$

This expression states that the differences in potential, pressure and kinetic energies between sections 1 and 2 must be zero. Of course, this relationship is true only if the flow is frictionless. In reality, all fluids have viscosity and, therefore, offer resistance to deformation.

During flow, this resistance creates shear stresses, which result in the conversion of mechanical energy to thermal energy, or heat. This thermal energy usually cannot be converted back to mechanical energy, resulting in a loss (E_{loss}) to the system. As compensation for this loss, a pump or fan is used to add energy (E_{pump}) to the flowing fluid.

Bernoulli's equation can now be rewritten to account for energy losses and additions between sections 1 and 2:

$$Z_1 + \frac{P_{s1}}{\rho} + \frac{V_1^2}{2g_c} + E_{pump} = Z_2 + \frac{P_{s2}}{\rho} + \frac{V_2^2}{2g_c} + E_{loss}$$

This expression can be simplified by introducing the concept of total pressure, P_T, and its components, static pressure, P_s, and velocity pressure or head. The relationship of these quantities is illustrated in Figure 53, which shows a section of ducting in which manometers are being used to measure local pressure levels.

In an actual ducting system, total pressure always decreases in the direction of flow because of mechanical energy losses. Static pressure

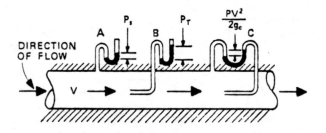

Manometer A (Top flush with wall of duct.)
Measures the static pressure (P.) which is a compressive unit force existing in the duct, and does not depend on the direction or magnitude of the fluid velocity.

Manometer B (Probe faces directly into direction of flow.)
Measures the total pressure (P₁) at a given point in the system. Total pressure is the sum of the static pressure and the velocity head ($P_T = P_s + \rho V^2/2g_c$).

Manometer C (Combination of manometers A and B.)
Measures the velocity head or velocity pressure $\rho V^2/2g$. which is directly related to duct velocity and represents kinetic energy.

Figure 53.   Duct pressure relationships.

and velocity head are mutually convertible; the magnitude of each is dependent on local duct cross-sectional area, which determines the flow velocity. Total pressure, which is the sum of static pressure and velocity head, is defined by

$$P_T = P_s + \frac{\rho V^2}{2g_c}$$

Incorporating this total pressure definition into the previous equation and simplifying gives

$$Z_1 + \frac{P_{T1}}{\rho} + E_{pump} = Z_2 + \frac{P_{T2}}{\rho} + E_{loss}$$

This equation can be simplified further for most gases (including air) flowing in a duct because the potential energy term Z (height of fluid above a datum line) effectively can be neglected. Then

$$\frac{P_{T1} - P_{T2}}{\rho} = E_{loss} - E_{pump}$$

This expression means, simply, that because the entrance and exit of a fluid ducting system are at atmospheric pressure, the loss (E_{loss}) in mechanical energy per pound of fluid flow must be balanced by pumping work (E_{pump}) on the system.

In fact, what happens is that the fluid flow through the duct adjusts itself until this condition is satisfied. For the purposes of this discussion, the duct fluid will be treated as incompressible. This assumption considerably simplifies the equations and is sufficient for liquids and most gases at low flow velocities.

Pressure-Flow Matching

When a ducting system is selected, the total pressure drop needs to be matched to the output of the pumping device. As duct resistance (and its associated pressure drop) is a function of cross-sectional area, length, surface roughness, turning radius, etc., it can be represented as

$$\Delta P_T = C_T Q^2$$

The application of this equation for matching three ducting system resistances to the output of an air-moving device is shown in Figure 54.

The procedure used to accomplish the match is actually quite simple. A flow, Q_{guess} (usually equal to the desired flow) is assumed, and the corresponding duct system pressure drop, $\Delta P_{T\,guess}$, is calculated. This determination allows the constant, C_T, in the previous equation to be evaluated and, then, the actual system pressure drop characteristic can be obtained (Figure 54). Superimposing the characteristic curve of the air-moving device on the system resistance plot locates the operating point of the intersection of the two curves.

At this point, identified as Q_A in Figure 54, the system requirements are matched exactly by the pump or fan output. If the fan is oversized and produces too much flow, the duct system resistance should be increased to balance the flow. For instance, if the resistance is increased so that system curve B or C is obtained, a reduced flow equal to Q_{guess} (also Q_B) or Q_C, respectively, results.

Calculating Duct Losses [50,53]

Calculating pressure losses in a plant's heating, ventilating and air conditioning ductwork involves analysis of several variables.

Nomenclature

A	= Area		P_T	= Total pressure
C_T	= Overall system loss constant		Q	= Volumetric flowrate
E_{loss}	= Energy loss to system		V	= Velocity
E_{pump}	= Input pumping power		Z	= Height of fluid above datum
g_c	= Gravitational constant			line
P	= Pressure		ΔP	= Difference in pressure
P_s	= Static pressure		ρ	= Density

Duct Losses from Friction

When long ducts are used, the effect of friction on pressure drop can be considerable. Frictional losses are a function of the duct surface condition and the type of fluid motion.

One type of duct flow is called laminar because the fluid particles move essentially along a streamline or laminae (thin layers) in the direction of flow. A second type of flow, called turbulent, is characterized by fluid particles moving in a random or eddying motion, while, on an average, still moving in the direction of flow. The type of motion that predominates in a duct is measured by the Reynolds number, N_{re}, which is defined as

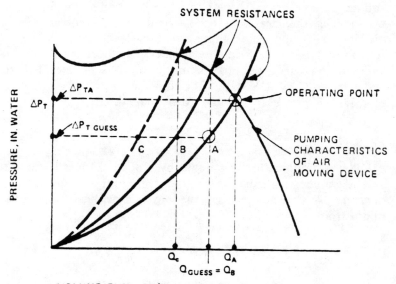

Figure 54.   Combination plot of system resistance and fan characteristics for analysis of pressure-flow matching.

$$N_{re} = \rho DV/\mu$$

The Reynolds number can be thought of as the ratio of the local inertial force per unit area, $\rho V^3 g_c$, to the local viscous force per unit area, $\mu V/gD$. A low Reynolds number indicates laminar flow and a higher number is characteristic of turbulent flow situations. The transition from one flow mechanism to the other does not occur at a specific duct Reynolds number, but rather over a range. For most ducts this range is $2000 \leq N_{re\ transition} \leq 3500$.

Duct pressure drop from frictional loss alone is given as a function of the velocity head ($\rho V^2/2g_c$) by

$$\Delta P_{friction} = f \frac{L}{D_H} \left(\frac{\rho V^2}{2g_c} \right)$$

where the hydraulic diameter, D_H, is defined as

$$D_H = \frac{4(\text{duct cross-sectional area})}{(\text{wetted duct perimeter})}$$

and the friction factor, f, is essentially a function of the Reynolds number and duct roughness (Figure 55). The straight line curves to the left are the laminar friction factors that depend on the duct cross-sectional ratio A/B as well as on the Reynolds number. For turbulent flows, the duct hydraulic diameter is used to obtain the Reynolds number from the earlier equation $N_{re} = \rho DV/\mu$, and the roughness to diameter ratio, ϵ/D, is estimated. Figure 55 then is used to estimate the friction factor.

Duct Dynamic Losses

Eddying motions, brought about by sudden changes in the direction and magnitude of the duct velocity, cause significant flow losses. These dynamic losses are a function of the local velocity head and can be determined from

$$\Delta P_{\text{dynamic loss}} = K_T \left(\frac{\rho V^2}{2g_c} \right)$$

The constant K_T, termed the dynamic loss coefficient, usually is determined experimentally. An enormous quantity of experimental data exists on the magnitude of this loss under a multitude of conditions—inlets, expansions, contractions, turning losses and the like. In this chapter, discussion will be limited to a few important cases that demonstrate the technique.

Dynamic Losses from Area Changes. Perhaps the most important duct area change is at the inlet point. Various internal-duct-inlet designs are shown in Figure 56. The importance of eliminating sharp entrance corners to reduce the loss coefficient, K_T, is indicated clearly.

Dynamic losses in excess of normal frictional losses also result when a fast-moving stream suddenly expands into an enlarged cross-sectional area or contracts into a reduced cross-sectional area. The effect of a sudden contraction in duct cross-sectional area is less important than that of an expansion. However, after the contraction, the flow continues to converge to an area smaller than the reduced duct size (called the vena contracta). In a sudden contraction, the dynamic loss is due largely to expansion of the flow filling the duct cross-sectional area after passing through the vena contracta. Dynamic loss coefficients for sudden changes in cross-sectional area are summarized in Figure 57.

Dynamic losses can be reduced by using transition pieces between ducts of different size. The effect a transition piece has on dynamic losses is illustrated in Figure 58.

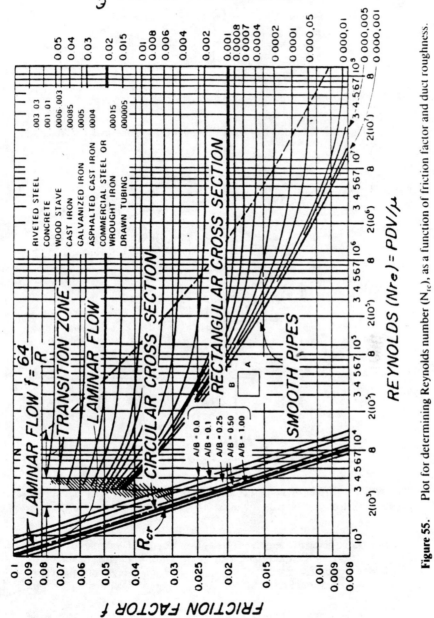

Figure 55.   Plot for determining Reynolds number (N_{re}), as a function of friction factor and duct roughness.

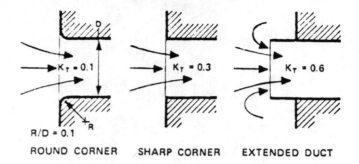

Figure 56.   Effect of inlet designs on dynamic loss coefficient.

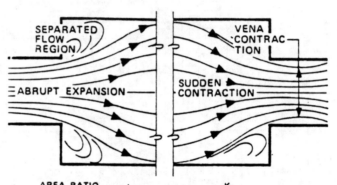

| AREA RATIO | K_1 | | |
Small Duct or Orifice Area ÷ Large Duct Area	Sudden Expansion	Sudden Contraction	Sharp-Edged Orifice
0.0	1.00	0.34	2.50
0.2	0.64	0.32	1.86
0.4	0.36	0.25	1.21
0.6	0.16	0.16	0.64
0.8	0.04	0.06	0.20
1.0	0.00	0.00	0.00

Figure 57.   Effect of sudden changes in cross-sectional area and corresponding dynamic loss coefficients for duct.

D = Characteristic length of system, ft (often the duct diameter)
f = Friction factor
g_c = Gravitational constant
K_T = Dynamic loss coefficient
L = Length of duct
N_{re} = Reynolds number
Q = Volumetric flowrate

Dynamic Losses from Changes in Flow Direction. Dynamic losses caused by changes in flow direction can be significant. If the flow cannot

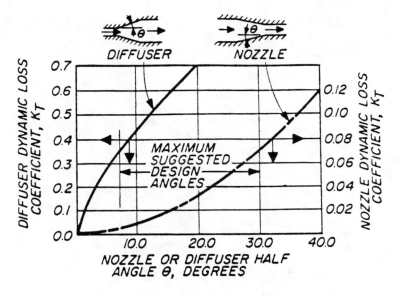

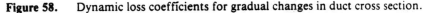

Figure 58.   Dynamic loss coefficients for gradual changes in duct cross section.

adjust quickly enough to follow a sharp duct turn smoothly, separation and turbulence result, and an additional pressure drop occurs.

Figure 59 summarizes the dynamic losses of circular and rectangular ducts for 90° smooth turns. A minimum value of R/D or R/A = 1.5 is suggested. When the ratio of mean turn radius to duct diameter (or area) is smaller than this value, the losses increase dramatically. Anything above this value improves airflow. If it is impossible to increase R/A to above 1.5, a flow splitter should be used. This device will divide the flow, reducing the effective width, A, and, consequently, increasing R/A. When using splitters, it is a good rule to make the R/A equal for all flow paths.

In some instances, the duct elbow is constructed of separate pieces that are joined with mitered corners. The greater the number of transition pieces, the smoother the air flow. For example, Figure 60 shows that when an additional transition piece is inserted into the three-piece mitered corner section, the dynamic loss coefficient, K_T, is reduced from 1.3 to 0.33. Thus, the value of the added piece is clear.

Predicting Flow and Pressure Drop in Multiple Branches

A ducting system with multiple flow paths can be evaluated easily when each branch is treated as a section of unbranched ducting. In this manner, the previous techniques for predicting frictional and dynamic

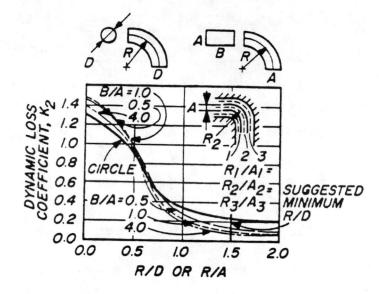

Figure 59.   Dynamic loss coefficient for 90° turns. Inset shows method of using turing vanes to balance airflow.

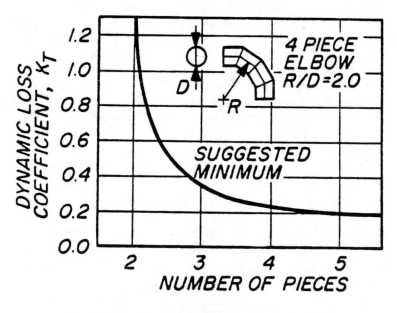

Figure 60.   Dynamic losses in a fabricated elbow.

losses are applicable. The procedure is illustrated by the example diagrammed in Figure 61. Here, a single fan supplies the flow for three individual ducts.

V   = Fluid velocity (ft/sec)
ΔP = Difference in pressure
ϵ/D = Roughness to diameter ratio
μ = Absolute viscosity (lb-mass/ft-sec)

ρ = Fluid density (lb-mass/ft^3)
D_H = Hydraulic diameter
Q_T = Total conditions

The pressure drop in each of the flow branches can be represented closely by

$$\Delta P = K_{Tn} Q_n^2$$

where n represents branch 1, 2 or 3.

For each assumed value of ΔP, individual flows Q_1, Q_2 and Q_3 can be obtained. Total flow, $Q_{total} = Q_1 + Q_2 + Q_3$, at this assumed ΔP then can be found. From these results, the total system characteristic of ΔP versus Q_T can be cross-plotted with a fan output curve. Once the operating pressure level is evaluated, the individual path flows can be determined from the foregoing equation.

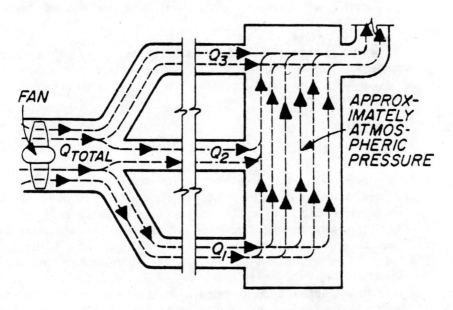

Figure 61.   Flow in a multiple-branch duct.

Summary

These general rules should be followed in designing a ducting system:

1. The flow medium should be conveyed as directly as possible at a velocity consistent with cost limitations imposed by materials, space and power.
2. Changes in flow direction should be minimized. When bends are required, a turning radius to duct diameter ratio not less than 1.5 should be used. If this requirement cannot be met, turning vanes or flow splitters should be used. If an elbow is of mitered construction, at least one transitional piece should be inserted.
3. The duct surface should be as smooth as possible, and steel or aluminum should be used. If surface roughness cannot be avoided, an allowance for it must be included in the estimated friction factor.
4. Abrupt increases in area should be avoided because they tend to cause flow separation and turbulence. When possible, expanding transitional segments should be utilized with a half angle not greater than 7.
5. Because acceleration tends to prevent separation, abrupt decreases in cross-sectional area are not as important as rapid expansions. However, contraction half angles should not exceed 30 degrees.
6. The fan or air-moving device selected must produce a pressure rise sufficient to match the total duct loss plus the losses caused by any other system components (filters, heat exchangers, washers, spray chambers, etc.).

In practice, it is often difficult to construct the ducting system exactly as designed. For this reason, fans should be selected with a factor of safety. A fan pressure level approximately 15% above the design prediction usually will suffice.

Simplified Duct Sizing [50,54]

When designing a dust collection system, it is necessary to determine the size of ductwork needed and find the friction loss encountered. Using a nomograph will simplify and speed up these calculations.

On the accompanying nomograph, Figure 62, draw a straight line from scale A (airflow, ft³/min) to scale D (velocity, ft/min). At the point of intersection with scale B will be found the minimum duct size needed to handle the air.

The nomograph also permits calculation of velocity pressure. Velocity pressure changes are proportional to changes of the velocity and can be read directly from scale D.

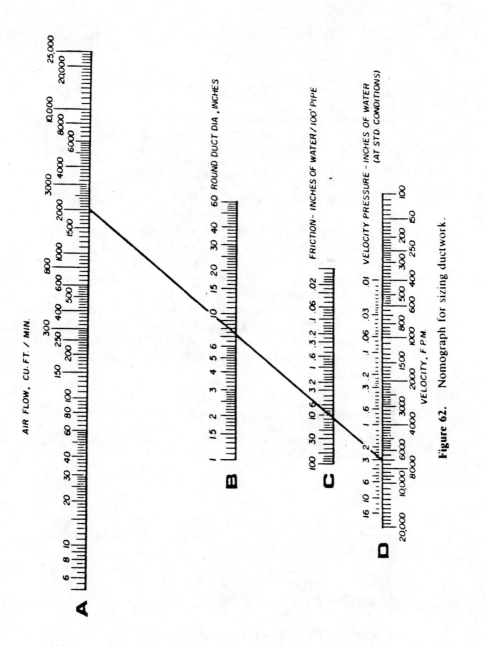

Figure 62. Nomograph for sizing ductwork.

Problem

Convey 2000 cfm of air at a velocity pressure of 3 in. H_2O. Determine the size of round duct required.

Answer

Connect 2000 on scale A with 3-in. D. Read the round duct size on scale B as 7½ in. The velocity of the air in the duct will be approximately 7000 fpm.

Duct Weight Calculation [50,55]

When designing a ventilation system for makeup air or pollution exhaust, it is usually necessary to calculate the total number of pounds of material required to determine the cost for the system. The nomograph provides a rapid and easy method for determining the weight per linear foot of galvanized sheet steel (Figure 63).

To calculate weight per linear foot, select either the diameter for round duct or the perimeter of rectangular duct on the A scale. On scale B select the required gage for the sheet steel of the duct. Draw a line from A to B extending it to scale C. Read the duct weight in pounds per linear foot on C.

Example

Find the total weight of a 25-in. round duct 35 ft long. Duct material is 24 gage sheet steel.

Solution

Align 25 on the round duct portion of Scale A with 24 on scale B, and read 8.7 lb per lin ft on scale C. Multiply 8.7 by 35, and find the weight of the duct to be 304.5 lb.

Sizing Roof Ventilators [50,56]

Roof ventilators can provide positive, effective control of the in-plant environment. These compact units remove heat and contamination efficiently at modest cost. In addition, the equipment can incorporate split or combined heating control, and room air can be recirculated.

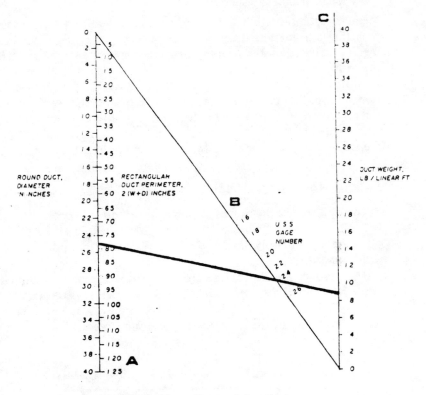

Figure 63.   Duct weight calculator.

Mechanical ventilation has other advantages. The unit's efficiency can be maintained regardless of weather conditions. Also, the equipment can be located in otherwise wasted space.

For best results, care should be taken to select equipment of the proper type and size, and with sufficient handling capacity. Several factors should be examined:

- Size of room or building that the system is to service
- Number of occupants and their jobs
- Heat gains from equipment and solar radiation
- Outside air temperature

Each of these factors provides basic data needed in the calculations for sizing and unit selection.

The amount of ventilation needed for a specified building or work area can be determined by one of two methods: (1) rate of air change or (2) heat load. Both procedures are used widely, but the rate of air change method is the simplest. It requires close examination of manufacturers' literature and measurement of the area to be ventilated. The heat load method is based on the quantity of air needed to remove heat generated in the work area.

Although there are no set rules for selecting the proper roof ventilation, two basic factors serve as guides. First, no matter what means is utilized to exhaust air from a space, equal quantities of makeup air must be provided. Second, the chosen system should be capable of handling the worst possible conditions for an indefinite length of time.

Rate of Air Change Method

The first step of the rate of air change method is to determine the total volume of air contained in the area to be ventilated. This is easily obtained by multiplying the dimensions of its boundaries: length × width × height.

The second step is to find the rate of recommended air changes. Table XI shows the estimated number of air changes per hour for various types of structures in temperature climate zones. In a hotter climate, at least a doubling of the air changes per hour is necessary.

Table XI. Air Changes per Hour Recommended

Situation	Air Changes per Hour
Boiler Rooms	30
Engine Rooms	45
Industrial Plant Buildings	
General	20
Fumes and moisture	30
Foundries	45
Forge Shop	45
Garages	15
Laboratories	15
Machine Shop	20
Mills (dye house)	30
(paper)	20
(textile)	15
Offices	10
Shops	
General	10
Paint	30
Waiting Rooms	15
Warehouses	6–20

Another factor affecting these values is the presence of contaminated air. For example, the number of changes should be increased if the plant has a large amount of smoke from any source, making sure that the air contamination is brought down to a safe level.

Multiplying the number of air changes required per hour by the volume of the building results in the cubic feet of air that must be withdrawn each hour. Further examination of the building—its size, shape, roof area—and reference to manufacturers' literature will indicate the correct number of ventilating units. A rule-of-thumb in finding the number of ventilators needed is to provide one unit for every 15- or 20-ft bay.

After determining how many units are required, all that remains is to find the handling capacity and size required for each unit. Capacity is obtained by dividing the total volume of air handled per hour by the number of systems required. For convenience and in general practice, the amount of air per hour is converted to cubic feet per minute by dividing by 60. With this information as a guide, examine manufacturers' capacity tables to select the size and speed of a system to meet specifications and conditions.

Example. A plant building, in which machinery generates irritable dust is 45 ft × 100 ft × 35 ft. Determine the amount of ideal ventilation required by the rate of air change method.

Solution. 1. Volume determination: Volume = 45 ft × 100 ft × 35 ft = 157,500 ft^3.

2. From Table XI (industrial plant buildings, fumes and moisture), the required air changes per hour are 30.

3. The amount of ideal ventilation is calculated as follows: volume (157,500) × air changes/hr (30) ÷ 60 min = 78,750 cfm.

4. The plant has five 20-ft bays; an installation of five roof ventilators would give ideal distribution.

Now the handling capacity of each ventilator can be determined by dividing the total ventilation by the number of units required: 78,750 cfm ÷ 5 units = 15,750 cfm per ventilator.

5. Refer to the manufacturers' capacity tables for selection of the unit.

Heat Loss Method

In this technique, the amount of heat generated in the plant is the chief factor to consider in determining the ventilation required.

The heat in an industrial plant comes from three primary sources:

- People (body heat)
- Equipment and heat-generating processes
- Sun rays

The first of these, body heat, is generated proportional to the body structure, size of individual, physical activity, age, sex, health, nutrition and working environment. Additional energy is expended as useful work. A person seated at rest generates 400 Btu/hr; during strenuous work, as much as 1400 Btu/hr per person is produced.

It is important, then, to know the number of people working in a specific area and the individual duties of each. Published guides listing heat dissipation rates of individuals for different occupations can help in determining heat loss to the environment.

Besides electric lights, which generate 3.4 Btu/hr/W, electrical motors, pumps, etc., give off sizable amounts of heat (see Table XII). Some plant processes may generate latent heat in the form of moisture. Total energy liberated as heat from any chemical or mechanical process may be determined from a knowledge of fuel consumption, efficiencies and other data.

Table XII.   Heat Generated by Electric Motors

Motor Size (hp)	
¼	Generates 4000 Btu/hr/hp
1	Generates 3400 Btu/hr/hp
5	Generates 3100 Btu/hr/hp
25	Generates 2900 Btu/hr/hp
100	Generates 2800 Btu/hr/hp

The final factor contributing to heat gain in the working environment is the sun's rays striking walls and roof. Solar heat gains in a room or building depend on several outdoor factors: atmospheric clarity, shading by trees or other structures, wind velocity and location. Finding such heat gains requires knowledge of solar heat transmitting values of building materials, along with corresponding heat transmission per square foot per hour for these materials. Values for several materials are given in Tables XIII and XIV.

Table XIII.   Solar Heat Gains Through Walls

Wall Construction	Wall Thickness (in.)	East and West (in.)	Southeast and Southwest Walls	South Wall
		Solar Heat Gain in Btu/ft²/hr Lat. 40° North or South		
Brick—Solid Unplastered	4½	23	16.6	8.8
	9	16	12.4	6.4
	13½	13	9.7	5.2
Brick—Solid Plastered ½ in.	4½	19	13.8	7.6
	9	15	11.0	6.0
	13½	12	8.3	4.8
	18	10	6.9	4.0
	22½	8	5.5	3.2
Brick—Hollow Plastered ½ in.	11	10	6.9	4.4
	15½	8	6.9	3.6
	20	7	4.1	3.2
Concrete	6	22	17.9	8.8
	8	19	13.8	7.2
	10	16	12.4	6.4
	16	14	11.0	6.0
Stone	12	17	12.4	6.8
	18	14	9.7	5.6
	24	11	8.3	4.8
Wood—Tongued and Grooved	1	17	12.4	6.8
	1½	14	9.7	5.6
Sheets				
Asbestos (flat)	¼	31	22	11.6
Corrugated asbestos	—	41	27	14.4
Corrugated iron	$^1/_{16}$	43	29	14.8
Corrugated iron on 1-in. boards	—	14	11	5.6
Glass				
Bare window glass	—	185	151.8	156.0
Windows with canvas awning	—	52	42.8	12.0

Not all the walls of a building are affected by solar radiation at the same time. For a rectangular structure, only one or two walls at a time are exposed fully to the sun's rays. If a room or building has two sun exposures, only the side with the largest exposure should be considered; if three sides undergo exposure, then only the side with the greatest exposure is considered.

Table XIV.   Solar Heat Gains Through Roofs—Maximum
Heat Transmission

Roof Construction	Btu/ft²/hr Lat. 40 deg N/S
Flat	
Asphalt on 6-in. concrete	26.7
Asphalt on 6-in. concrete with 1-in. cork	9.2
Asphalt on 6-in. concrete with 2-in. cork	5.5
Asphalt on 6-in. hollow tile	22.1
Asphalt on 6-in. hollow tile with 1-in. cork	9.2
Asphalt on 6-in. hollow tile with 2-in. cork	5.5
Asphalt, 1-in. cork, 1¼-in. boards, joist and plaster ceiling	6.4
Pitched	
Corrugated asbestos	68.1
Corrugated asbestos lined ½-in. boards	23.9

Calculations are based not only on the one wall receiving the greatest solar energy, but also on the hottest time of the day. Figure 64 gives a rough estimate of the percentage of surface area that should be included in calculations for solar effects. These percentages apply only to northern latitudes; in southern latitudes, maximum radiation falls on the north wall from 10 A.M. to 2 P.M.

After heat generated by the working environment and surroundings has been determined, the proper fan can be selected. The amount of ventilation needed can be calculated by tabulating the total heat gained through the structure's walls and roof along with heat generated by employees and machinery, and applying this figure to the following:

$$\text{Air flow (cfm)} = \frac{\text{Total energy or Btu/ft}^2\text{/hr}}{\text{Temperature difference} \times 1.08}$$

The temperature gradient in the above expression is the difference between actual indoor and outdoor temperatures (which must be a minimum for the calculations).

In general, the rate of ventilation required increases as the temperature difference decreases. It is thus impossible to cool a building below the outside temperature by ventilation alone. By examining the structure's dimensions and noting the number of bays, the engineer can estimate how many units are required. The capacity of each discharge roof ventilator is determined by dividing the total ventilation amount (cfm) by the

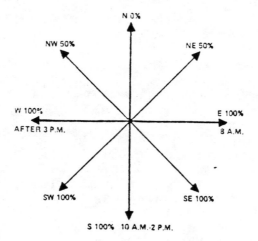

Figure 64. Arrows indicate solar intensity at various times of the day in different directions. The percentages shown can be used to calculate solar heat transmitted through wall areas.

number of units required. Then, by referring to capacity tables, ventilators meeting the desired specifications can be chosen.

Example. A building has these specifications:

- Dimensions are 60 ft × 120 ft × 30 ft high.
- Walls are 8-in.-thick concrete.
- The longer walls have four windows 8 ft × 3 ft, and shorter walls have two windows 4 ft × 10 ft with corrugated asbestos awning covers and heavy drapes or shades.
- The roof is made of asphalt on 6-in. concrete.
- The shorter walls face east and west.
- There are 75 people employed in the building, with 50 engaged in light work and 25 in heavy work.
- The following sources generate electrical heat: twelve 1-hp electric motors and thirty 5-hp motors.

Determine ventilation by Heat Load method.

Solution. The hottest time of the day will occur around 4 P.M. Thus, calculate the solar heat gain for the west wall and roof. The average difference between indoor and outdoor temperatures is 7°F.

- Area of concrete portion of wall: 60 ft × 30 ft   = 1800 ft²
- Area of windows: 4 ft × 10 ft × 2 windows   =   80 ft²

- Area of concrete − windows = 1800 − 80   =   1720 ft²
- Area of roof = 60 ft × 120 ft   =   7200 ft²

Heat gains (Tables XIII and XIV):

- Through concrete: 1800 sq ft × 19 Btu/ft²/ft   =   34,200 Btu/hr
- Through windows (taken as corrugated asbestos rather than glass): 80 ft² × 41   =   3,280 Btu/hr
- Through roof: 7200 ft² × 16.7 Btu/ft²/hr   = 192,240 Btu/hr
- From occupants:
  - Light work: 50 people × 600 Btu/hr/person   =   30,000 Btu/hr
  - Heavy work: 25 people × 1400 Btu/hr/person   =   35,000 Btu/hr
- From electric motors (Table XII)
  - 12 × 1 hp × 3400 Btu/hr/hp   =   40,800 Btu/hr
  - 30 × 5 hp × 3100 Btu/hr/hp   = 465,000 Btu/hr
  - Total heat gain   800,520 Btu/hr

Assume that inside temperature can exceed outside temperature by 7°F. Ventilation required will be

$$\frac{\text{Total heat gain in Btu/ft}^2\text{/hr}}{\text{Temperature difference} \times 1.08} = \frac{800,520}{7 \times 1.08} = 105,889 \, \text{cfm}$$

Building has six 20 ft bays   6 units needed

Therefore, 105,889 cfm ÷ 6 units = 17,648 cfm per ventilator.

Manufacturers' capacity tables will indicate the proper unit, in this case an 18,000-cfm unit. However, it may be more desirable to use two 9000-cfm units per bay instead to get a more uniform air movement. In that case, twelve 9000-cfm units are needed.

CHAPTER 6

RESPIRATOR FILTERS
AND CHEMICAL CARTRIDGES

PARTICULATE FILTERS

Much confusion has arisen over the way in which OSHA regulations are presented for the manufacturer or user to follow. In OSHA Section 1910.134 (Respiratory Protection) Subpart(a)(1) [8] (the control of those occupational diseases caused by breathing air contaminated by harmful dusts, fogs, fumes, mists, gases, smokes, sprays or vapors), the primary objective shall be to prevent atmospheric concentration. This is accomplished as much as is feasible, by accepted engineering control measures (for example, enclosure or confinement of the operation, general and local ventilation and substitution of less toxic materials). When effective engineering controls are not feasible, or while they are being instituted, appropriate respirators shall be used according to specified requirements [8].

As discussed in earlier chapters, the materials in question must be examined for toxicity, levels of contamination and respirable nature. Sampling must be conducted to determine whether overexposure exists. Overexposure can be defined as exposed to air contaminants at a level greater than that specified in Section 1910.1000 [8]—Air contaminants—a list of 400 substances that appeared in 1971, or special standards in the 1000 series.

Once sampling is conducted and the level of overexposure to the air contaminant determined, the type of respirator is chosen. We will examine a uniform method of approach entitled, "Joint NIOSH/OSHA Standards Completion Program: Respirator Decision Logic," after the relative terminology and considerations involved in components that make up a respirator have been described. Our approach will center on

151

the research conducted by the Bureau of Mines, now called the Mine Health and Safety Administration.

MECHANICAL FILTERS

Mechanical filter respirators are based on the principle that particulate matter is retained when air is passed through a filter of fibrous or other material [57]. Currently, all respirator standards for filtration are specified in the literature [1].

None of the testing requirements are printed in the OSHA standards and few, if any, OSHA offices have a copy of Title 30 Subpart B, Part II, in their reference sections. Yet all filter respirators must meet the specified criteria [1]. Some filter media can vary widely in construction and design, so the separation mechanisms must be considered carefully. The effectiveness of all separation mechanisms is related primarily to particle size. The most widely used references on the size of particles and their typical properties are the "Frank Chart" (Figure 65) and the "Sylvan Chart" (Figure 66), which specify the range of particle sizes, concentration, and collector performance. Both are distributed by American Air Filter Co.

Materials used in early respirators were of cellulose fiber. More recently, cellulose, plastic, glass, wool and combinations of two or more of these materials have been tried. In early designs, asbestos floc was added to provide high initial efficiencies. A controlling factor is cost. As the filters have a limited life span and reuse is impossible because there is no way to clean them, disposability is a key factor. With the more modern wire drawing and filament in continuous-length drawing operations, most dust sizes can be filtered or screened adequately by even wire screens in the Tyler mesh screen sizes of the No. 325 to 400 range. Two items come into consideration at this point; resistance to flow by clogging and channeling.

Channeling is the physical occurrence in which large openings exist due to nonuniform filter media. The incoming particles take the path of least resistance and all tend to flow or channel through the opening. There are five criteria that must be considered for a filter medium to provide good filtration [58]:

- Direct interception
- Impaction (inertial contact)
- Diffusion (Brownian motion)
- Electrostatic attraction
- Gravity

DIAM. OF PARTICLES IN MICRONS	U.S. STD MESH	SCALE OF ATMOSPHERIC IMPURITIES	RATE OF SETTLING IN F.P.M. FOR SPHERES SPEC. GRAV. 1 AT 70°F.	DUST PARTICLES CONTAINED IN 1 CUB. FT. OF AIR (See Foot Note)		LAWS OF SETTLING IN RELATION TO PARTICLE SIZE (Lines of Demarcation approx.)
				NUMBER	SURFACE AREA IN SQ. IN.	
8000 6000			1750			PARTICLES FALL WITH INCREASING VELOCITY
4000						
2000	10		790	.0125	61×10^{-6}	
1000 800 600	20		555	.1	12×10^{-5}	
400	60					
200						
100	100 150		59.2	12.5	61×10^{-5}	STOKES LAW
80 60	200 250		14.8	100	12×10^{-4}	
40	325 500					
20			.592	12,500	61×10^{-4}	
10 8 6	1000		.148	100,000	12×10^{-3}	FOR AIR AT 70°F.
4						
2			.007 = 5" PER HR.	125×10^{6}	61×10^{-3}	CUNNINGHAM'S FACTOR
1 .8 .6			.002 = 1.4" PER HR.	10×10^{7}	12×10^{-2}	
.4						
.2			.00007 = 1/2" PER HR.	125×10^{9}	61×10^{-2}	
.1			0	10×10^{10}	1.2	PARTICLES MOVE LIKE GAS MOLECULES
			0	12.5×10^{12}	6.1	BROWNIAN MOVEMENT
.01			0	10×10^{13}	12	
.001			0	12.5×10^{15}	61	

Laws of Settling column:

PARTICLES SETTLE WITH CONSTANT VELOCITY

$$C = \sqrt{\frac{2gds_1}{3Ks_2}}$$

$$C = 24.9\sqrt{Ds_1}$$

C = Velocity cm/sec
C = Velocity ft/min.
d = Diam. of particle in cm.
D = Diam. of particle in Microns
r = Radius of particle in cm.

STOKES LAW

$$C = \frac{2r^2 g}{9}\frac{s_1 - s_2}{\eta}$$

$g = 981$ cm/sec^2 acceleration
$s_1 =$ Density of particle
$s_2 =$ Density of Air (Very small relative to s_1)

FOR AIR AT 70°F.

$C = 300,460 s_1 d^2$

$C = .00592 s_1 D^2$

$\eta =$ Viscosity of air in poises $= 1814 \times 10^{-7}$ for air at 70°F.

$\lambda = 10^{-5}$ cm. (Mean free path of gas molecules)

CUNNINGHAM'S FACTOR

$$C = C'\left(1 + K\frac{\lambda}{r}\right)$$

C' = C of STOKES LAW
K = .8 TO .86

BROWNIAN MOVEMENT

A = Distance of motion in time t
R = Gas constant $= 8.316 \times 10^{7}$
T = Absolute Temperature
N = Number of Gas molecules in one mol $= 6.06 \times 10^{23}$

$$A = \sqrt{\frac{RT}{N}\frac{t}{3\pi\eta r}}$$

IT IS ASSUMED THAT THE PARTICLES ARE OF UNIFORM SPHERICAL SHAPE HAVING SPECIFIC GRAVITY ONE AND THAT THE DUST CONCENTRATION IS 0.1 GRAINS PER 1000 CU. FT. OF AIR, THE AVERAGE OF METROPOLITAN DISTRICTS.

Figure 65. The Frank Chart—size and characteristics of airborne solids (courtesy American Air Filter Co.).

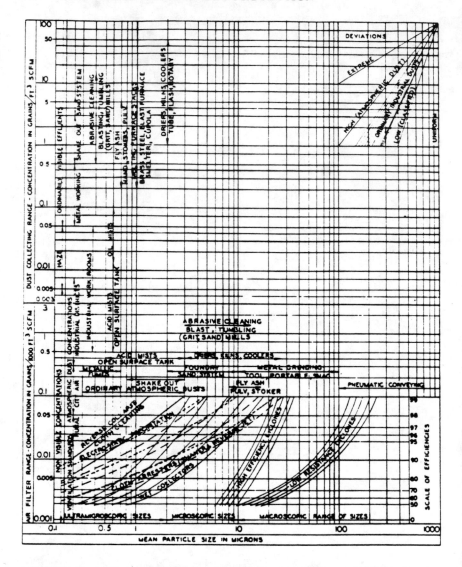

COMPILED BY S. SYLVAN APRIL 1952 : COPYRIGHT 1952 AMERICAN AIR FILTER CO. INC.
ACKNOWLEDGEMENTS OF PARTIAL SOURCES OF DATA REPORTED :
1 FRANK W.G. - AMERICAN AIR FILTER - SIZE AND CHARACTERISTICS OF AIR BORNE SOLIDS - 1931
2 FIRST AND DRINKER - ARCHIVES OF INDUSTRIAL HYGIENE AND OCCUPATIONAL MEDICINE - APRIL 1952
3 TAFT INSTITUTE AND AAF LABORATORY TEST DATA - 1961 - '63
4 REVERSE COLLAPSE CLOTH CLEANING ADDED 1964

Figure 66.   The Sylvan Chart—range of particle sizes, concentrations and collector performance (courtesy American Air Filter Co.).

The particle size range for the respirating mechanism for each of these is shown in Table XV [58].

Direct interception of a particle occurs (Figure 67) when a particle of radius "r" approaches a fiber along a streamline that passes more closely to the fiber than the distance "v." The particle strikes the fiber and is collected. The formula is:

$$R = \frac{r}{r_v} = \frac{dp}{df}$$

where
- R = direct interception parameter
- r = particle radius (μ)
- rf = fiber radius (μ)
- dp = particle diameter (μ)
- df = fiber diameter (μ)

The target efficiency of the interception mechanism is a function of R and the Reynolds number.

Inertial impaction occurs when a particle has sufficient mass to deviate by inertia from the line of flow as the airstream passes around the fiber. Stein, et al. [59] derived the classic inertial parameter (see Figure 68):

$$\psi = \frac{C\rho v d_p^2}{18\mu df}$$

where
- ψ = inertial parameter (dimensionless)
- C = Cunningham Correction Factor (dimensionless)
- p = density of aerosol particle (g/cm^3)
- v = velocity of airflow (cm/sec)
- μ = viscosity of gas (air) (g/cm-sec)
- dp = particle diameter (cm)
- df = fiber diameter (cm)

These forces are important for larger than submicron particles.

Diffusion (Brownian motion) depends on the size of the particles being comparable to the mean free path of gas molecules (0.06 μ). Their motion is more violent, and the collisions with filter fibers are more likely to occur. The diffusion parameters expressed by Stein et al. [59] can be expressed as

$$D = \frac{1}{vd_f}\left(\frac{CkT}{3\pi\mu d_p}\right)$$

Table XV.   Particle Size Range for Separating Mechanisms

Force	Particle Size Range (μ)
Direct Interception	>1
Impaction (inertial contact)	>1
Diffusion (Brownian Motion)	<0.1 to 0.2
Electrostatic Attraction	>0.01
Gravity	>1

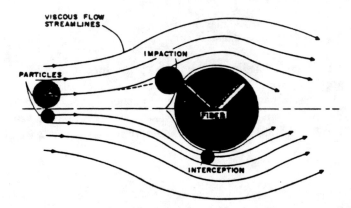

Figure 67.   Particle removal by fibrous filter through mechanisms of interception and impaction [58].

where   D = diffusion parameter

$$\frac{CkT}{3\pi\mu d_p} = \text{diffusion coefficient (sec/cm}^2)$$

k = Boltzmann constant 1.38×10^{-16} erg/°K
T = absolute temperature of air (°K)
v = velocity of airflow (cm/sec)
df = fiber diameter (cm)
dp = particle diameter (cm)
μ = viscosity of gas (air) (g/cm-sec)

The importance of diffusion for removing fine particulates increases considerably as the velocity of the air passing through the filter decreases, as at the beginning and end of an inhalation cycle. The longer the time in the filter, the greater the chance for capture.

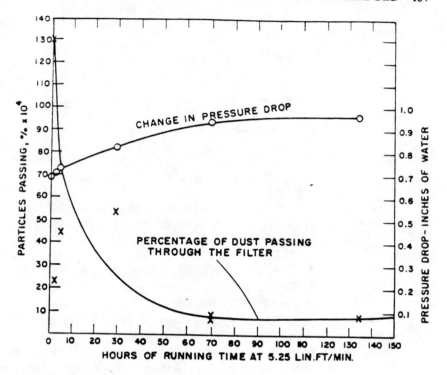

Figure 68. Effect of running time on efficiency of AEC filter paper at a flow-rate of 5 linear fpm [62].

Electrostatic attraction of particulates has been achieved by carding the fibers and adding a coating of resin to them. Certain dielectric waxes, resins and plastics have been used to generate an electrostatic charge to attract and hold particulate matter.

Gravity, as a force for removal of particulates by a fibrous bed, is a function of terminal velocity:

$$G = \frac{u}{v} = \frac{C\rho dp^2 g}{18\mu v}$$

where G = settling parameter (dimensionless)
  u = terminal settling velocity of the particle (cm/sec)
  v = velocity of airflow (cm/sec)
  μ = viscosity of gas (air) (g/cm-sec)
  ρ = density of aerosol particle (g/cm³)
  g = acceleration of gravity (cm/sec²)

Gravitational force is usually small in nature and generally is not considered. The overall efficiencies of a filter, based on the work of Davies [60] is

$$\eta_o = 0.16(R + (0.5 + 0.8R)(\psi + D) - 0.1052R(\psi + D)^2)$$

where η_o = total target efficiencies
  R = direct interception parameter
  ψ = inertial parameter
  D = diffusion parameter

The overall efficiency of a mass of fibers comprising a filter mat can be calculated from η_o, the packing density of the mat and the filter thickness, using Davies' method.

Filter performance characteristics of a filter medium used for a respirator are efficiency and pressure drop. Efficiency is influenced by filtration velocity, fiber diameter, loading and particle size.

To increase the efficiency of small particle removal and to decrease the resistance to airflow, the velocity of air passing through the filter medium must be kept as low as possible. Velocity reduction is achieved by folding or by manipulating the slope of the filter to provide greater surface areas, resulting in a low pressure drop and a greater ability to collect or improve loading characteristics. Once the filter is used, the particles themselves act as a filter medium; however, with the vibration and pulsation of breathing, no accurate measurement of this phenomenon can be accomplished. In studies by Jordan and Silverman [61], the efficiency of collection for a filter subjected to pulsating flow is about the same as results obtained by steady-state flow. The range of velocities encountered by the wearer would cause the efficiency of collection to be increased.

Fiber size technology has increased greatly during the last few years, but probably the "HEPA" filters are the most notable advance. Loading of the filters, as with any physical screening type operation, increases filtration, but at what pressure loss? Figure 68 illustrates the effect of running time on efficiency of AEC filter paper [62]. Figure 69 illustrates the clogging of various types of filter material [60]. Materials such as cotton sheeting suffer a large pressure drop due to loading and are not practical as a filter medium for respirator cartridges. The key to filter design is to be sufficiently strong to be handled or, in the case of throw-away design filters, to be able to last the whole day (duration of test). Particle size is so varied in many operations that for any given filtration velocity there is a particle size that will penetrate a filter (Figure 70) [58]. For this reason, medical tests must be used to examine the effectiveness of respiratory protection.

Pressure drop is changed as the respirator filter becomes more effec-

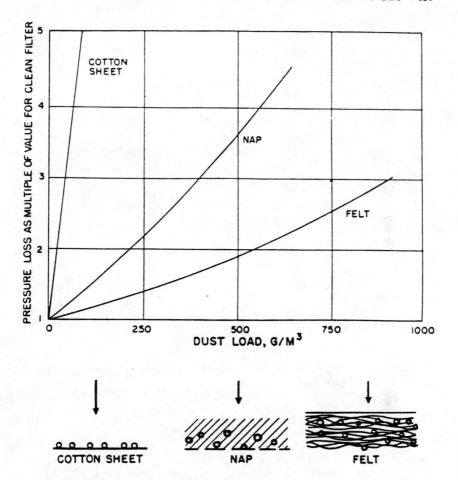

Figure 69.   Clogging of various types of filter material [60].

tive or loaded with material. Particle size, shape, density, surface characteristics, packing characteristics of deposited material, air contaminant
levels and related density, and humidity all have an effect on the pressure
drop.

Silverman [63] related the resistance due to the presence of loading by
the following formula:

$$R_f - R_i = R = \frac{k_1 LTV^2}{7000}$$

where R_f = final resistance (in. H_2O)
        R_i = initial resistance (in. $H_2O = k_0 V$)

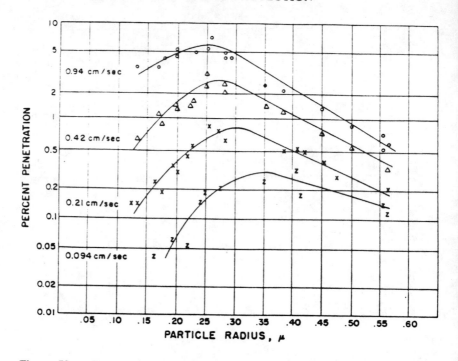

Figure 70.   Penetration of homogeneous DOP aerosols through a fiberglass FG-50 filter mat [64].

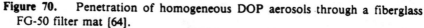

R = net resistance due to dust
k_o = resistance coefficient for clean filter
V = filtering velocity (ft/min)
L = dust load in air to filter (gr/ft³)
T = time (min) for filter resistance to increase R in. of H_2O
k_1 = specific resistance of the dust (in. H_2O/lb dust/ft² of cloth area/fpm filtering velocity

The next step is to measure the breakthrough of the filter medium and set minimum efficiencies for approval performance. Currently, the Mine Safety & Health Administration, under Section 11.140-1 to 12 [1], specifies the tests required for performance. Silica dust, silica mist, lead fume and dioctyl phthalate (DOP) are the substances used. Table XVIa summarizes the results. Tables XVIa and XVIb specify the maximum resistance measured in millimeters of water column height allowable.

CHEMICAL CARTRIDGE RESPIRATORS

Chemical cartridge respirators use a cartridge to remove gases and vapors from the air by sorption. Sorption is the attraction and holding to

Table XVIa.   Air-Purifying and Powered Air-Purifying
Respirator Filter Tests Required for Approval
[30 CFR Part 11, Subpart K, § 11.140–4, et seq.]

	Silica Dust Tests			Lead Fume Test	Silica Mist Test	DOP Test
Respirator Types	11.140–4	11.140–5	11.140–12	11.140–6	11.140–7	11.140–11
Dusts: Air contamination level not less than 0.05 mg/M^3 or 2 mppcf	X					
Fumes: air contamination level not less than 0.05 mg/M^3				.X		
Mists: air contamination level not less than 0.05 mg/M^3 or 2 mppcf					X	
Dusts, fumes, and mists: air contamination level less than 0.05 mg/M^3 or 2 mppcf, and radionuclides			X			X
Radon daughters	[a]X				[b]X	
Asbestos-containing dusts and mists	[b]X				[c]X	
Single use dust and mist respirators		[c]X			[c]X	

[a] For resistance only.
[b] For penetration only.
[c] Test required only where applicable.

Table XVIb.   Maximum Allowable Resistance Requirements
for Dust, Fume and Mist Respirators

Maximum Resistance
[mm. water-column height]

Type of Respirator	Initial Inhalation	Final Inhalation	Exhalation
Single use	12	15	15
Dust, fume and mist, with single-use filter	30	50	20
Dust, fume and mist, with reusable filter	20	40	20
Radon daughter	18	25[a]	15
Asbestos dust and mist	18	25	15

[a] Measured after silica dust test described in § 11.140–4.

the surface of a solid as molecules of vapor and gases come into contact with that surface at room temperatures. The solid substance is the sorbent, and the gas or vapor being sorbed is the sorbate. If the molecules of the sorbate are held to the surface by physical forces, similar to condensation, the process is termed adsorption. If electron transfer takes place between the sorbate and surface of the sorbent, the phenomenon is chemisorption. In adsorption, the sorbate does not remain on the surface but enters into the solid and reacts with it chemically, changing the chemical nature of each. In 1976 the NIOSH/Mine Enforcement Safety Administration Method for Approval of Respirator Cartridges and Canisters [65] for use in organic vapor atmospheres required exposure to carbon tetrachloride alone, under controlled conditions, as specified in 30 CFR. Cartridges were subjected to 1000 ppm of carbon tetrachloride in air at a flowrate of 64 liter/min (three tests using cartridges as received) and 32 liter/min (four tests using cartridges equilibrated in humid air.) Service life was defined as the length of time required to reach 5 ppm breakthrough. A service life of at least 50 minutes was required for approval.

Successful performance by a cartridge against these tests resulted in its approval for all organic vapors. Nelson and Harder [66], in a five-year respirator cartridge study at the Lawrence Livermore Laboratory at Los Alamos, New Mexico, published the results on the performance of commercially available organic vapor respirator cartridges tested against 121 different organic vapor and gases. Of these gases and vapors, 51 produced shorter service lives than carbon tetrachloride. This included vinyl chloride, a known carcinogen, which gave a service life of 3.8 minutes. In a similar study carried out by Freedman [67] at the Bureau of Mines, approved cartridges were tested against 1000 ppm each of 29 organic vapor and gases. Of these gases, 16 had service lives shorter than the 50 minutes required by the MESA-30CFR Section 11.

One should note that odor detection is different for each individual, depending on time of the year and humidity. The section on quantitative and qualitative fit testing will discuss odor detection, but research shows that equipment that was labeled as certified and thought to be sufficient did not provide the protection as required.

ADSORPTION CAPACITY

The equation for the capacity of a charcoal to adsorption of a solvent vapor is based on the Polanyi potential theory [65]:

$$A = \frac{T}{V_m} \log\left(\frac{P_s}{P}\right)$$

where   A = adsorption potential
        T = temperature (°K)
        V_m = molar volume at normal boiling point (cc/mol)
        P_s = saturation vapor pressure (torr)
        P = partial pressure (torr)

This was modified further by Dubinin [68] and co-workers to produce a straight-line graph:

$$W_s = \rho W_o \exp\left(-\frac{BT^2}{\beta^2}\left(\log\left(\frac{p_s}{p}\right)\right)^2\right)$$

where W_s = adsorption capacity (g solvent/g adsorbent)
        ρ = solvent density (g/cc)
        W_o = maximum adsorption space (cc)
        B = microporosity constant
        T = temperature (°K)
        β = affinity coefficient
        P_s = saturated vapor pressure of the solvent at temperature T (torr)
        P = equilibrium partial pressure of the solvent (torr)

The question arose, however, concerning how long the cartridge would be effective at a certain level of contamination. Jonas and Rehrmann [69] modified the Wheeler equation into the present form:

$$t_b = \frac{W_s}{C_oQ}\left[W - \frac{\rho Q}{k}\ln\left(\frac{C_o}{C_b}\right)\right]$$

where t_b = breakthrough time (min)
        W_s = adsorption capacity (g/g)
        C_o = input concentration (g/l)
        Q = volumetric flowrate (liter/min)
        W = weight of charcoal (g)
        ρ = density of charcoal (g/cc)
        k = adsorption rate constant (min^{-1})
        C_b = breakthrough concentration (g/cc)

Humidity is the next area that must be considered. Burrage and Allmand [70] studied the effect of moisture on the sorption of carbon tetrachloride and reported the following empirical relationship:

$$\frac{t_m}{t_d} = \frac{k}{w + k}$$

where t_m = breakthrough time using moist charcoal and moist air
t_d = breakthrough time using dry charcoal and dry air
w = weight of water adsorbed
k = a constant

The most comprehensive work on humidity has been done by Nelson et al. [71]. They concluded that storage (preconditioning) and use in humidities above 65% greatly reduce the service life of respirators. They made the following four generalizations:

1. Both the precondition and use humidity alter the cartridge service life.

2. The use humidity has a greater effect than the preconditioning humidity.

3. The service life is approximately the same between 0 and 50% humidity.

4. Humidity has a greater effect on cartridge performance at lower concentrations of solvent vapor.

At this point, a review of the reports by Nelson et al. [71] is appropriate. The reports took five years to complete and were summarized and published in the *American Industrial Hygiene Association Journal* [72]. It was felt that a respirator cartridge user might be misled by the words printed on the cartridge—"Permissible Cartridge for Organic Vapor." MESA did not guarantee its effectiveness against all organic vapors. As a typical organic vapor half-mask respirator cartridge is a plastic or metal case that contains approximately 25–40 g of adsorbing media, the products tested were noted as to whether the carbon originated from a petroleum or a coconut base. Table XVII lists the various manufacturers tested. Various other factors, such as breathing rate, boiling points and correction factors for humidities also were taken into account. Table XVIII illustrates the wide range in breathing rates as a function of work rate. As conditions of humidity vary both in storage and seasonal changes in the workplace, Table XIX illustrates the variation. Concern about how much the use of humidity affects the service life is illustrated in Figure 71. Test conditions include a flowrate of 53.3 liter/min at 50% relative humidity. Decreasing the concentration by a factor of 10 generally increases the service life four to five times [72]. The results of the work are shown in Table XX and Figure 72. Test conditions include a flowrate of 53.3 liter/min at 50% relative humidity. Decreasing the concentration by a factor of 10 generally increases the service life four to five times [72]. Decreasing the concentration by a factor of 10 generally increases the service life four to five times.

The cartridge service life (the 10% breakthrough time) now can be estimated from the following empirical expression:

Table XVII.   Manufacturing Specifications of Organic
Vapor Half-Mask Respirator Cartridges [72][a]

Manufacturer	Model No.	Total Carbon Weight[b] w_c[a] (g)	Carbon Density ρ_c (g/cm³)	Carbon Base
American Optical Co.	R-51	74	0.43	Petroleum
Bausch and Lomb	Organic Vapor	80	0.43	Petroleum
Glendale Optical Co.	GR-4021, GR-2021	80	0.43	Petroleum
Mine Safety Appliance Co.	44135	52	0.38	Coconut
	459315	68	0.40	Coconut
	76883[c]	51	0.43	Various
Safeline Products	5961	74	0.43	Petroleum
Scott Aviation	800-OV	80	0.40	Petroleum
	502-OV[c]	85	0.46	Petroleum
Welch Manufacturing Co.	7500-1	69	0.44	Petroleum
Willson	R-21	97	0.44	Petroleum

[a]Each mask uses two cartridges except where otherwise indicated.
[b]Weight of both cartridges.
[c]Single-cartridge respirator.

Table XVIII.   Breathing Rate as a Function
of Work Rate [72]

Work Rate Description	Work Rate (kg-m/min)	Average Breathing Rate (liter/min)
Sitting	0	14
Light	208	21
Moderate	415	30
Moderately heavy	622	37
Heavy	830	55
Extremely heavy	1107	75

$$t\ 10\% = \frac{2.4 \times 10^6 W_c(a + bt)}{C^{2/3}MQ}$$

where
W_c = carbon weight
a, b and t = relative solvent volatility
c = concentration
M = molecular weight
Q = breathing rate

Table XIX.   Breakthrough Time Correction Factors
at Various Humidities at 1000 ppm [72][a]

Use Relative Humidity (%)	Breakthrough Time Multiplier at 1000 ppm					
	Storage Relative Humidity (%)					
	0	20	50	65	80	90
0	0.94	0.95	0.99	0.97	0.95	0.95
20	1.02	1.02	1.03	1.04	1.01	1.00
50	0.98	0.99	1.00	0.99	0.95	0.77
65	0.97	0.98	0.99	0.94	0.84	0.66
80	0.87	0.91	0.88	0.83	0.72	0.50
90	0.84	0.85	0.83	0.78	0.67	0.48

[a]The data have been normalized to the 50% use and storage humidities.

With a substance of methanol at a concentration of 1000 ppm, and at 50% relative humidity, the calculated time averaged 6 minutes and the experimental time lasted 3.2 minutes. NIOSH and the National Aeronautics and Space Administration (NASA) jointly contracted with the Bendix Launch Support Division to begin development of an improved certification program for organic vapor cartridges and canisters. Published as the "Development of Improved Respirator Cartridge and Canister Test Method" [65], Table XXI presents the estimated service lives of the reusable cartridges against selected organic vapors. Further changes in the testing procedure are recommended. Table XXII lists maximum use concentrations for cartridges; Table XXIII gives the maximum resistance for cartridges; and Table XXIV specifies bench tests for cartridges considering relative humidity concentration, number of tests, allowable penetration and minimum life in minutes.

Figure 73 shows a facepiece with a single-cartridge unit, which provides respiratory protection against radionuclides and dusts, fumes and mists having a TLV of less than 0.1 mg/μ^3, where the contaminant concentration does not exceed 100 times the concentration limit for the radionuclide involved or 100 times the TLV. The full facepiece provides unobstructed vision from side to side and downward. The oval filter cartridge is designed with a large effective area to provide low breathing resistance with high loading capacity. Figure 74 shows a welding application in which a filter cartridge and canister have been adapted to the welder's shield.

Table XX.   Comparison of Experimental and Calculated 10% Breakthrough at 22°C [72]

Solvent	Concentration (ppm)	Flowrate (liter/min)	Test Relative Humidity (%)	10% Breakthrough Time			
				Calculated			Experimental
				Mecklenburg Equation (min)	Wheeler Equation (min)	Equation 16 (min)	(min)
Benzene[a]	125	53.3	50	440	418	377	355
	500	53.3	50	169	161	150	134
	2000	53.3	50	59.3	56.4	59.4	41.9
Benzene[b]	1000	53.3	20	114	110	126[c]	101
	1000	53.3	50	114	110	127	101
	1000	53.3	80	114	110	112[c]	87.4
Toluene[a]	1000	20.6	50	328	322	255	288
	1000	36.7	50	180	174	143	164
	1000	53.3	50	121	116	98.7	114
Methanol[a]	1000	53.3	50	8.6	7.9	-0.5	3.2
Isopropanol[a]	500	53.3	50	170	160	77.5	126
	2000	53.3	50	75.1	63.3	30.7	54.7
Butanol[a]	1000	53.3	50	150	143	120	141
Pentanol[a]	1000	53.3	50	137	134	139	130
Vinyl Chloride[b]	50	40	50	99.2	96.2	-69.1	77.0
	250	40	50	58.5	56.8	-23.6	52.5
	1000	40	50	32.4	31.4	-9.4	22.7
Ethyl Chloride[a]	1000	53.3	50	21.5	18.5	26.5	10.7
1-Chlorobutane[a]	1000	53.3	20	89.9	87.2	75.5[c]	86.3
	1000	53.3	50	89.9	87.2	73.3	87.3
	1000	53.3	90	89.9	87.2	61.0[c]	68.0

Table XX, continued

Solvent	Concentration (ppm)	Flowrate (liter/min)	Test Relative Humidity (%)	10% Breakthrough Time			
				Calculated			Experimental
				Mecklenburg Equation (min)	Wheeler Equation (min)	Equation 16 (min)	(min)
Chlorobenzene[a]	1000	53.3	50	132	128	97.9	131
Dichloromethane[a]	500	53.3	50	30.3	28.5	44.5	30.0
	2000	53.3	50	21.1	19.7	17.7	17.3
o-Dichlorobenzene[a]	1000	53.3	50	132	130	124	132
Chloroform[a]	1000	53.3	50	69.9	66.6	51.9	52.4
Methyl Chloroform[a]	250	53.3	50	251	242	149	207
	2000	53.3	50	51.3	49.5	37.2	56.1
Trichloroethylene[a]	1000	53.3	50	108	103	72.6	83.0
Carbon Tetrachloride[a]	1000	53.3	20	82.4	79.1	89.4[c]	84.9
	1000	53.3	50	82.4	79.1	86.8	68.8
	1000	53.3	90	82.4	79.1	71.3[c]	66.0
Perchloroethylene[a]	1000	53.3	50	128	123	112	129
Methyl Acetate[a]	100	53.3	50	373	353	248	146
	1000	53.3	50	73.9	81.8	53.4	45.9
Ethyl Acetate[b]	1000	53.3	20	115	111	83.1[c]	88.4
	1000	53.3	65	115	111	79.9[c]	90.4
	1000	53.3	90	115	111	67.2[c]	68.4
Propyl Acetate[a]	1000	53.3	50	110	106	72.4[c]	99.0
Butyl Acetate[a]	1000	53.3	50	106	104	87.1	96.9
Acetone[b]	100	53.3	50	504	484	499	245
	500	53.3	50	160	154	170	96.7

Acetone[b]	1000	53.3	50	94.4	90.8	107	66.3
	1000	53.3	20	94.4	90.8	110[c]	61.1
	1000	53.3	80	94.4	90.8	94.3[c]	54.5
	1000	53.3	90	94.4	90.8	89.0[c]	53.1
2-Butanone[d]	1000	53.3	50	136	132	103	94.4
Diisobutyl Ketone[d]	1000	53.3	50	97.4	97.2	103	83.3
Pentane[d]	1000	53.3	50	86.2	83.8	67.5	71.3
Hexane[b]	100	53.3	50	646	631	420	565
	500	53.3	50	156	152	144	143
	2000	53.3	50	44.1	43.0	57.0	37.9
Hexane[a]	1000	53.3	0	77.6	75.4	66.7[c]	76.7
	1000	53.3	65	77.6	75.4	66.7[c]	68.1
	1000	53.3	90	77.6	75.4	56.6[c]	64.0
Cyclohexane[d]	1000	53.3	50	124	122	90.4	82.3
Heptane[d]	1000	53.3	50	106	104	86.9	80.5
Methylamine[d]	1000	53.3	50	49.1	46.7	13.4	17.9
Ethylamine[d]	1000	53.3	50	99.9	96.1	57.1	49.7
Diethylamine[a]	250	53.3	50	117	110	179	92.5
	1000	53.3	50	52.7	49.8	71.0	35.6
	2000	53.3	50	33.7	31.9	44.7	20.6
Dipropylamine[d]	1000	53.3	50	141	140	110	105

[a] MSA cartridges, coconut base, 52.2 g/pair.
[b] AO cartridges, petroleum base, 70.5 g/pair.
[c] Use humidity correction.
[d] AO cartridges, coconut base, 62.2 g/pair.

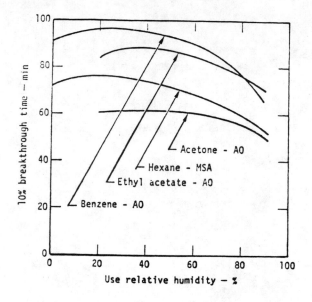

Figure 71.   Service life as a function of concentration.

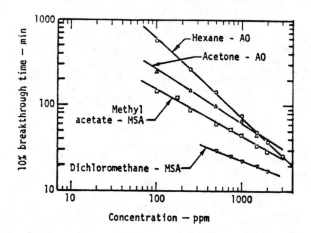

Figure 72.   Service life as a function of concentration.

Table XXI.   Estimated Service Lives of the Reusable
Cartridge Against Selected Organic Vapors [65]

	TLV (ppm)	$C_0 \times 10^3$ (g/l)	w_s (g/g)	A^2	Service Life (min)[a]
Benzene	10	0.325	0.167	99.7	244
Toluene	100	3.83	0.387	16.7	96.1
Ethylbenzene	100	4.42	0.438	5.6	93.4
m-Xylene	100	4.41	0.438	4.9	94.5
Cumene	50	2.50	0.439	4.1	167
Mesitylene	—	4.99	0.455	0.6	86.8
p-Cymene	—	5.57	0.453	0.2	77.4
Methanol	200	1.33	0.036	240	12.9
Ethanol	1000	1.92	0.181	80.6	44.8
2-Propanol	400	2.50	0.275	40.3	105
Allyl Alcohol	2	0.048	0.063	190	624
Propanol	200	2.50	0.322	24.4	122
Sec-Butanol	150	3.08	0.365	15.7	113
Butanol	50	1.54	0.370	14.6	229
2-Pentanol	—	3.67	0.411	4.3	107
3-Methyl-1-butanol	100	3.67	0.421	1.9	109
4-Methyl-2-pentanol	25	1.07	0.386	9.4	343
Pentanol	—	3.67	0.425	1.1	110
2-Ethyl-1-butanol	—	4.25	0.437	0.6	97.8
Methyl Chloride	100	2.10	0.009	395	2.1
Vinyl Chloride	1	0.026	0.001	578	18.3
Ethyl Chloride	1000	2.68	0.080	174	14.2
2-Chloropropane	—	3.27	0.200	80.5	29.1
Allyl Chloride	1	0.032	0.027	283	402
1-Chloropropane	—	3.27	0.106	145	15.4
2-Chloro-2-methylpropane	—	3.85	0.280	46.9	69.2
1-Chlorobutane	—	3.85	0.334	33.3	82.5
2-Chloro-2-methylbutane	—	4.43	0.370	21.1	79.5
1-Chloropentane	—	4.43	0.407	13.6	87.4
Chlorobenzene	75	3.51	0.516	12.4	140
1-Chlorohexane	—	5.02	0.445	4.5	84.3
o-Chlorotoluene	50	2.63	0.547	4.6	198
1-Chloroheptane	—	5.60	0.463	0.8	78.7
Dichloromethane	200	3.53	0.145	155	19.6
t-1,2-Dichloroethylene	200	4.03	0.249	96.2	29.4
1,1-Dichloroethane	200	4.12	0.312	67.6	36.1
c-1,2-Dichloroethylene	200	4.03	0.297	80.3	35.1
1,2-Dichloroethane	50	2.06	0.330	69.2	76.0
1,2-Dichloropropane	75	3.52	0.438	32.5	118
1,4-Dichlorobutane	—	5.28	0.597	2.8	108
o-Dichlorobenzene	50	3.06	0.685	0.9	213
Chloroform	25	1.24	0.235	118	180

Table XXI.   Continued

	TLV (ppm)	$C_0 \times 10^3$ (g/l)	w_s (g/g)	A^2	Service Life (min)[a]
Methylchloroform	350	5.55	0.465	41.8	79.7
Trichloroethylene	100	5.46	0.518	39.2	90.3
1,1,2-Trichloroethane	10	0.555	0.423	57.8	725
1,2,3-Trichloropropane	50	3.06	0.707	4.4	220
Carbon Tetrachloride	10	0.640	0.334	90.7	248
Perchloroethylene	100	6.90	0.748	13.6	103
1,1,2,2-Tetrachloroethane	5	0.349	0.854	35.3	2328
Methyl Acetate	200	3.08	0.217	84.5	33.5
Vinyl Acetate	—	3.58	0.312	45.0	80.3
Ethyl Acetate	400	3.66	0.327	36.8	85.0
Isopropyl Acetate	250	4.16	0.373	20.9	85.3
Propyl Acetate	200	4.25	0.402	15.4	90.0
Butyl Acetate	150	4.83	0.443	5.4	87.3
Isopentyl Acetate	100	5.41	0.452	1.9	79.5
Pentyl Acetate	100	5.41	0.457	1.4	80.4
Acetone	1000	2.41	0.133	112	26.2
2-Butanone	200	3.00	0.276	42.9	87.5
2-Pentanone	200	3.58	0.350	20.3	93.0
3-Pentanone	—	3.58	0.355	19.1	94.4
4-Methyl-2-pentanone	100	4.16	0.384	10.0	87.8
Mesityl Oxide	25	1.02	0.379	17.8	354
2,4-Pentanedione	—	4.16	0.478	7.3	109
2-Heptanone	100	4.75	0.424	1.4	84.9
Cyclohexanone	50	2.04	0.486	8.3	227
Pentane	600	3.00	0.197	50.5	62.5
2,3-Dimethylbutane	—	3.58	0.257	30.2	68.3
Hexane	100	3.58	0.270	25.2	71.8
Methylcyclopentane	—	3.50	0.283	32.8	76.9
Cyclohexane	300	3.50	0.302	30.7	82.1
Cyclohexene	300	3.41	0.305	33.5	85.1
2,2,4-Trimethylpentane	—	4.75	0.333	9.5	66.7
Heptane	400	4.17	0.322	11.5	73.5
Methylcyclohexane	—	4.08	0.348	15.4	81.2
Nonane	—	5.33	0.376	1.1	67.1
Methyl Iodide	5	0.295	0.033	357	53
Acrylonitrile	20	0.441	0.097	143	104
1,2-Dibromoethane	20	1.56	0.791	36.7	482
Epichlorohydrin	5	0.192	0.244	91.5	604

[a] Calculated from the modified Wheeler equation.

Table XXII.   Subpart L—Chemical Cartridge Respirators

§ 11.150 Chemical cartridge respirators: description.

Chemical cartridge respirators including all completely assembled respirators designed for use as respiratory protection during entry into, or escape from, atmospheres not immediately dangerous to life and health are described according to the specific gases or vapors against which they are designed to provide respiratory protection, as follows:

Type of Chemical Cartridge Respirator[a]	Maximum Use Concentration (ppm)
Ammonia	300
Chlorine	10
Hydrogen Chloride	50
Methyl Amine	100
Organic Vapor	1000[b]
Sulfur Dioxide	50
Vinyl Chloride	10

[a]Not for use against gases or vapors with poor warning properties (except where MESA or OSHA standards may permit such use for a specific gas or vapor) or those that generate high heats of reaction with sorbent material in the cartridge.

[b]Maximum use concentrations are lower for organic vapors that produce atmospheres immediately hazardous to life or health at concentrations equal to, or lower than, this concentration.

NOTE: Chemical cartridge respirators for respiratory protection against gases or vapors not specifically listed with their maximum use concentration, except pesticides, may be approved if the applicant submits a request for such approval, in writing, to the Institute. MSHA and the Institute shall consider each such application and accept or reject the application after a review of the effects on the wearer's health and safety and in the light of any field experience in use of chemical cartridge respirators as protection against such hazards.

POWERED AIR-PURIFYING RESPIRATORS

The idea of combining an air line portable blower respirator and a filter respirator resulted in the powered air-purifying respirator. The development of the respirator was suggested by William Burgess [73] in discussing the modification of respirators to use a tight-fitting respirator

Table XXIII.   Maximum Resistance (mm water column
height) (37 FR 6244, Mar. 25, 1972, as amended at
42 FR 65167, Dec. 30, 1977)

| Type of Chemical-Cartridge Respirator | Inhalation | | Exhalation |
	Initial	Final[a]	
Other than single-use vinyl chloride respirators			
For gases, vapors, or gases and vapors	40	45	20
For gases, vapors, or gases and vapors, and dusts, fumes and mists	50	70	20
For gases, vapors, or gases and vapors, and mists of paints, lacquers and enamels	50	70	20
Single-use respirator with valves			
For vinyl chloride	20	25	20
For vinyl chloride and pneumoconiosis- and fibrosis-producing dusts	30	45	20
Single-use respirator without valves			
For vinyl chloride	15	20	b
For vinyl chloride and pneumoconiosis- and fibrosis-producing dusts	25	40	b

[a]Measured at end of service life specified in Table 11 and 11a.
[b]Same as inhalation.

enclosure with a portable continuous-flow air supply. He concluded that the concept had not been accepted in America, but had proved successful in French mines.

In 1978 the Safety in Mines Research Establishment (SMRE), the British version of the U.S. Bureau of Mines, developed the SMRE dust helmet, which protests head, eyes and lungs in a single comfortable unit. It combines a hard hat face shield and powered air supply in one unit. The Racal Amplivox Company of England commercialized the unit and markets it through Racal Airstream Inc., Rockville, Maryland [74]. The unit is illustrated in Figure 75. The Bureau of Mines examined the unit under both laboratory and mine conditions [57]. The unit draws power from a portable battery that is pack-belt mounted; this powers a small battery-powered fan to force environmental air through two filters. The air then is channeled over the head of the wearer and directed behind a full face shield over the miner's face.

The helmet was evaluated in a 30-inch-diameter fiberglass section wind tunnel test to simulate the efficiencies of the helmet on coal longwall faces, where velocities as high as 1200 fpm might be encountered. Air-

Table XXIV. Cartridge Bench Test and Requirements
[30 CFR Part 11, Subpart L, § 11.162-8]

Cartridge	Test Condition	Test Atmosphere			Number of Tests	Penetration (ppm)	Minimum Life[b] (min)
		Gas or Vapor	Concentration (ppm)	Flowrate (lpm)			
Ammonia	As received	NH_3	1000	64	3	50	50
Ammonia	Equilibrated	NH_3	1000	32	4	50	50
Chlorine	As received	Cl_2	500	64	3	5	35
Chlorine	Equilibrated	Cl_2	500	32	4	5	35
Hydrogen Chloride	As received	HCl	500	64	3	5	50
Hydrogen Chloride	Equilibrated	HCl	500	32	4	5	50
Methylamine	As required	CH_3NH_3	1000	64	3	10	25
Methylamine	Equilibrated	CH_3NH_3	1000	32	4	10	25
Organic Vapors	As received	CCl_4	1000	64	3	5	50
Organic Vapors	Equilibrated	CCl_4	1000	32	4	5	50
Sulfur Dioxide	As received	SO_2	500	64	3	5	30
Sulfur Dioxide	Equilibrated	SO_2	500	32	4	5	30

[a] Minimum life will be determined at the indicated penetration.
[b] Where a respirator is designed for respiratory protection against more than one type of gas or vapor, as for use in ammonia and in chlorine, the minimum life shall be one-half that shown for each type of gas or vapor. Where a respirator is designed for respiratory protection against more than one gas of a type, as for use in chlorine and sulfur dioxide, the stated minimum life shall apply.

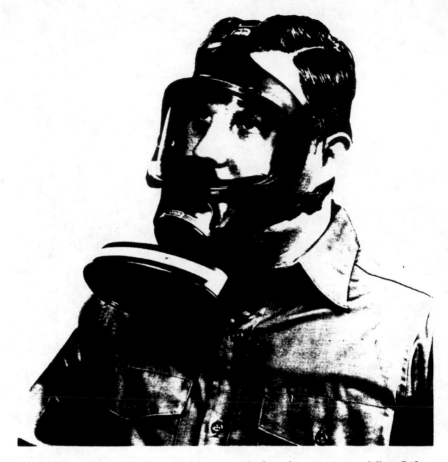

Figure 73.   Cartridge filter respirator with facepiece (courtesy Mine Safety Appliance Co.).

flow velocities in this tube were varied to 400, 800, 1200 and 1600 fpm. The effects of air velocity, helmet position and breathing were studied. Figure 76 illustrates the mannequin used in the sampling, along with the testing port locations. Methane was used as a tracer gas to simulate respirable dust in the laboratory condition. The efficiency of the helmet in actual mine tests, under normal air velocities (400 fpm), averaged a rating of 84%.

The air helmet is covered under Mine Safety & Health Administration Section 11.130, which concerns Dust, Fume and Mist Respirators [58].

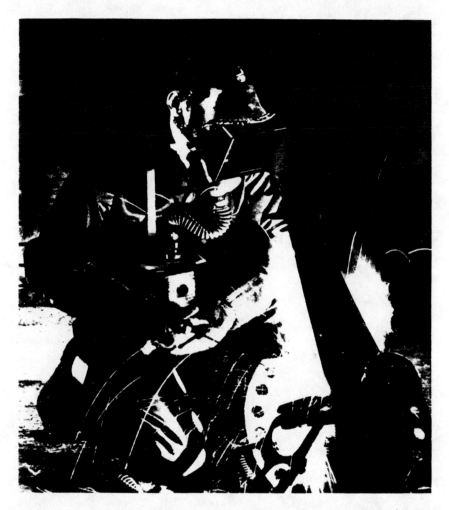

Figure 74.   Welding application in which cartridge has been adapted to welding shield (courtesy Mine Safety Appliance Co.).

All the applicable parts of this system must apply to these respirators, with the added requirement that the noise level generated by the respirator measured inside the hood or helmet at maximum airflow shall not exceed 80 dBA. A second type of powered filter respirator is mounted on a belt with the complete motor and filter unit. Figure 77 illustrates a typical design. The hose from the filter unit extends to a full-face respirator style and provides a sufficient flowrate.

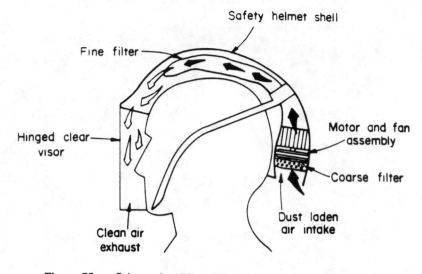

Figure 75. Schematic of Racal-Amphivox "airstream" helmet.

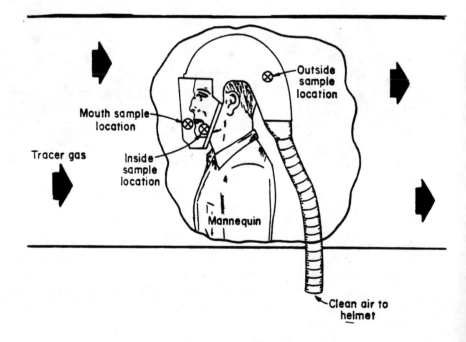

Figure 76. Airstream helmet testing in wind tunnel.

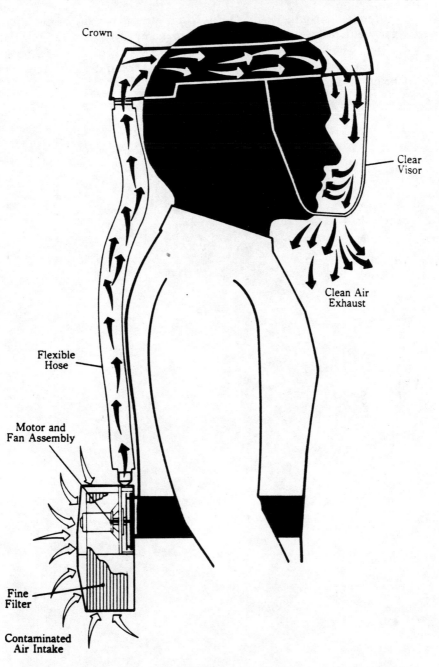

Crown

Clear Visor

Clean Air Exhaust

Flexible Hose

Motor and Fan Assembly

Fine Filter

Contaminated Air Intake

Figure 77. Powered air-purifying respirator, providing eye, face and respiratory protection (courtesy Racal Airstream Inc.).

Powered air-purifying respirators have the advantage of mobility and can be used by people who have minor impairment to the respiratory system when approved by a physician. The supply of air places no strain on the lungs, and only the cost and maintenance of the unit keeps it from being used more widely.

CHAPTER 7
SUPPLIED AIR RESPIRATORS

INTRODUCTION

The history of air line respirators dates back to the Assyrians (900 B.C.), who used air inhaled from inflated animal skins. The first hard-hat style diving suit (1840) is the more direct ancestor to the modern air line respirator. Most publications on respirators do not give credit to the early researchers who developed the technique of supplied air, either by lung pressure or external pump to the respirator user. We will examine OSHA and MSHA regulations, and currently used systems for supplied air respirators. The factor that makes the supplied air system of such great use is the unlimited supply of breathing air; however, it also is its greatest drawback.

The method used to supply the air is a hose system, which can be tangled, tripped on and damaged. The authors feel that the use of supplied air respirators will increase in many industrial operations in years to come for the following reasons:

1. Their cost, the cost of maintenance and powered supply of air are less than for the filter or self-contained types.
2. The filter type will be used less as unions and employee groups negotiate for spirogram and lung testing programs.
3. Management will realize that the effort used to breathe through filter types could be better spent on production.
4. Engineers faced with tough environmental and heat stress and cold weather energy problems will use vortex heating-cooling devices. The cost of fan-type ventilation systems will be replaced by fully enclosed process systems.
5. Manufacturers will spend more to give people such comforts as AM-FM radio, heating, cooling and emerging warning lights, where distractions are permitted.

6. Legal action and lawsuits due to lung diseases contracted by non-smokers will increase the desire to better protect those exposed to hazardous materials.
7. The present design will be incorporated more fully into protective clothing to give a total protection factor approach.

REGULATIONS

Before we examine the systems themselves, it is helpful to review the regulatory sections in OSHA and MSHA and explain the background of the standards. According to the OSHA Respiratory Protection Section [8], 1910.134(d)(1), air shall meet at least the requirements of the specifications for Grade D breathing air, as described in Compressed Gas Association Commodity Specification [75] G7.1-1966. Oxygen must never be used with air line respirators.

The Compressed Gas Association describes Grade D breathing air with the following limiting characteristics:

1. Percentage oxygen (v/v) balance predominantly nitrogen atm 19–23. Note that the term atm (atmospheric) denotes the oxygen content normally present in atmospheric air; the numerical values denote the oxygen limits for synthesized air.
2. The water content of compressed air required for any particular grade may vary with the intended use from saturated to very dry. If a specific water limit is required, it should be specified as a limiting dewpoint or concentration in ppm (v/v). Dewpoint is expressed in °F at 1 atm abs. (760 mm Hg).
3. Hydrocarbons (condensed) is 5 mg/m^3.
4. Carbon monoxide is 20 ppm.
5. Carbon dioxide is 1000 ppm.
6. Odor—reference is made to Section 5.1.5.

Specific measurements of odor in Type I air are impractical. Air normally may have a slight odor. The presence of a pronounced odor should render the air unsatisfactory for breathing.

There are nine grades of breathing air—A to J—referred to as Type I. In Type II, or the liquid state, there are two types—A and B. Atmospheric air is naturally occurring, and it is impractical to set limits for trace elements. That oxygen must never be used with air line respirators is placed in the standards because if a welder or worker had a slight burn in his uniform, for example, the oxygen could turn him into a ball of fire.

In Section (d)(2), breathing air may be supplied to respirators from cylinders or air compressors. Cylinders shall be tested and maintained as prescribed in the Shipping Container Specification Regulations of the Department of Transportation (49CFR Part 178) [76]. Figure 78 shows the typical markings for a cylinder display. The importance of this section in the regulation is that the materials for a certain size cylinder must be safely contained by the cylinder, and proper labeling must be followed by the supplier. A standard cylinder contains more than 2000 psi of air and, if knocked over, can rocket through a brick wall or kill someone.

Section (d)(2)(ii) deals with compressors used to supply breathing air through an air line. A breathing air-type compressor shall be used. Com-

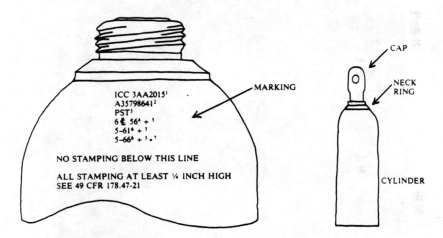

1. DOT or ICC marking may appear-new manufacture must read "DOT" 49CFR171.14
   "3AA" indicates spec in 49CFR178.37.
   "2015" is the marked service pressure.

2. Serial number—no duplicates permitted with any particular symbol-serial number combination.

3. Symbol of manufacturer, user or purchaser.

4. "6 56" date of manufacture. Month and year.
   "L" disinterested inspector's official mark.

5. Plus mark (+) indicates cylinder may be 10% overcharged per 49CFR173.302(C).

6. Retest dates.

7. 5 pointed star indicates ten year retest interval
   See 48CFR173.34(e)(15).

CAUTION: This is a training aid and does not include all provisions of the regulations.

Figure 78.   Marking requirements for a cylinder display (from the OSHA Training Institute).

pressors shall be constructed and situated to avoid entry of contaminated air into the system, and suitable inline air-purifying sorbent beds and filters installed to further assure breathing air quality. A receiver of sufficient capacity to enable the respirator wearer to escape from a contaminated atmosphere in the event of compressor failure, as well as alarms to indicate compressor failure and overheating, shall be installed in the system. If an oil-lubricated compressor is used, it must have a high-temperature or carbon monoxide alarm, or both.

If a high-temperature alarm is used, the air from the compressor shall

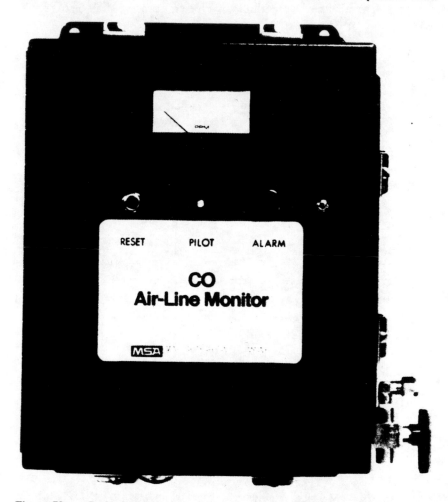

Figure 79.   Carbon monoxide monitor for respiratory air lines (courtesy Mine Safety Appliance Co.).

be tested frequently for carbon monoxide to ensure that it meets the specification (see Figures 79 and 80) of the Compressed Gas Association [75].

The new CO air line monitor is an economical instrument for continuously monitoring compressed air lines for carbon monoxide in the toxic range. The air line monitor provides audible and visual alarms when a predetermined CO concentration is reached. Its features include the following:

- No pump; flow-controlled diffusion sampling
- Long-life electrochemical cell

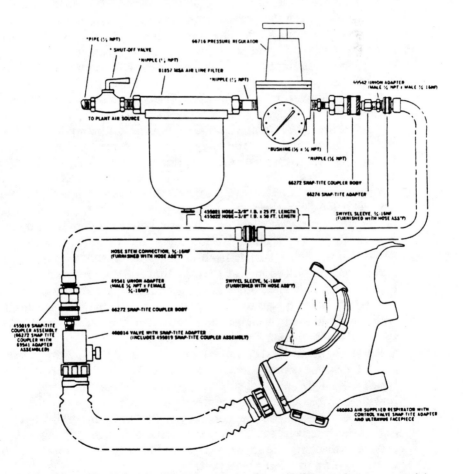

Figure 80. Typical assembly of constant-flow air line respirator as used in conjunction with a compressor system (courtesy Mine Safety Appliance Co.).

- No humidifier or reagents
- Audible alarm
- Visual alarm
- Instrument flow failure alarm
- Adjustable alarm point
- Remote alarm relays
- Linear meter readout
- NEMA-type steel enclosure
- Simple calibration

The detector is an electrochemical, polarographic cell that oxidizes carbon monoxide in proportion to its concentration in the line being sampled. Gas from the line enters the sensor cell by diffusion, thus eliminating the need for a sampling pump. Sample flow is regulated by the instrument's flow system; no flow adjustments are required. If the flow of sample gas is stopped, the instrument flow failure alarm is activated automatically.

In reviewing various equipment suppliers' literature, one finds claims such as, "only at 3000 psi and mechanical separation can air for breathing be purified." A Compressed Gas Association pamphlet [77] reviews the various methods of producing compressed air for humans and the various factors involved. The OSHA standard specifying a clean area for compressors to draw air for use is based on common sense. The problem most plants face is whether to use a portable pump or tap off the existing air lines running in their plant. The concern for possible contamination in the air line is a very real one. Most plants have compressed air, but insufficient air filters, refrigeration units or dryer units to remove condensate in the line and scale from piping units. As many painters inside tanks use compressed air for the painting, they merely tap off for the respirator as well. The statement about the right type of compressor does not specify which type is to be used. It states only that if an oil-lubricated compressor is used, a high-temperature alarm must be installed when testing the supplied air for carbon monoxide.

Rotary or centrifugal compressors are suitable for 150 psi or less. Coaxial screw-type compressors are available for up to 300 psi, and piston type, with single and dual stages, are very common for a wide range of pressures. More important problems occur with the water vapor compressed during the compression stages; this must be drained from the lines and reservoir (or receivers) constantly. Maintaining the compressors, checking the safety valves by blowing them down and being watchful for corrosion are important.

The following guide is provided to assist in the proper selection of a compressed air source.

1. For low volume and short times, bottled air is easier to locate, and no maintenance is required.
2. For average-volume jobs that require a short time period a portable compressor for one or two users provides better performance.
3. High volumes must be supplied by a compressor piping system.

Figure 80 illustrates a typical air-supplied respirator. The drawing may be deceptive because the quality of the air, impurity content and filter may not provide sufficient removal of material. Another reason is the air termperature. When air is compressed it gets hot, and moisture or water vapor levels are raised. These problems can be eliminated for the most part by passing the air through air dryers, refrigerated air dryers or air purifiers.

Air purifiers have been used with good results in many plants. Figures 81a and b illustrate a typical unit. The filters trap solids, oil, oil mists, water vapor, taste or odor, water vapor and carbon monoxide in various stages. As they are reduced in capacity above 100 °F, the graph provided gives the users a method to estimate life expectancy. The factors that influence volume are:

1. type of breathing mask, helmet and full hood,
2. air pressure required,
3. air flowrate and temperature,
4. vortex cooler or heater units, and
5. section of the country (weather conditions).

It should be noted that compressed air costs vary with types of motors, compressors, and the overall system. Such sources as "Compressed Air and Gas Data" [78] should be consulted for long-term and efficient installations.

MSHA REGULATIONS

Although OSHA has a section on basic respiratory aspects, specific requirements for air line respirators are specified in Mine Safety and Health Regulations Section 11.110 [1]. There are three basic types:

Type A. This is a hose mask respirator for entry into, and escape from, atmospheres not immediately dangerous to life or health. It consists of a motor-driven or hand-operated blower that permits the free entrance of air when the blower is not operating; a strong large-diameter hose having a low resistance to airflow; a harness to which the hose and lifeline are attached; and a tight-fitting facepiece.

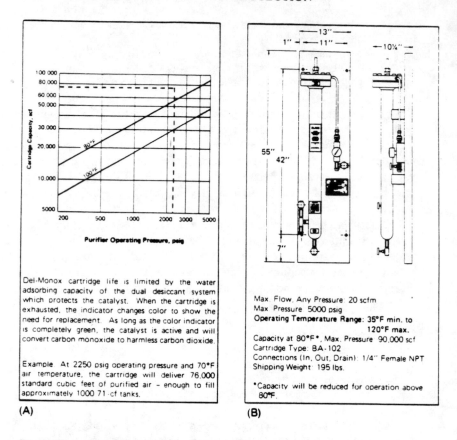

Del-Monox cartridge life is limited by the water adsorbing capacity of the dual desiccant system which protects the catalyst. When the cartridge is exhausted, the indicator changes color to show the need for replacement. As long as the color indicator is completely green, the catalyst is active and will convert carbon monoxide to harmless carbon dioxide.

Example At 2250 psig operating pressure and 70°F air temperature, the cartridge will deliver 76,000 standard cubic feet of purified air – enough to fill approximately 1000 71-cf tanks.

(A)

Max. Flow, Any Pressure: 20 scfm
Max. Pressure: 5000 psig
Operating Temperature Range: 35°F min. to
                                    120°F max.
Capacity at 80°F *, Max. Pressure: 90,000 scf
Cartridge Type: BA-102
Connections (In, Out, Drain): 1/4" Female NPT
Shipping Weight: 195 lbs.

*Capacity will be reduced for operation above 80°F.

(B)

Figure 81.   Examples of air purifier and results: (A) cartridge life; (B) specifications (courtesy Deltech Engineering Inc.).

Type B. This is similar to Type A, the major exception being that the user draws inspired air by means of his lungs alone.

Type C. An air line respirator for entry into, and escape from, atmospheres not immediately dangerous to life or health, it consists of a source of respirable breathing air, a hose, a detachable coupling, a control valve, orifice, demand valve or pressure demand valve, an arrangement for attaching the hose to the wearer, and a facepiece, hood or helmet.

Types AE, BE and CE supplied-air respirators are primarily the same as Types A, B and C except that they have been modified with devices designed to protect the wearer's head and neck against impact and abrasion from rebounding abrasive material, and with shielding material such as plastic, glass, woven wire, sheet metal or other suitable material to protect the window(s) of facepieces, hoods and helmets. These do not interfere unduly with the wearer's vision and permit easy access to the external surface of such window(s) for cleaning. Although these are the 1981 and present standards, they first appeared in a Bureau of Mines Information Circular [57].

The type of air supplied to the respirators must contain 19.5 vol % oxygen and meet the Compressed Gas Association G.7 specification discussed earlier. MSHA requires the following air-supply-line requirements and tests for Types A, B and C respirators.

1. Type A specifies the length of hose to be 300 feet long in 25-foot sections.
2. Type B specifies the length of hose to be 75 feet long in 25-foot sections.
3. Type C specifies the length of hose to be a maximum of 300 feet long in 25-foot sections.
4. The air-supply hose with air-regulating valve or orifice shall permit a flow of not less than 115 liters/min (4 ft^3/min) to tight-fitting, and 170 liters/min (6 ft^3/min) to loose-fitting respiratory-inlet coverings. The maximum flow shall not exceed 425 liters/min (15 ft^3/min). Other tests specify noncollapsibility, nonkinkability, strength, tightness, permeation of hose by gasoline and detachable couplings.
5. The respirators must be fit-tested with 25 feet of hose maximum length in an isoamyl acetate atmosphere containing 1% or 10,000 ppm.

VORTEX TUBES®

Vortex tubes [79] run on compressed air and, with adjustment, can produce either cool air or warm air. Operations requiring heavy protective clothing build up the wearer's body temperature. Some workers tire from heat stress or the inability of the body to remove the heat buildup due to physical activity, lack of ventilation, radiation or all three. The standard suit provides cooling for up to 200°F, but specialty suits and different styles are sold by various manufacturers.

The way in which the air is distributed over the body is of importance and should be noted. The Vortec man cooling system uses air cooled by the vortex tube conducted into the vest at an entrance fitting located at the small of the back. The air fills the vest, causing it to puff into a swollen appearance. The inner lining of the vest has hundreds of tiny holes that allow the air to escape all over the trunk area of the body.

Figure 82 illustrates a small amount of the air leaving the vest: (1) it flows downward into the trousers and along the legs, so the legs are cooled without separate tubes running into the pants; (2) the air leaves the vest, moves upward and fills the inner jacket area at the arm holes of

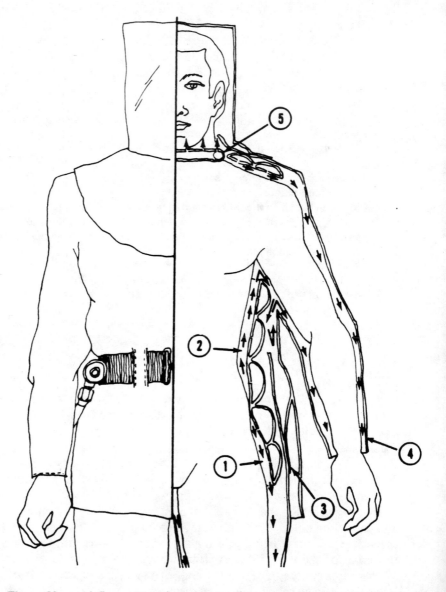

Figure 82.   Airflow pattern in a man cooling system (courtesy Vortec Corp.).

the vest; and (3) the elastic band seal at the bottom of the shirt prevents the air from falling out of the bottom of the jacket. As the passage of air is blocked from the bottom, the air is forced to flow out through the sleeves. It should be noted that the suit can be set up for left-handed workers as well.

Figure 83 illustrates a typical heat stress application. The limitation on the amount of heat depends on the hose system supplying the air. Normal hoses can burn up and are of no use in high-temperature applications. Welding and abrasive blasting operations lend themselves very well to this device. Figure 84 shows a man cooling system on a worker.

USING MAN COOLING SYSTEMS TO BEST ADVANTAGE

Vortec's man cooling systems [79] are designed to provide worker comfort and safety from heat stress in moderate-to-hot industrial environments up to 200°F. Certain systems should be used only up to about 130°F. Specifically, these are:

- Coverall systems
- Any man cooling system without head cooling
- Any system with the lightweight hood (Model 850)

The full suit system is well designed for use up to 200°F.

In selecting the proper man cooling equipment, the source of heat is as important as the amount. Whenever the heat is primarily radiant, a reflectorized system is indicated. For example, workers near furnaces, forging presses, ovens, etc., should use the reflectorized clothing. The reflective coating will reflect up to 90% of incident radiant heat. Of course, any heat reflected does not have to be offset by the vortex tube air conditioner. Systems are not intended to be used in severe heat situations, such as oven entry and fire entry applications. Highly specialized, very expensive equipment is made for these applications, but it is not available from Vortec. Note: man cooling systems are for worker cooling only—*they do not offer protection from hazardous atmospheres.*

THE AIR SUPPLY

Pressure

Man cooling systems are designed to use a normal shop air supply of 80–110 psig pressure. Unless pressures run considerably higher than 110

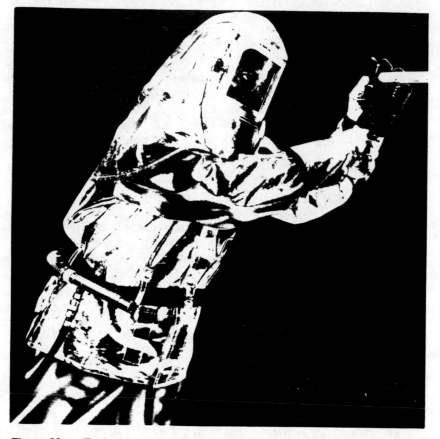

Figure 83.   Typical heat stress application of a man cooling system (courtesy Vortec Corp.).

psig, one must not use a regulator to reduce the inlet pressure. Pressures higher than 200 psig must not be used. Pressures lower than 80 psig still will produce some cooling; however, the flow of air and amount of cooling reduce rapidly as supply pressure falls.

Line Sizes

For piping air up to the air purifying filter, ⅜-inch pipe or larger should be used. Runs of this pipe over 50 feet should be ½-inch in size. If the air purifying filter is to be used for two workers, the pipe supplying it should not be smaller than ½ inch in size, and it should be ¾ inch in size

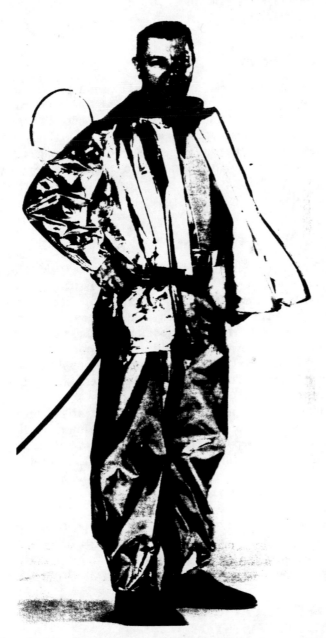

Figure 84.   Man cooling system especially engineered to ensure uniform cooling of the worker with maximum comfort and freedom. The design is an integrated cooling system to provide comfort, convenience and mobility (courtesy Vortec Corp.).

for runs of 50 feet or longer. Do not use compressed air hoses longer than 50 feet on the downstream side of the air purifying filter.

Compressor Size

In most large plants, the size of the compressor is adequate to handle several man cooling systems operating simultaneously. For smaller plants, one should estimate required horsepower based on the rated capacity of the man cooling systems. Systems for body cooling only consume 15 scfm at 100 psig. Systems for body and head cooling consume 25 scfm each. It takes one horsepower to compress 4 scfm of air to 100 psig. Divide total scfm required by four to obtain compressor horsepower required.

FILTERS

The use of an air purifying filter, such as the Clemco Model CPF-80, is recommended for all Vortec man cooling systems. It will serve two men in full suit systems (total flow of 50 scfm). The filter contains several filter materials, including activated charcoal, and will remove mists (including oil mist), water vapor and particles (down to 0.5 μ in size) from the compressed air supply. Most important, it cleanses the air of any objectionable odor. *Note: the air purifying filter will not remove carbon monoxide.* The compressed air system should be tested for CO content.

Because the air purifying filter removes nearly all the water and dirt, it is not essential to use any other filters. However, if a Vortec Model 701S-36A filter separator is installed just ahead of the air purifying filter, it will act as a prefilter, and the life of the air purifying filter cartridges will be extended several times. The technique has the added advantage that water is drained automatically from the system by the float-operated valve in the 701S-36A.

Standard-sized Vortec man cooling clothing items will fit a wide range of workers up to 6 ft 3 in. and 210 lb. For heavier workers, one also should order the Model 863 vest extension. Special sizes are available on special order at extra cost (and with longer delivery times).

DRESSING PROCEDURE
(FULL SUIT SYSTEMS)

Vortec man cooling systems are designed for use over workers' clothing. For best results, workers should wear light shirts and pants. The vest is attached inside the jacket by means of the small Velcro® patch at the back of the neck. These two garments, along with the Vortec tube air conditioner and the belt normally are kept together and handled as one assembly. This assembly is put on first, and the front closures of the Diffuse-Air® Vest are fastened loosely, but the front of the jacket is not closed. Next, the trousers are put on and attached by Velcro patches to the corresponding patches on the inside of the jacket. Care should be taken to make these attachments at the right height, so the entire suit is sized to the height of the man. When the trousers are fastened properly, the vest will be inside. Next, one should take the front, lower corners of the inner skirt in each hand, pull the elastic band sewn into the bottom of the inner skirt and snap the skirt together at the front. Then one should fasten the front closure of the jacket and buckle the Vortex Tube belt. One can snap the cuffs of sleeves and trousers if desired.

The neckring now can be brought into place over the head. The high temperature hood should be placed on the head and, finally, the neckring can be held in the optimum position using the Velcro strap inside the hood. To remove the hood, just release this Velcro strap. The hood then can be rotated up or removed.

The hood, which incorporates a standard hard hat, should be adjusted to the proper hat size for the man, using the markings on the straps inside the hat as a guide. When the hat size is adjusted properly, the chin brace attached to the face shield will fit comfortably under the chin and prevent the entire hood from falling off if the worker bends over. The many small holes in the neckring face upward, but are not intended to blow directly on the face. When assembled at the factory, the neckring holes direct the air at the inside of the face shield, keeping it clear of fog. Thereafter, it is reflected off the face shield, onto the face and around the head.

THE AIR DISTRIBUTION SYSTEM

Man cooling systems depend on their unique design to provide even distribution of air over the entire body. In the full suit systems, all parts of the body are cooled by the combined action of several elements, as shown in Figure 82.

Cold air from the Vortex Tube is conducted into the vest at an entrance fitting located at the small of the back. It fills the vest, causing it to puff into a quilted appearance. The inner lining of the vest has hundreds of tiny holes that allow the air to escape all over the trunk area of the body. A small amount of the air leaving the vest (1) flows downward into the trousers and along the legs, so the legs are cooled without tubes running into the trousers; (2) most of the air leaving the vest moves up along the body and spills into the inner jacket area at the armholes of the vest; (3) the air is prevented from falling out the bottom of the jacket by the elastic band seal at the bottom of the skirt; and (4) it is forced to flow out of the jacket through the sleeves, which is how the arms are cooled.

At the small of the back, where the cold air enters the vest, is a small manifold. This directs some of the cold air up the tube, which runs up the center of the back of the jacket and feeds the neckring. The entire suit system can be reassembled for left-handed workers by reversing this manifold. This will place the vortex tube air conditioner with its controls conveniently at the worker's left hand.

ADJUSTMENTS DURING USE

The vortex tube air conditioner is attached to the compressed air hose by a quick connector. The worker should familiarize himself with this connector so that he can release it easily with one hand without looking at it. In an emergency situation the worker is attached to his hose; swift disconnection is the easiest way to free oneself. One should not attempt to remove the jacket in an emergency. The valve at the hot end of the vortex tube air conditioner controls the amount of cold air and the temperatures produced. When it is screwed all the way into the tube, no air will leave the hot end. Then the air flowing into the suit will be at maximum flow, but the temperature will only be about 4°F below the compressed air line temperature. This setting, if line temperature is moderate, still will produce some cooling for the workers, because the air flowing is dry and the body's perspiration system will help.

As the control valve is opened, the flow into the suit decreases, but the air gets much colder. Maximum refrigeration is produced at about 1-1½ turns open. If the system has been operating with cold air flowing for a period of time and the valve is suddenly closed in an attempt to reduce the cooling, the air flowing into the suit will, of course, increase. Momentarily, the worker will feel even colder as the increased flow brings in the refrigeration that has been stored in the hose and vest materials. Thus, after any adjustment of the valve, the workers should allow the system a short time, perhaps a minute, to stabilize at the new setting. Initially, workers will adjust the control valve frequently, but as one becomes familiar with the system, there is a tendency to set it once and forget it.

CARE OF MAN COOLING EQUIPMENT

As there are no moving parts in the vortex tube air conditioner, it requires little maintenance. Likewise, the suit needs little maintenance if handled correctly. Only these few simple procedures are required:

1. Change filter cartridges if any odor is noticed in the air.
2. Drain filter after each two-hour use, using the drain cock at the bottom.
3. Hang suit carefully *on a hanger* between uses.
4. Never machine-wash aluminized clothing. Both inside and outside surfaces can be cleaned easily by hand washing with a mild soap.
5. Use Model 858 aluminized touchup spray lightly to restore silver appearance whenever needed. This will be required only after repeated use at elbows, knees and frequently flexed locations.
6. Vortex tube air conditioners will be restored by Vortec Corporation to new condition for a flat fee of $50, regardless of condition. Units intended for this service should be marked "for restoration service" and returned prepaid to Vortec Corporation. This service is available *only* for vortex tubes, Models 20815 and 20825. It is not available for clothing items.

ABRASIVE BLASTING

Probably the most common use of air-supplied respirators has been the application in abrasive blasting. In OSHA Section 1910.94, Ventilation [8], an abrasive-blasting respirator is defined as a continuous-flow air line respirator constructed to cover the wearer's head, neck and shoulders to protect him from rebounding abrasives. The air supply must meet ANSI Z 9.2 -1960 [80], a standard no longer published. A letter by the manufacturers of Del-Monex air purifiers to OSHA resulted in OSHA Code 1910.134(D)(i) or Compressed Gas Association Code being used to define air for breathing. NIOSH has contracted out for reports on the conditions of abrasive blasting, and the first report [81] covers the period from June 1971 to August 1973. It was conducted by the Boeing Aerospace Company, Seattle, Washington. The abstract section of the report states:

> The results of this study indicated there are approximately one hundred thousand abrasive blasters with personnel exposure to silica dust environments with up to sixty million man-hours per year. The

protection afforded these workmen is, on the average, marginal to poor. Equipment deficiencies and lack of maintenance are the rule rather than the exception. The average sand blaster would appear to have an excellent chance of receiving above the threshold limit values for quartz exposures and extreme noise exposures.

The survey concentrated on the monument industry, shipyards, painting/sandblasting contractors, primary metal (dry blasting) and primary metals (airless blasting). Included in the report were field survey observations and summary conclusions and recommendations. Field survey observations included such statements as, "the floor in front of the average wheelabrator is a sea of ball bearings making walking a first magnitude hazard, and storage of respirators is generally where convenient: in the corner, on a hook, in a work bench, but generally where last used."

Recommendations for improvement stated that "NIOSH and OSHA could remedy many of the deficiencies by concentrating on the local equipment suppliers. These are the men upon whom the average blaster depends for advice on selection, fit, use maintenance, and all aspects of safety."

To gauge the extent of abrasive blasting operations, the amount of abrasive material was surveyed. Sand usage was reported as 372,000 ton/yr; mineral aggregate, 53,000 ton/yr; and steel shot, 150 ton/yr. This gives one an idea of the extent of the problem.

NIOSH studied this area in another survey [82]. In this survey, many of the plant problems were discussed with the aid of manufacturers of equipment, trade unions and various engineering groups and companies. The results concluded that many changes in equipment must be made, but also that respirator users should be provided with, and instructed to wear, a dust control breathing respirator. Such a device also should be worn by all workers servicing any phase of the dust collecting system. Of most importance are engineering controls to limit the exposed number of workers and to ease materials handling, and a reclamation system for the abrasive material. Figure 85 illustrates a typical portable abrasive blast cleaning unit.

Figures 86 and 87 illustrate a typical setup for moving pieces into the work area. Corresponding ventilation data are provided. The idea shown most readily points to engineering controls to limit the spread of material in the workplace, as well as to collect the material. Respiratory equipment for the individual is more specialized and more easily controlled. Also, the materials with which one comes into contact in many cases involve lead grinding, such as in the automobile industry and lead paint

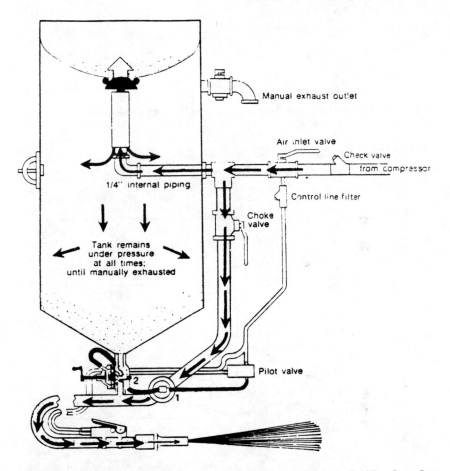

Figure 85. Portable blast-cleaning unit (courtesy Paul & Griffin Co., San Francisco, California).

type operations. Figure 88 illustrates an air line respirator, and Figure 89 illustrates an abrasive mask, typical of those used in many plants today. Designed for complete protection against lead exposures encountered in grinding, the MSA Leadfoe air line respirator (Figure 88) provides a minimum of 6 ft^3/min of fresh air through a hose inlet in the back of a rigid aluminum helmet. The helmet has an adjustable suspension for comfort over long periods of use. A 54 in.^{2} semirectangular lens provides unobstructed vision. The helmet has been designed scientifically to ensure a low noise level. A control valve is available for users who want precise individual control over the rate of airflow. For those who want a

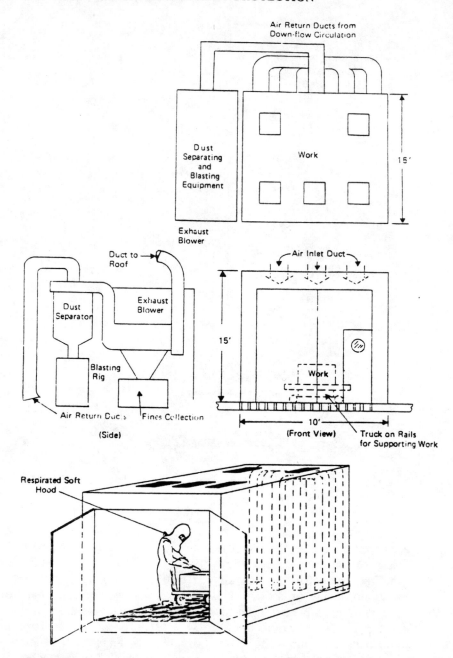

Figure 86a.   Schematic of installation of abrasive blasting room with downdraft ventilation.

1. Air flow determined by average downflow velocity within enclosure at 3 feet above floor:

$$\frac{\text{Average Downflow Velocity}}{\text{(eight data points)}} \times \frac{\text{Enclosure Cross-}}{\text{Sectional Area}} = \frac{\text{Average Air}}{\text{Flow}}$$

$$18 \text{ lfm} \times (10' \times 15' = 150 \text{ ft}^2) = 2700 \text{ cfm}$$

2. Air flow determined by average velocity through exhaust duct (12-inch diameter):

$$\frac{\text{Average Exhaust Velocity}}{\text{(five data points)}} \times \frac{\text{Duct Cross-}}{\text{Sectional Area}} = \frac{\text{Average Air}}{\text{Flow}}$$

$$3300 \text{ lfm} \times 0.785 \text{ ft}^2 = 2590 \text{ cfm}$$

3. Air flow determined by average velocity through ceiling air inlet ports (five total):

$$\frac{\text{Average Inlet Centerline}}{\text{Velocity (five data points)}} \times \frac{\text{Roof Inlet}}{\text{Area (five ports)}} = \frac{\text{Average Air}}{\text{Flow}}$$

$$286 \text{ lfm} \times 0.9^a \times (18 \text{ in.} \times 18 \text{ in.} \times 5 = 11.25 \text{ ft}^a) = 2896 \text{ cfm}$$

[a] 0.9 is an averaging factor for centerline velocity measurements to given an approximate overall average velocity.

Figure 86b.   Installation air flowrate data.

central control of flow, a quick-disconnect is provided. Either a cape or a collar is available with the unit. The MSA Leadfoe air line respirator has USBM Approval 19B-53.

A specially designed air line respirator for use in shotblasting or sand-blasting operations (Figure 89) is a complete assembly weighing only four pounds. It consists of a facepiece with connecting tube, control valve, web belt and a hood to protect the head and trunk of the wearer. The all-rubber facepiece adjusts quickly to various face shapes and sizes. Air is fed into the facepiece through a corrugated tube and flows over the lens to inhibit fogging; exhaled air is vented through twin valves. The wide-vision safety lens is protected by an alloy steel screen cover, which can be lifted for close inspection of work. Lightweight and heavy-duty hoods are available. Adjustment knob adjusts airflow. It has Bureau of Mines approval 19B-38.

ABRASIVE BLAST/CLEANING OPERATIONS— SUMMARY

Abrasive blast cleaning operations offer an excellent industry example of some problems that may result in respiratory hazards to workers.

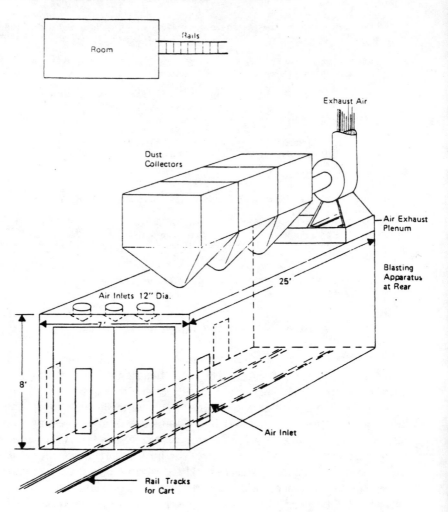

Figure 87a. Schematic of installation of abrasive blast-cleaning room crossflow ventilation.

Dust, as generated by abrasive breakdown and pulverized surface materials, develops serious safety problems. Dense dust formed in the immediate vicinity of hand-held/operated abrasive blast nozzles reduces visibility and often obscures the work area. Production time is lost in shutdowns for dust clearance or when operations continue under adverse conditions. If enclosures are not cleared of airborne dust, blast operators may be exposed to harmful dust concentrations on removal of respirator

1. Air flow determined by average velocity through exhaust vent:

Average Exhaust Velocity (five data points)	$\times$	Vent Open Flow Area	$=$	Average Air Flow
3100 lfm	$\times$	(60% $\times$ 16 in. $\times$ 16 in. = 1.07 ft^2)	$=$	3307 cfm

2. Air flow determined by average velocity through exhaust duct (downstream of blower):

Average Exhaust Velocity (fifteen data points)	$\times$	Duct Cross- Sectional Area	$=$	Average Air Flow
827 lfm	$\times$	3.4 ft^2	$=$	2819 cfm

3. Air flow determined by average velocity through inlet slots:

Average Inlet Velocity (four data points) (lfm)		$\times$	Duct Cross- Sectional Area	$=$	Average Air Flow (cfm)
Right Wall	550	$\times$	(8 in. $\times$ 30 = 1.7 ft^2)	$=$	917
Right Door	500	$\times$	(20% $\times$ 8 in. $\times$ 30 = 0.34 ft^2)	$=$	170
Left Door	287	$\times$	(8 in. $\times$ 30 in. = 1.7 ft^2)	$=$	488
Left Wall	487	$\times$	(8 in. $\times$ 30 in. = 1.7 ft^2)	$=$	829
Ceiling Cones (Estimated)	350	$\times$	(3 $\times$ .78 ft^2 = 2.34 ft^2)	$=$	819
			TOTAL		3223

Figure 87b.   Installation air flowrate data.

helmets. Dust accumulations also create slippery floor conditions. Therefore, it is necessary to control generated dust through engineering controls, such as well-maintained ventilation systems, enclosing the operation for both dust control and removal.

Vision impairment can be expected during such work operations, and adequate controls and protection must be provided to the worker. Operator vision tests should be conducted as part of any safety program.

In addition to dust and ventilation problems, other potential problems are noise, personal injury and exposures from various machines as well as from the hazardous work location.

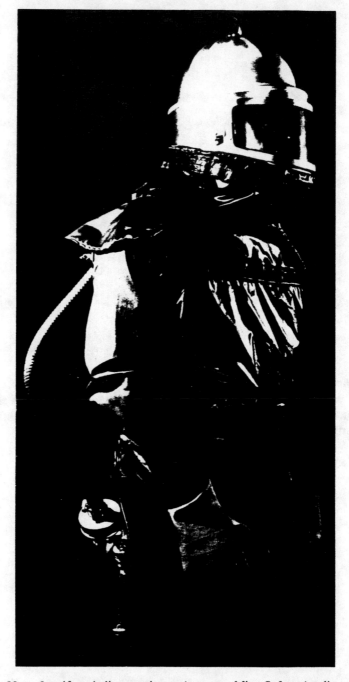

Figure 88. Leadfoe air line respirator (courtesy Mine Safety Appliance Co.).

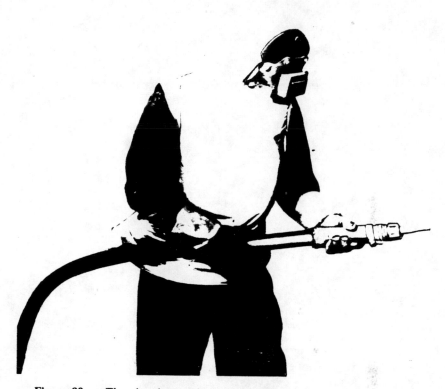

Figure 89.   The abrasive mask (courtesy Mine Safety Appliance Co.).

CHAPTER 8

SELF-CONTAINED BREATHING APPARATUS

INTRODUCTION

The first commercially practical self-contained breathing apparatus was developed by H. A. Fleuss in 1878 [5]. Designed for underwater diving, it was operated on a closed circuit basis and used 100% oxygen for breathing. However, the improper use of oxygen caused oxygen poisoning at depths greater than 25 feet, a fact that was not known until the knowledge of underwater physiology advanced with man's desire to explore the oceans. In 1903 the first Draeger apparatus was designed and manufactured by Bernhard Draeger, of Lubeck, Germany [83]. Self-contained (closed circuit) oxygen breathing apparatus was introduced into the United States during the summer of 1907. The first equipment was purchased by the Boston and Montana Mining and Smelting Co. (later a part of Anaconda Copper) of Butte, Montana [84]. At this time, the Technologic Branch of the Federal Geological Survey, Pittsburgh, Pennsylvania (which later became the U.S. Bureau of Mines), purchased several Draeger units. The Westphalia unit, manufactured in Germany, was followed in 1911–12 by the Fleuss-Proto unit, manufactured by Siebe, Gorman & Co. of London, England. After the Bureau of Mines was established, it began to equip railroad cars and stations with units and train miners in their use and care as part of the campaign for greater mining safety and efficiency.

The self-contained breathing units were used in mines to fight fires. With the outbreak of World War I, the Gibbs apparatus was developed by the Bureau of Mines and the U.S. Army at Edison Laboratories, Orange, New Jersey. The rights to manufacture the apparatus were bought by Mine Safety Appliances Co. of Pittsburgh. With the outbreak of World War II, Captain Jacques-Yves Cousteau and Emile Gagnan combined an improved demand regulator and high-pressure air tanks to create the first truly efficient and safe open-circuit, self-contained underwater breathing apparatus (SCUBA) tank to the world. After the war, the aqualung was used to depths of 180 feet without significant difficulty. What is noteworthy about the apparatus, is that it was adapted successfully for use in fire fighting and worker respiratory protection, although designed and developed primarily for the diving industry. Attempts to generate oxygen by chemical reaction led to the development of the CLEMOX, a ¼-hour self-generating oxygen breathing apparatus. The Mine Safety Appliance Company developed it during World War II for the U.S. Navy to use in fighting ship fires.

REGULATORY REVIEW

In the general respiratory protection section 1910.134, Section (d), Air Quality [8], OSHA refers to the same specification for air line respirators and self-contained respirators as were discussed in the section on air line respirators. With few exceptions, it is treated as any other respirator. Section (e)(3) (Use of Respirators) states: "Written procedures shall be prepared covering safe use of respirators in dangerous atmospheres that might be encountered in normal operations or in emergencies. Personnel shall be familiar with these procedures and the available respirators." Section (f) states that self-contained breathing apparatus shall be inspected monthly. Air and oxygen cylinders shall be fully charged according to the manufacturer's instructions. It shall be determined that the regulator and warning devices function properly because OSHA considers self-contained respirators as a device used primarily for emergency situations, fire fighting and those areas in which entry into an area may be made only for purposes of life rescue or to prevent a greater hazard from release of a product. Section 1910.1017, Vinyl Chloride [8] is an example of such a section.

The Mine Safety and Health Administration uses Subpart H, entitled "Self-Contained Breathing Apparatus" [1], to describe the many types of equipment. There is a tremendous difference in standards due to applications. Firemen, divers and emergency personnel can leave the area or are supplied by reserves. In a mine collapse, the time period is greater between changes of supply; for example, 4 hours for an oxygen rebreathing-type apparatus to 30 minutes for a typical pressurized tank containing breathing air. MSHA defines this type of respirator as a type used during entry into, or escape from, hazardous atmospheres. There are several types designed to suit specific atmospheric conditions.

A closed-circuit apparatus is one in which the exhalation is rebreathed by the wearer after the carbon dioxide has been effectively removed. A suitable oxygen concentration is restored from sources composed of (1) compressed oxygen, (2) chemical oxygen, and (3) liquid oxygen.

The development of the techniques employed to provide the wearer with a long-lasting supply of oxygen is described in the literature [85]. The problems encountered with liquid oxygen, mainly the rate of evaporation and supply of liquid oxygen in mining areas, forced most users to compressed oxygen systems. With modern stainless steel technology and better understanding of cryogenic properties, liquid oxygen may be rediscovered. Figure 90 shows the Mine Safety Appliance McCaa® (four-hour) oxygen rebreathing-type apparatus. Figure 91 shows how the apparatus works. High-pressure oxygen from the cylinder is reduced in pressure to a breathing level. The exhaled breath travels by one tube through a carbon-dioxide-removing chemical and into a cooler. The purified exhalation flows into the breathing bag, where it mixes with incoming oxygen from the cylinder. The original device, the McCaa two-hour apparatus, was designed by G. S. McCaa, mine safety and district engineer of the Bureau of Mines (1918–1929), in charge of testing oxygen breathing apparatus. Figures 92 and 93 illustrate the circulatory system of the device.

The Chemox apparatus was approved on October 3, 1946 and rated for ¼ of an hour. In May, 1959, it was modified further to cover the use of an MSA mine rescue communication system. Figure 94 shows a Mine Safety Appliance Chemox® apparatus, which generates its own oxygen and provides complete respiratory protection in any area of oxygen deficiency or concentration of toxic gases. It has USBM Approval 1307 for up to one hour (based on test procedures of Bureau of Mines Approval Schedule 13). In use, a lesser or longer protection period may result based on the user and his level of exertion. The Chemox oxygen breathing apparatus utilizes a replaceable chemical canister, which removes the carbon dioxide from the wearer's exhaled breath and evolves oxygen. This continues automatically in accordance with the wearer's breathing requirements. Figure 95 shows the 1961 version of the Chemox ¼-hour apparatus circulatory system [84].

The oxygen for breathing is generated in the canister section of the Chemox apparatus by the chemical reaction of moisture in the exhaled breath and the potassium superoxide (KO_2), following the chemical equation

$$4KO_2 + 2H_2O = 4KOH + 3O_2$$

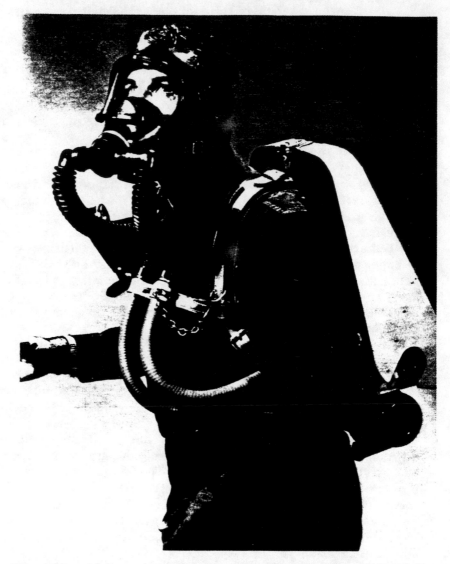

Figure 90.   McCaa oxygen rebreathing-type apparatus (courtesy Mine Safety
Appliance Co.).

The exhaled carbon dioxide is retained in accordance with the equation

$$2KOH + CO_2 = K_2CO_3 + H_2O$$

The rate of oxygen liberation is governed by the rate of breathing of the
wearer. Once the chemical in the canister is activated, oxygen is liberated

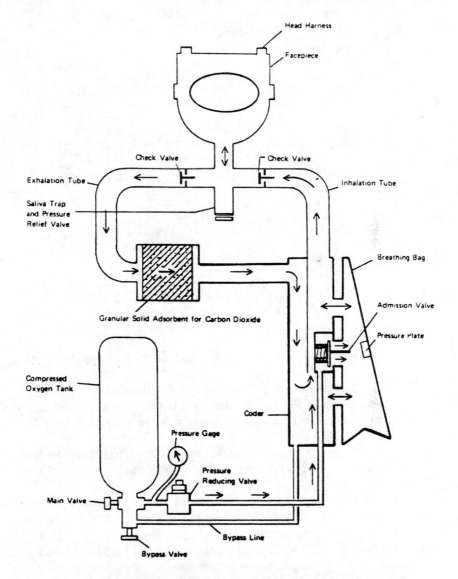

Figure 91.   SCBA closed-circuit device using gaseous oxygen.

at a somewhat faster rate than it is consumed, ensuring an adequate supply to the wearer, regardless whether he is breathing normally or rapidly. Eventually, excessive pressure will build up in the apparatus and be released through the valve in the facepiece. The service time is approximately 45 minutes of hard work; a warning timer signals the end of the time period. There are two warning properties if the timer does not signal

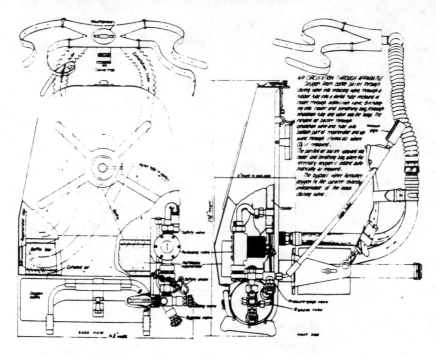

Figure 92.   Circulatory system of McCaa two-hour apparatus [84].

the end of the service life. The first is the failure of the fogging on the facepiece lenses to clear on inhalation; the second is increased resistance to breathing on exhalation, which cannot be alleviated by using the pressure-release valve.

The open-circuit apparatus vents the exhalation to the atmosphere and does not rebreathe it. There are two types; demand type and pressure-demand type.

The demand type apparatus is one in which the pressure inside the facepiece in relation to the immediate environment is positive during exhalation and negative during inhalation.

The pressure-demand type is an apparatus in which the pressure inside the facepiece in relation to the immediate environment is positive during both inhalation and exhalation. This style would allow no outside atmospheric contaminants into the respirator's facepiece.

The term "demand regulator" indicates that airflow is on inhalation demand, automatically regulating itself to the desired level to compensate for variations in breathing needs. The difference in the two regulators is that the pressure-demand type has additional controls on the regu-

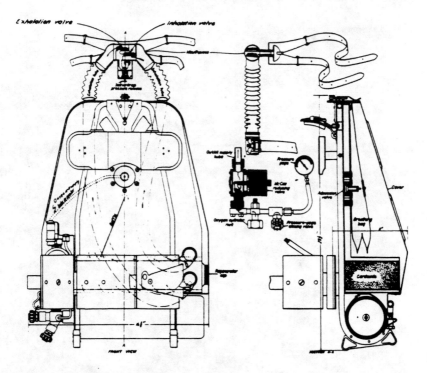

Figure 93.   Details of McCaa two-hour apparatus [84].

lator to supply positive pressure to the face mask at all times, yet still has the demand feature. The service time of the positive pressure-demand regulator would be the same as that of the demand regulator if the seal on the facepiece does not leak. Any leakage would increase air consumption, but since the pressure is positive, no contaminants seep into the respirator and decrease service time.

Demand type regulators are adequate in oxygen-deficient atmospheres; however, in hazardous atmospheres immediately dangerous to life or health, the manufacturers recommend they not be used. Figure 96 shows the demand regulator being worn, while Figure 97 shows another view of the apparatus. The mask provides a high flowrate to meet breathing demands, even during extreme exertion. It has NIOSH-Bureau of Mines Approval TC 13F-29 for up to 30 minutes, a time period based on USBM testing procedure. The less exertion on the part of the wearer, the longer the period of service, but exertion in excess of USBM testing standard results in shorter service life. The fast-action mask slips on quickly and adjusts in seconds. The demand regulator has a flow capacity in

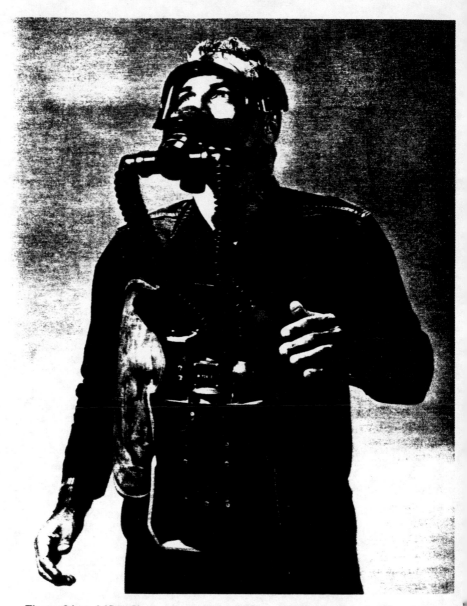

Figure 94.   MSA Chemox oxygen breathing apparatus (courtesy Mine Safety Appliance Co.).

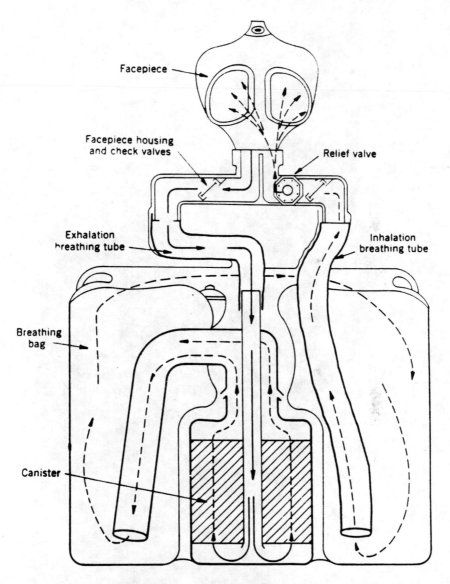

Figure 95. Circulatory system of Chemox ¼-hour apparatus [84].

excess of 400 l/min, which is more than that required for hard work. The Model 401 responds precisely to varying lung demands by metering the flow for each inhalation. The wearer opens the cylinder valve, adjusts his facepiece and breathes normally. The Model 401 air mask can be used by

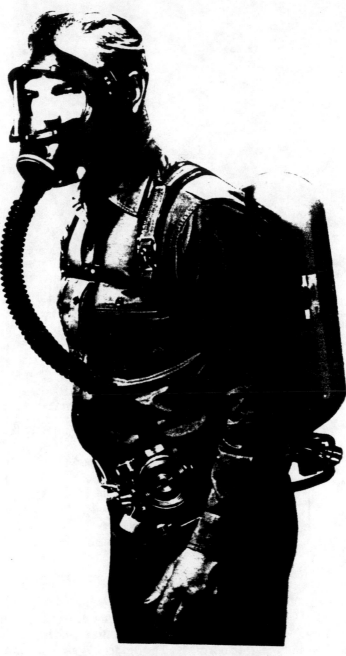

Figure 96.   Model 401 air mask.

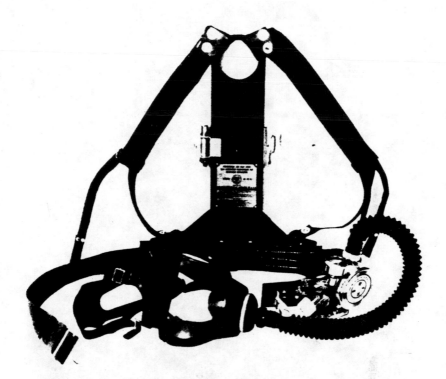

Figure 97. Model 401 air mask off the wearer (courtesy Mine Safety Appliance Co.).

firefighters and industrial workers in oxygen-deficient atmospheres and hazardous concentrations of toxic gases.

Figure 98 illustrates a pressure-demand regulator. This mask is designed for use in atmospheres of potential toxicity so severe that a slight positive pressure in the facepiece is necessary. The MSA pressure demand unit maintains a slight positive pressure during inhalation and, through a unique pressure-balanced exhalation valve, provides low exhalation resistance. The unit is supplied with an Audi-Larm audible signal device to indicate when to leave a toxic atmosphere. Its features include:

- Single-lens Clearvue facepiece with wide visibility
- Cylinder carried comfortably with readily adjustable harness
- Standard belt-mounted demand regulator and Audi-Larm

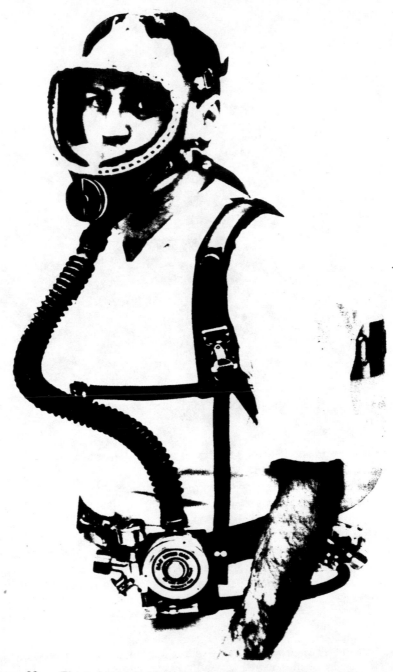

Figure 98.   The pressure-demand mask (courtesy Mine Safety Appliance Co.).

A modified third type combination of respirators also is recognized by MSHA, mostly for industrial use during emergency entry into a hazardous atmosphere. The code states that a self-contained breathing apparatus and a Type "C" or Type "Ce" air line respirator or air line respirator approved for abrasive blasting combined with a self-contained breathing apparatus supplied by 3, 5 or 10-minutes of breathing air must be used, provided the air line supply is used during entry. A second method used is to classify the self-contained unit for a 15-minute or longer service time and not more than 20% of the rated capacity of the air supply used during entry.

Section 11.70(c) of MSHA prohibits use of self-contained breathing apparatus classified for less than one hour service time during underground mine rescue and recovery operations.

General Requirements, MSHA Section 11.85(1–19) [1], specify the general requirements for the various methods of testing. Notably, the weight shall not be greater than 16 kg (35 lb). The length of breathing time (service time) for open-circuit apparatus is measured with a breathing machine, with a workrate of 622 kg-m/min, based on the research of Silverman [86] in 1945. Service time is classified according to length in hours (4, 3, 2, 1) or minutes (45, 30, 15, 10, 5, 3). Service time tests for closed-circuit apparatus are classified according to the length of time the apparatus supplies adequate breathing gas to the wearer during man-test No. 4, described in Tables XXV–XXVIII.

In man tests, a man in a respirator performs such various functions as crawling, running, climbing and pulling various weights, reflecting the weight of the respirator apparatus and the wearer's own weight in a simulated mine rescue operation. As illustrated by the tables for the 3-minute approval, the wearer would: (1) climb a vertical treadmill for 1 minute; (2) pull a 20-kg (45 lb) weight to 5 ft at the rate of 15 times/min; and (3) walk at 4.8 kmh (3 mph) for 1 minute. The treadmill shall be inclined 15° from vertical and operated at a speed of 30 cm/sec (1 fps) as specified by the footnote.

Although MSHA requires various types of tests for service life, manufacturers generally consider the service life to be dependent on the wearer. Its booklet [87] generally considers the following items:

1. degree of physical activity of the user;
2. physical condition of the user;
3. degree to which the user's breathing is increased by excitement, fear or other emotional factors;
4. degree of training or experience the user has had with this, or similar, equipment;
5. possible presence in the compressed air of carbon dioxide to increase breathing rate; and

Table XXV.   Duration and Sequence of Specific Activities for Test 1
[30 CFR Part 11, Subpart H, § 11.85, et seq.]

Activity	Service Time							
	3 minutes	5 minutes	10 minutes	15 minutes	30 minutes	45 minutes	1 hour	2, 3 and 4 hours
Sampling and Readings				2	2	2	2	Perform 1 hour test 2, 3, or 4 times respectively.
Walks at 4.8 km (3 mi) per Hour	3	5	3	4	8	12	18	
Sampling and Readings			2	2	2	2	2	
Walks at 4.8 km. (3 mi) per Hour			3	5	8	12	18	
Sampling and Readings				2	2	2	2	
Walks at 4.8 km. (3 mi) per Hour			2	2	6	13	16	
Sampling and Readings					2	2	2	

**Table XXVI. Duration and Sequence of Specific Activities for Test 2
[30 CFR Part 11, Subpart H, § 11.85, et seq]**

Activity	Service Time							
	3 minutes	75 minutes	10 minutes	15 minutes	30 minutes	45 minutes	1 hour	2, 3 and 4 hours[a]
Sampling and Readings				2	2	2	2	2
Walks at 4.8 km. (3 mi) per Hour			1	1	3	4	6	10
Carries 23 kg. (50 lb) weight over Overcast			1 time in 2 minutes	2 times in 2 minutes	2 times in 4 minutes	3 times in 6 minutes	4 times in 8 minutes	5 times in 10 minutes
Walks at 4.8 km (3 mi) per Hour				1	3	3	3	5
Climbs Vertical Treadmill[b] (or equivalent)	1	1		1	1	1	1	1
Walks at 4.8 km (3 mi) per Hour		1	1			2	3	5
Climbs Vertical Treadmill (or equivalent)		1	1			1	1	1
Sampling and Readings				2	2	2	2	2
Walks at 4.8 km (3 mi) per Hour				2	2	3	5	11
Climbs Vertical Treadmill (or equivalent)				1	1		1	1
Carries 23 kg (50 lb) weight over Overcast				1 time in 2 minutes	3 times in 6 minutes	4 times in 8 minutes	5 times in 10 minutes	5 times in 10 minutes
Sampling and Readings			2			2	2	2
Walks at 4.8 km (3 mi) per Hour				1	3	3	3	
Climbs Vertical Treadmill (or equivalent)			1	1	1	1	1	Then repeat above activities once

Table XXVI, continued

Activity	Service Time							
	3 minutes	75 minutes	10 minutes	15 minutes	30 minutes	45 minutes	1 hour	2, 3 and 4 hours[a]
Walks at 4.8 km (3 mi) per Hour			2			2	3	
Climbs Vertical Treadmill (or equivalent)						1	1	
Carries 20 kg (45 lb) Weight and Walks at 4.8 km (3 mi) per Hour	1						2	
Walks at 4.8 km (3 mi) per Hour		2				1	4	
Sampling and Readings				2	2	2	2	

[a]Total test time for Test 2 for 2-hours, 3 hour and 4-hour apparatus is 2 hours.
[b]Treadmill shall be inclined 15° from vertical and operated at a speed of 1 fps.

Table XXVII. Duration and Sequence of Specific Activities for Test 3
[30 CFR Part 11, Subpart H, § 11.85, et seq]

Activity	Service Time							
	3 minutes	75 minutes	10 minutes	15 minutes	30 minutes	45 minutes	1 hour	2, 3 and 4 hours[b]
Sampling and Readings				2	2	2	2	(b)
Walks at 4.8 km (3 mi) per Hour		1	1	1	2	2	3	
Runs at 9.7 km (6 mi) per Hour	1	1	1		1	1	1	
Pulls 20 kg (45 lb) Weight to 5 ft		15 times in 1 minute		30 times in 2 minutes	30 times in 2 minutes	30 times in 2 minutes	60 times in 6 minutes	
Lies on Side	½	1		2	3	4	5	
Lies on Back	½	1		2	2	3	3	
Crawls on Hands and Knees	1	1	1	2	2	2	2	
Sampling and Readings			2		2	2	2	
Runs at 9.7 km (6 mi) per Hour				1	1	1	1	
Walks at 4.8 km (3 mi) per Hour					2	8	10	
Pulls 20 kg (45 lb) Weight to 5 ft			30 times in 2 minutes	60 times in 6 minutes		60 times in 6 minutes	60 times in 6 minutes	
Sampling and Readings				2		2	2	
Walks at 4.8 km (3 mi) per Hour			1		3	4	10	
Lies on Side						2	4	
Lies on Back						2	1	
Sampling and Readings					2	2	2	

[a]Perform test No. 3 for 1 hour apparatus; then perform test 1 for 1 hour apparatus.
[b]Total test time for test 3 for 2-hour, 3-hour and 4-hour apparatus is 2 hours.

Table XXVIII.   Duration and Sequence of Specific Activities for Test 4
[30 CFR Part 11, Subpart H, § 11.85, et seq]

Activity					Service Time					
	3 minutes	5 minutes	10 minutes	15 minutes	30 minutes	45 minutes	1 hour	2 hours	3 hours	4 hours
Sampling and Readings				2	2	2	2	[a]	[b]	[c]
Walks at 4.8 km (3 mi) per Hour				1	2	2	2			
Climbs Vertical Treadmill[d] (or equivalent)	1	1	1	1	1	1	1			
Walks at 4.8 km (3 mi) per Hour		1	1	1	2	2	2			
Pulls 20 kg (45 lb) Weight to 5 ft		30 times in 2 minutes	30 times in 2 minutes	30 times in 2 minutes	60 times in 5 minutes	60 times in 5 minutes	60 times in 5 minutes			
Walks at 4.8 km (3 mi) per Hour			1	1	1	2	3			
Carries 23 kg (50 lb) Weight Over Overcast				1 time in 1 minute	1 time in 1 minute	2 times in 3 minutes	4 times in 8 minutes			
Sampling and Readings			2		2	2	2			
Walks at 4.8 km (3 mi) per Hour				1	3	3	4			

Runs at 9.7 km (6 mi) per Hour	1		1	1	1	1
Carries 23 kg (50 lb) Weight Over Overcast		1 time in 1 minute	1 time in 1 minute	2 times in 3 minutes	4 times in 6 minutes	6 times in 9 minutes
Pulls 20 kg (45 lb) Weight to 5 ft	15 times in 1 minute		15 times in 1 minute	60 times in 5 minutes	30 times in 2 minutes	36 times in 3 minutes
Sampling and Readings			2	2	2	2
Walks at 4.8 km (3 mi) per Hour	1	1			2	6
Pulls 20 kg (45 lb) Weight to 5 ft				60 times in 5 minutes	60 times in 5 minutes	
Carries 20 kg (45 lb) Weight and Walks at 4.8 km (3 mi) per Hour					3	3
Sampling and Readings				2		2

a Perform test No. 1 for 30-minute apparatus; then perform test No. 4 for 1-hour apparatus; then perform test No. 1 for 30-minute apparatus.
b Perform test No. 1 for 1-hour apparatus; then perform test No. 4 for 1-hour apparatus; then perform test No. 1 for 1-hour apparatus.
c Perform test No. 1 for 1-hour apparatus; then perform test No. 4 for 1-hour apparatus; then perform test No. 1 for 1-hour apparatus twice (i.e., two one-hour tests).
d Treadmill shall be inclined 15° from vertical and operated at a speed of 30 cm. (1 foot) per second.

6.   atmospheric pressure; if used in a pressurized tunnel or caisson at 2
     atm pressure, the duration will be one-half as long as when used at 1
     atm, and, at 3 atm, will be one-third as long.

For self-contained respirators, the tests for carbon dioxide in inspired
gas are discussed in Section 11.85–12, based on the work of E. T. Kloos
and J. Lamonica [88]. Open-circuit apparatus specifies that the breathing rate will be 14.5 respirations per minute, with a minute volume of
10.5 liters. Closed-circuit apparatus specify measurement of carbon
dioxide at the mouth of the test dummy. Figure 99 illustrates the test procedure. Table XXIX specifies the values.

In considering this section we must reflect on the material in the earlier
chapters on toxicology and lung physiology. Although carbon dioxide is
of a low order of toxicity, its current TLV = 5000 ppm [6]. The most
common effect of inhaling carbon dioxide in any amount above the
normal content of the atmospheric air is an increase in arterial CO_2 partial
pressure. This causes breathing to become faster and deeper. Any CO_2
increase in the inhaled air also increases CO_2 in the blood. Therefore, the

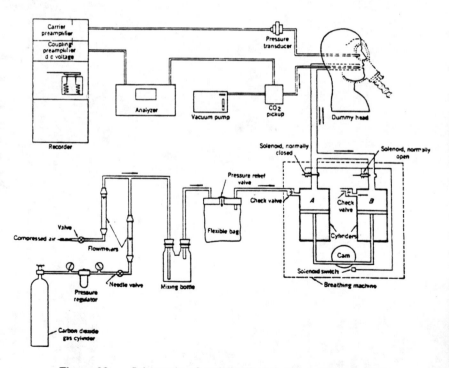

Figure 99.   Schematic of carbon dioxide test equipment [88].

Table XXIX.   Carbon Monoxide Concentration and Service
Time

Maximum Allowable Average Concentration of Carbon Dioxide (inspired air percent by volume)	Service Time
2.5	Not more than 30 minutes
2.0	1 hour
1.5	2 hours
1.0	3 hours
1.0	4 hours

body sensors will detect even a small imbalance in arterial CO_2 and will trigger an increase in lung ventilation to restore equilibrium. To state it more simply, the respirator wearer will use up his air supply at a faster rate, which decreases his chances of escape or successful rescue. The Bureau of Mines (MSHA) found a disturbing factor in testing self-contained breathing apparatus—even the breath-to-breath variation of the most experienced wearer prevented accurate evaluation of the apparatus. Therefore, the Bureau of Mines developed a test method that eliminated human breathing variations. Section 11.815–12 specifies that the sedentary breathing machine cam will be used in the test. The sedentary rate was chosen because it gave the greatest average concentration of CO_2 in the inspired air. Any increase above sedentary breathing rate also would increase tidal air volume and dead space air volume. As dead-space air is a fixed volume, an increase in tidal volume will dilute the CO_2 in the dead space and give a lower average concentration of CO_2 in the inspired air.

MSHA section 11.85–13 is entitled "Tests During Low Temperature Operations," in which the manufacturing company is required to specify the minimum temperature for safe operation. "Two persons shall wear the apparatus in a low temperature chamber for 30 minutes or the supposed service time." During the test period, the wearers will exercise and rest. Exercise will consist of stepping onto and off of an 8.5-inch-high box at the rate of 30 cycles per minute.

Low-temperature factors are important because of rescue work and firefighting in winter field conditions. E. T. Kloos examined the performance of open-circuit self-contained breathing apparatus at $-25°F$ [89]. The tests compared room temperature results of respirators to the apparatus being stored in a freezer (air cylinder and regulator). A dummy head was used for one set of tests, which later were compared to two men using a 6 foot × 9 foot × 7 foot-high walk-in temperature-controlled chamber. Figure 100 illustrates the apparatus. Temperatures as low as −30° were maintained within ±5°F. It was noted that many serious functional changes in apparatus performance occurred at low temperatures. Pressure regulators malfunctioned when diaphragms lost flexibility. Under certain conditions, frozen condensed moisture sealed exhalation valves and fogged eyepieces. High-pressure leaks not encountered at ordinary temperatures (75°F) developed at low temperature. The following 10 recommendations were made as a result of the report.

1. Use a facepiece fitted with a nosecup.
2. If possible, avoid storing or precooling the apparatus at low temperatures.
3. Use special parts for low-temperature operations whenever necessary.
4. Additional tightening of valve packings and threaded connections may be necessary to stop high-pressure leaks.
5. Do not overtighten cold valve packings and threaded connections. This will avoid damage when brought back to room temperature.
6. Dry off exhalation valves before exposure to low temperatures to prevent them from freezing shut.
7. Do not add additional air to a cylinder after pressure in a fully charged cylinder has dropped, owing to a decrease in temperature.

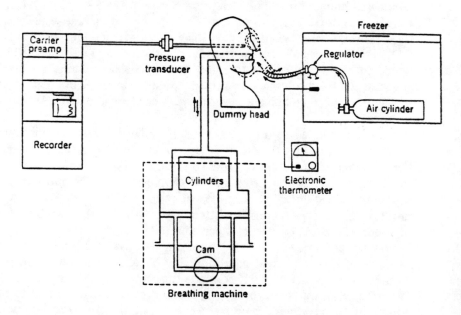

Figure 100.   **Schematic of breathing machine tests.**

8. Check the operation of the apparatus at low temperatures before using it in a dangerous atmosphere.
9. Enter toxic atmospheres cautiously. If any difficulty occurs, return to fresh air immediately and determine the cause.
10. Persons who wear apparatus should be trained thoroughly in its function, performance and limitations.

MSHA Section 11.82—Timers; elapsed time indicators (e) states that service-life indicators or warning devices shall be provided in addition to a pressure gauge on compressed gas self-contained breathing apparatus, except that the apparatus used will be for escape only and will operate automatically without preadjustment by the wearer. Each service life indicator or warning device shall sound an alarm when the remaining service life of the apparatus is reduced within a range of 20–25% of its rated service time.

INTRODUCTION

For respirators to provide the protection for which they were designed, users must be fit-tested. Since the OSHA Act was passed, many people responsible for respirator selection simply have handed out respirators. Users were not measured or fitted, and considerations such as glasses, speech amplification and protector factors were not considered.

This chapter considers the user's physical requirements and examines how protection factors to safeguard the user's health are determined. OSHA Section 1910.134(e)(5)(i) states: "Every respirator wearer *shall* receive fitting instructions including demonstrations and practice in how the respirator should be worn, how to adjust it, and how to determine if it fits properly" [8].

ANTHROPOMETRIC MEASUREMENTS

As most respirator facepieces are manufactured from rubber, plastic or combinations of the two, what size of facial structure is the model used to mold the facepiece and how many different sizes of facepieces do the manufacturers produce? How many respirators are designed to fit women? These questions are under regulatory review, but few, if any, such questions were asked when OSHA was passed in 1970.

Anthropometry, a study of human body size variability, was published by NIOSH [90] in April 1972. The report concluded that an adequate source of head and face anthropometry measured on civilian industrial workers does not exist. Data compiled by the U.S. Air Force in 1967 and a U.S. Air Force Women's survey of 1968 could be compared to the civilian population. The study resulted in the publication of a report entitled "Human Variability and Respirator Sizing" [91], which was developed to assist designers in understanding human facial variability, quantifying that variability and describing a design concept to effectively use the existing data in sizing respirator facepieces. The methods of measurement also were considered in designing respirator test panels. Also, the Los Alamos Scientific Laboratory of the University of California [92] published a report entitled "Selection of Respirator Test Panels Representative of U.S. Adult Facial Sizes," which describes aspects of fit testing and selection.

FITTING TESTS

There are two types of fitting tests presently used: qualitative and quantitative. Qualitative tests are generally fast and inexpensive. They rely on wearer's odor threshold or ability to smell a test substance. Isoamyl acetate, a liquid with a banana-like odor, is used widely in testing the facepiece fit for organic vapor cartridge and organic vapor canister respirators. There is presently no accepted method of vaporizing the isoamyl acetate, but either a 1.5-inch-diameter stencil brush or cotton wad is saturated for this purpose. The respirator wearer dons the respirator in an isolated area. NIOSH recommends the user perform the following [23]:

1. The user should breathe normally.
2. The user should breathe deeply, as during heavy exertion. This should not be done long enough to cause hyperventilation.
3. Side-to-side and up-and-down head movements should be exaggerated, but should approximate those that take place on the job.
4. The user should talk, which is accomplished most easily by reading a prepared text loudly enough to be understood by someone standing nearby.
5. Other exercises, such as bending and stretching, should be done, depending on the job the wearer must perform.

The major drawback of the isoamyl acetate test is that the odor threshold varies widely among individuals. Furthermore, the sense of smell is dulled easily and may deteriorate during the test so that the wearer can detect only high vapor concentrations. If the respirator is comfortable, the wearer may say that it fits, although it has a large leak. Conversely, a wearer may claim that a particular respirator leaks, simply because it is uncomfortable.

As odor threshold is the criterion, if the odor threshold of a compound is greater than its TLV, overexposure of the respirator user is possible because breakthrough may not be detected. In a study by Reist and Rex [93], the investigators found that individuals respond differently to the same odor. At a certain odor concentration, one person may detect the odor but not be able to recognize it; another may recognize and detect it. A third might not even sense it at all. Table XXX compares 100% recognition thresholds with TLVs for selected compounds.

The initial smoke test using stannic chloride or titanium tetrachloride as the test substance is used for fit testing the facepiece of particulate filter respirators. This test can be used both for air-purifying and atmosphere-supplying respirators, but an air-purifying respirator must have a high efficiency filter. A squeeze bulb pushes air through a tube filled with either substance, emitting a dense cloud of the irritating smoke. The user steps into a test enclosure and the irritant smoke is "sprayed" into the test hole. If the user detects any of the irritant smoke, a defective fit is indicated. The user must adjust or replace the respirator and/or filter when this happens. The irritant smoke must be applied with caution because the aerosol is highly irritating to the eyes, skin and mucous membranes. The user generally responds in a positive manner when a leak occurs by coughing or sneezing, indicating a more positive approach.

The negative and positive pressure tests use slight pressure by the lungs. They are used to give gross estimates of fit and usually are performed first. In the negative pressure test, the wearer closes off the inlet of the canister, cartridge(s) or filters by covering the breathing tube with the palm(s) or squeezing so that it does not pass air. He inhales gently so that the facepiece collapses slightly and holds his breath for about 10 seconds. If the facepiece remains slightly collapsed and no inward leakage is detected, the respirator is probably tight enough (Figure 101).

In the positive pressure test, the wearer closes off the exhalation valve and exhales gently into the facepiece. The fit is considered satisfactory if slight positive pressure can be built up inside the facepiece without any evidence of outward leakage. For some respirators, this method requires that the wearer remove the exhalation valve cover, which often disturbs the respirator fit even more than does the negative pressure test.

Other tests, such as the respirator qualitative/quantitative fit test method [94], refer to a Bureau of Mines technique of blowing a stream of talcum powder or coal dust directly around the face to facepiece seal. The user then would remove the respirator and the leakage would be revealed by telltale streaks of the dust or powder. This method is rarely used at present. Uranine (a fluorescein dye) was sprayed around the

Table XXX. Comparison of 100% Recognition Odor
Thresholds and 1976 TLV's for Selected Compounds [93][a]

Group 1 – Odor Threshold and TLV approximately the same

	Odor Threshold[b] (ppm)	TLV (ppm)	Ratio
Acrylonitrile	21.4	20 S	1.07
Arsine	0.21	0.05	4.20
Cyclohexene	300	300	1.00
Cyclohexanol	100	50	2.00
Epichlorhydrin	10	5 S	2.00
Ethyl Benzene	.200	100	2.00
Ethylene Diamine	11.2	10	1.12
Hydrogen Chloride	10	5	2.00
Methyl Acetate	200	200	1.00
Methylamine	10	10	1.00
Methyl Chloroform	500	350	1.43
Nitrogen Dioxide	5	5	1.00
Propyl Alcohol	200	200	1.00
Styrene, Monomer	200	100	2.00
Turpentine	200	100	2.00

Group 2 – Odor Threshold from 2 to 10 times the TLV

Acrolein	0.21	0.1	2.10
Allyl Alcohol	7	2	3.50
Carbon Tetrachloride	75	10 S	7.5
Chloroform	200	25	8.00
Crotonaldehyde	7.32[c]	0.1	10.8
1,2 Dichloroethylene	500	200	2.50
Dichloroethyl Ether	35	5 S	7.00
Dimethyl Acetamide	46.8	10 S	4.68
Hydrogen Selenide	0.3	0.05	6.00
Isopropyl Glycidyl Ether (IGE)	300	50	6.00

Group 3 – Odor Threshold equal to or greater than 10 times the TLV

Bromoform	530	0.5 S	10.60
Camphor (synthetic)	1.6–200	2	0.8–100
Carbon Disulfide	d	20	–
a-Chloroacetophenone	1.34[c]	0.05	26.8
Chloropicrin	1.08[c]	0.1	10.8
Diglycidyl Ether (DGE)	5.0	0.5	10.0
Dimethylformamide	100	10 S	10.0
Ethylene Oxide	500	50	10.0
Mercury Vapor	d	0.05 mg/m^3	–
Methyl Bromide	d	15	–
Methyl Chloride	d	100	–

Table XXX, continued

Methyl Formate	2000	100	20.0
Methanol	2000	200	10.0
Methyl Cyclohexanol	500	50	10.0
Phosgene	1.0	0.1	10.0
Phosphine	d	0.3	–
Radioactive Gases and Vapors	d	–	–
Toluene 2,4 Diiocyanate (TDI)	2.14	0.02	107.
Vinyl Chloride	d	(200)e	–

[a]As odor recognition threshold varies from individual to individual, this table should be used only as a rough guide. Also, it is not necessarily complete.
[b]Recognition threshold, except where noted.
[c]Detection threshold.
[d]Little or no recognition threshold in range of concentration where cartridge or cannister use is indicated.
[e]New standard pending.

respirator sealing surface and, when removed, the leakage was detected by a fluorescent light source. The U.S. Army has experimented with a method that uses a 1450 mg/m³ concentration of chloropicrin (trichloronitromethane (PS)) as an odor-sensitive, vapor-challenge agent. A leak is considered to have occurred if the wearer can detect the odor.

Currently, OSHA does not specify how the respirator is to be fit tested, but the U.S. Department of Labor MSHA specifies the test condition in Section 11.140 [6]:

1. The respirator is modified with efficient activated charcoal-filled canister or cartridge(s) without interference to the facepiece or seal.
2. The modified respirator will be worn by persons for at least 2 minutes each in a test chamber containing 100 parts (by volume) of isoamyl acetate vapor per million parts of air.
3. The odor of isoamyl acetate shall not be detected by the wearer of the modified respirator while in the test atmosphere.

QUANTITATIVE RESPIRATOR FIT TESTS

Quantitative respirator performance tests [94] require the wearer to stand in an artificially generated atmosphere, in which a relatively nontoxic gas, vapor or aerosol is easily detectable. The atmosphere inside the respirator is sampled continuously through a probe in the respiratory inlet covering. The leakage is expressed as a percentage of the test atmosphere outside the respirator, called "percentage of penetration" or,

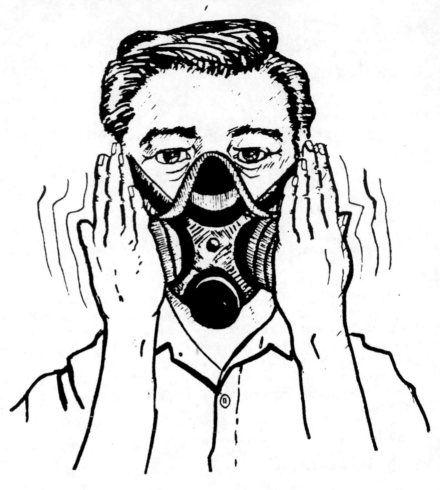

Figure 101.   Negative pressure test.

simply ''penetration.'' As the test does not rely on subjective response and the results are given numerically, the results are very accurate. This is important where facepiece leakages must be minimized in areas of highly toxic atmospheres or those immediately dangerous to life or health.

The major drawback is the cost. The tests are expensive, requiring specialized equipment and highly trained operators. Each test respirator must be equipped with a sampling probe to allow continued removal of an air sample from the facepiece; therefore, the same facepiece cannot be worn in actual service because the test orifice negates the approval of the respirator.

As no definite method of, or procedure for, quantitative fit testing presently is specified by OSHA or MSHA, a review of current practice techniques is outlined. The British Safety in Mines Research Establishment uses argon for testing full-face respirators. The wearer dons a respirator with two breathing tubes and is positioned in a transparent plastic hood sealed around the waist. Pure argon is supplied into the top of the hood from a regulated cylinder supply. The hood pressure is maintained slightly above atmospheric. Argon is used because it is inexpensive, available in pure form and physiologically inert. To implement the test, the user inhales oxygen of medical quality via a cylinder supplied and fitted with a pressure reducer and demand valve.

The oxygen breathing tube is fitted with a sampling port and a valve to control the direction of flow. A spirometer measures the volume of oxygen used. The amount of argon in the exhaled gas is measured with a mass spectrometer. This instrument can measure the differential amount of argon present in the exhaled breath to a concentration of 10 ppm. A multiway tap is connected to a mass spectrometer and the various sampling ports. Sampling is accomplished using a small suction pump. This method has been implemented to measure respirator leakage on the order of 0.001%.

National Dreager Inc., manufacturer of detector tubes and respiratory equipment, has developed two versions of the Model 80 facemask fit-test device using 2% by volume ethylene as the test gas. This method uses either a detector tube or an electronic leak detector to measure the concentration of test gas exhaled in the breath. With detector tubes, 0.5–10 ppm of ethylene leakage tests can be detected in the range of 0.0025 to 0.05%.

In the use of an electronic leak detector method, a 2% mixture of sulfur hexafluoride in air is used as the test gas. Detector sensitivity is approximately the same as the detector tube method of test. The presence of the radiation source in this detector, however, requires a special operator's license and a testing supervisor trained in handling radiation sources.

A number of commercial companies and the U.S. Bureau of Mines have developed a procedure for using dichlorodifluoromethane (Freon-12) as a test gas. The sampled mixture is photometrically analyzed on a Davis-Halide meter, and the output is displayed on a strip-chart recorder. The measurable leakage is in the range of 0.2%.

The Scott Aviation Division of ATO Inc. uses helium as a test gas for fit testing. The concentration of helium used is 10%, and the wearer breathes medical-grade oxygen. The helium leak detection method can measure penetrations in the range of 1.0 to 0.001%.

The Federal Aviation Administration, Survival Research Unit, uses N-pentane as a test gas. A slight negative sampling port is used from which a gas sample is drawn and evaluated by a Perkin Elmer dual column gas chromatograph with a hydrogen-flame ionization detector. Operation tests using this leak detection scheme have measured leakages as low as 1.0%.

The Los Alamos Scientific Laboratory has developed a method to use sulfur hexafluoride at 50 ppm concentration. The system uses a hydrogen-flame photometer. Sulfur emits a characteristic luminescence at the 394-Nm wavelength, and the intensity of luminescence is a direct function of the sulfur concentration. The lower detection limit of the system is 0.5 ppm, and at 50 ppm the sensitivity of the system is 1.0%. Los Alamos Scientific Laboratory also developed an aerosol, di-2-ethylhexyl phthalate (DEHP). Two aerosol generators and a special fan for mixing the DEHP and room air produce a concentration of 25 ± 5 mg/m^3 and a mass median aerodynamic diameter (MMAD) of 0.6 ± 0.2 μm, with a geometric standard deviation of 2.00 ± 0.2. The amount of DEHP aerosol in a sample is quantified by measuring the intensity of light scattered from the aerosol particles as they pass through a conical scattering chamber using a photomultiplier tube with results displayed on a strip-chart recorder. Leakages as low as 0.0001% have been measured.

Sodium chloride as a test substance has been experimented with in several countries and the United States. Los Alamos Scientific Laboratory is the group credited with the development. The concentration in the test hood is 15 ± 2 mg/m_3, and the particles have an MMAD of 0.66 ± 0.12 μm, with a geometric standard deviation of 2.15 ± 0.19. Calibration is done with a flame photometer using propane supplied by an external tank. The photomultiplier analyzes the flame, and the results are processed electronically, with information displayed on a strip-chart recorder. Sensitivities have been recorded as low as 0.0001%.

The U.S. Army has developed a method of using *bacillus subtilis*, or *bacillus globigii* spore-forming bacterium, as the test agent. Rather sophisticated in nature, respirator leakage can be measured to 1%.

The Harvard School of Public Health has developed a uranine method of fit testing. Uranine is a commercial dyestuff that is used as a tracer in medical and environmental air pollution studies. The disodium salt of fluorescein is readily soluble in water and excited by blue light ranging from 4400 to 5100 A. A 2.35% solution of uranine is generated using a nebulizer for the test concentration. Leakages are measured by a strip-chart recorder, and sensitivities as low as 0.05% are measured.

Dioctyl phthalate is a similar test substance to NaCl. The aerosol is generated using a nozzle-type atomizer; however, being an oil, DOP does not dry into solid particles when injected into a diluting airstream. Leakages of less than 0.01% can be detected.

HOW SAFE ARE THE FIT TEST AGENTS?

It is important for the testing group to be able both to make highly accurate measurements and to examine the agent's toxicity. Although the person being tested is exposed for a few minutes, the people who set up the equipment may be exposed to adverse health effects in the research, demonstration and calibration stages. Therefore, we have provided a quick review of the materials used in quantitative and qualitative fit testing programs, as outlined by the Aero Medical Review [94].

Isoamyl acetate ($C_7H_{14}O_2$) has a molecular weight of 130.21. Its lowest lethal dose is 500 mg/kg, estimated by oral administration to humans. Its TLV is 100 ppm, or 525 mg/m^3 [6].

Stannic chloride ($SnCl_4$) has a molecular weight of 260.49. There is no present TLV listed by ACGIH. NIOSH [28] gives 700 mg/kg as the lethal dose (LD_{50}) for rats by oral route of administration.

Titanium tetrachlorine ($TiCl_4$) has a molecular weight of 189.7. There is no present listing by ACGIH for TLV. NIOSH [28] lists 10 mg/m^3 as the lowest lethal concentration for mice by oral route of inhalation. It is highly corrosive and presents a special hazard because it reacts violently with water to liberate heat and produce hydrochloric acid. When it comes in contact with the skin, the chemical should be wiped dry. A splash of the liquid in an eye may lead to permanent eye structure damage.

Talcum powder is a finely pulverized hydrous magnesium silicate.

Coal dust varies with the area of the country mined. As both talcum powder and coal dust are used rarely in present methods, they will be mentioned only briefly.

Chloropicrin (trichloronitromethane) is used as a fumigant and tracer gas. The vapor is intensely irritating to skin, eyes, mucous membranes and stomach. The formula is CCl_3NO_2 and its molecular weight is 164.37. ACGIH lists the current TLV [6] at 0.1 ppm and 0.7 mg/m^3 for airborne concentration.

Uranine ($Na_2(C_{20}H_{10}O_5)$) is a disodium salt of fluorescein. Its molecular weight is 376.78. It is a commercial/medical dyestuff red-orange powder readily soluble in water. No ACGIH TLV is avilable at present, and it should be noted that it causes nausea and vomiting in some cases.

Clinical applications include the diagnosis of eye disorders, determination of blood circulation time and study of blood flow.

QUANTITATIVE TEST MATERIALS

Argon has a molecular weight of 39.95 and is a 1% constituent of the earth's atmosphere. As it is an inert nonflammable gas, it could be a simple asphyxiant. No ACGIH data are available, but care in handling should be emphasized.

Ethylene (C_2H_4) is a colorless flammable gas. The molecular weight is 28.05. The ACGIH 1981 threshold limit values [6] list ethylene as a simple asphyxiant. NIOSH]28] lists ethylene's lowest lethal concentration at 95,000 ppm for a 5-minute inhalation exposure to some mammals.

Dichlorodifluoromethane (CCl_2F_2), or Freon-12, is a nonflammable gas used mainly for its air-conditioning and refrigeration properties. Its molecular weight is 120.91. Most firemen are familiar with the fact that Freon-12 decomposes to phosgene at or around 500°F. The ACGIH TLVs [6] for airborne concentrations are 1000 ppm or 4950 mg/m^3.

Helium is a trace component of the earth's atmosphere and is used for deep diving underwater atmospheres. ACGIH [6] lists helium as a simple asphyxiant. As it is an inert nonflammable gas, no problems have been noted with its use.

N-Pentane (C_5H_{12}) is a flammable gas with a molecular weight of 72.17. ACGIH [6] lists the threshold limit values for airborne concentrations at 600 ppm, or 1800 mg/m^3. NIOSH [28] lists the lowest lethal concentration at an estimated 130,000 ppm for an inhalation exposure to a human subject.

Sulfur hexafluoride (SF_6) is an odorless, colorless, nonflammable gas. The impurities in it are sulfur tetrafluoride and sulfur pentafluoride, which have TLVs [6] of 0.1 ppm and 0.025 ppm, respectively. In the pure form, sulfur hexafluoride is considered pharmacologically inactive. ACGIH [6] lists the 1981 TLVs at 1000 ppm, or 6000 mg/m^3 for airborne concentrations.

AEROSOLS USED AS FIT TEST AGENTS

Di-2-ethylhexyl phthalate is an ester of phthalic acid and used commercially as a softener in rigid polymers like PVC. Extensive research by NIOSH [28] basically has revealed no problems as far as inhalation is concerned. The ACGIH [6] currently recommends a TLV of 5.0 mg/m³ for DEHP in air.

Sodium chloride (NaCl), or table salt, has a molecular weight of 58.4. The ACGIH [6] recommends a TLV of 10 mg/m³. This material is probably considered the safest to use, although it contributes to hypertension and may have some carcinogenic properties.

The *Bacillus subtilis/Bacillus globigii* aerosol test methods using spores of nonpathogenic bacteria are in the experimental stages by government and medical specialists and are mentioned to give depth to the various technologies explored in testing.

SIMULATING WORK CONDITIONS

In the fit testing of respirators, normal operations such as breathing, deep breathing, moving the head from side to side (slowly) or up and down, talking or reading a short message were discussed. OSHA section 1910.134 [8] does not specify how well the respirator shall fit. Additions such as 1910.1017 [8], the Vinyl Chloride Standard, used the level of atmospheric concentration the employee could be exposed to as the rationale for the respirator used. For example, if the employee were exposed to concentrations not over 10 ppm, the required apparatus could be any one of three types:

- combination Type C supplied-air respirator, demand type, with half facepiece and auxiliary self-contained air supply,
- Type C supplied-air respirator, demand type, with half facepiece; or
- any chemical cartridge respirator with an organic vapor cartridge that provides a service life of at least 1 hour for concentrations of vinyl chloride up to 10 ppm.

Unknown concentrations, or those above 3600 ppm, required an open-circuit, self-contained breathing apparatus, pressure-demand type, with full facepiece.

In the Cotton Dust Standard section (1910.1043) [8], OSHA used the level of exposure ratio to specify the type of protection required. In 1910.1043(f), Table 1(A), with a cotton dust concenration of not greater than five times the applicable permissible exposure limit the user can use any dust respirator, including single use. In a cotton dust concentration of 10 times the applicable permissible exposure limit, the user can use (1) any dust respirator, except single use or quarter-mask; (2) any supplied-air respirator; or (3) any self-contained breathing apparatus.

Basically, each section of the OSHA Standards 1910.1046 [8] specifies how the respirator will be selected based on concentrations of contaminants present, and not specifically on the job performed.

The purpose of presenting the preceding information was to state current legal requirements, but three groups—NIOSH, MHSA and the Los Alamos Scientific Laboratories—are having a direct effect on the respirator fit testing of the future. In 1975 Edwin C. Hyatt [95] stated that in 1965 the Bureau of Mines did not use the term "protection factor," but implied it in its approval schedules for gas masks and chemical cartridge respirators by using the term "maximum use concentrations." Half-mask respirators equipped with high-efficiency filters were approved for use up to 10 times the TLV. In 1967 the Atomic Energy Commission (now Nuclear Regulatory Commission) Director of Regulations published proposed protection factors in the *Federal Register* that ranged from 10 for high-efficiency particulate removing half-mask respirators to 10,000 for positive-pressure self-contained breathing apparatus.

Example: If the ACGIH TLV were 20 ppm and the TWA concentration measured were 2000 ppm, the protection factor required would be 100. In fit testing the respirator during quantitative fit testing, the concentration of the air inside the booth, hood or test enclosure is divided by the material measured leaking into the facepiece or enclosure:

$$\text{Protection factor} = \frac{1000 \text{ ppm of test substance}}{1 \text{ ppm of measured test}}$$

Based on the test substance, concentration in the booth is 1000 ppm. The amount of test material that leaked into the respirator and was drawn into the vacuum pump for analysis is 1 ppm.

NIOSH [96] lists protection factors for different types of respirators. Table XXXI gives protection factors to be noted in the use of respirators. It should be noted that this table is based on Mine Enforcement and Safety Administration rules, which have been changed to some extent by the new Mine Safety and Health Administration.

Presently, MSHA rules [1] specify man tests, test conditioning and general requirements. Man tests describe the duration and sequence of specific activities. These tests will be conducted to (1) familiarize the wearer with the apparatus during use; (2) provide for a gradual increase in activity; (3) evaluate the apparatus under different types of work and physical orientation; and (4) provide information on the operating and breathing characteristics of the apparatus during actual use. Tables XXXII-XXXV show the duration of the tests for various activities.

Table XXXI.   Protection Factors in the Use of Respirators [96]

A. Protection Factors for Particulate Filter Respirators

Protection Factor	Permissible Respiratory Protection
5X	Any dust and mist respirator (30 CFR 11.130)
5X	Any dust and mist respirator, except single use (30 CFR 11.130)
10X	Any dust and mist respirator, except single-use or quarter-mask respirator (30 CFR 11.130)
10X	Any fume respirator (30 CFR 11.130)
10X	Any high-efficiency particulate filter respirator (30 CFR 11.130)
50X	A high-efficiency particulate filter respirator with a full facepiece (30 CFR 11.130)
1000X	A powered air-purifying respirator with a high-efficiency particulate filter (30 CFR 11.130)

B. Protection Factors for Chemical Cartridges and Gas Masks

Protection Factor	Permissible Respiratory Protection
10X	Any chemical cartridge respirator with a **Name** cartridge(s) (30 CFR 11.150)
50X	A chemical cartridge respirator with full facepiece and **Name** cartridge(s) (30 CFR 11.150)
50X	A gas mask with a full facepiece and **Name** canister (30 CFR 11.90(a))
1000X	A powered air-purifying chemical cartridge respirator with a **Name** cartridge (unlisted device)*
Escape	Any gas mask providing protection against **Name** vapors (30 CFR 11.90)

* Classes of respirators are only included in situations in which at least one device has been approved.

NOTE: The approval **Name** may consist of acid gases or organic vapors as a class or specific acid gases, ammonia or organic vapors. It also may consist of combinations of acid gases, organic vapors and other gases and vapors.

C. Protection Factors for Combination Chemical Cartridges and Particulate Filters and Gas Masks and Particulate Filters

Protection Factors	Permissible Respiratory Protection
10X	Any chemical cartridge respirator with **Name** cartridge(s) and **Name** filter(s) (30 CFR 11.150 and 11.130)
50X	A chemical cartridge respirator with a full facepiece, **Name** cartridge(s) and high-efficiency filter(s) (30 CFR 11.150 and 11.130)
50X	A gas mask with a full facepiece and **Name** canister and high-efficiency filter (30 CFR 11.90(a) and 11.130)
1000X	A powered air-purifying chemical cartridge respirator with a **Name** cartridge and high-efficiency particulate filter
Escape	Any gas mask providing protection against **Name** and particulates (30 CFR 11.90 and 11.130)

Table XXXI, continued

Name refers to any acid gas, alkaline gas, organic vapor or other specific gas or vapor.

Type refers to dust and mist, fume or high-efficiency particulate.

NOTE: A pesticide respirator is a special type of chemical cartridge respirator or gas mask with a combination sorbent and particulate filter. Where a substance is a pesticide, the following phrase is added as a footnote to the respirator tables. "Including pesticide respirators which meet the requirements of this class."

D.   Protection Factors for Supplied-Air Respirators

Protection Factor	Permissible Respiratory Protection
10X	Any supplied-air respirator (30 CFR 11.110(a))
50X	Any supplied-air respirator with a full facepiece, helmet or hood (30CFR 11.110(a))
1000X	*A Type C supplied-air respirator operated in pressure-demand or other positive-pressure or continuous-flow mode (30 CFR 11.110(a))
2000X	A Type C supplied-air respirator with a full facepiece operated in pressure-demand or other positive pressure mode or with a full facepiece, hood or helmet operated in continuous flow mode (30 CFR 11.110(a))

*This category is not covered fully by preceding category.

E.   Protection Factors for Self-Contained Breathing Apparatus

Protection Factor	Permissible Respiratory Protection
10X	Any self-contained breathing apparatus (30 CFR 11.70(a))
50X	Any self-contained breathing apparatus with a full facepiece (30 CFR 11.70(a))
10,000 + X	Self-contained breathing apparatus with a full facepiece operated in pressure-demand or other positive-pressure mode (30 CFR 11.70(a))
10,000 + X	A combination respirator, which includes a Type C supplied-air respirator with a full facepiece operated in pressure-demand or other positive-pressure or continuous-flow mode and auxiliary self-contained breathing apparatus operated in pressure-demand or positive pressure mode (30 CFR 11.70(b))
Escape	Any escape self-contained breathing apparatus (30 CFR 11.70(a))

SPECIAL AREAS

With the specific plant in mind and the current trends for various facial hair designs, the question of fit testing often arises. Hyatt [97] discussed the problems and classified the various styles of facial hair (Figure 102). He concluded that quantitative aerosol respirator man tests

Table XXXII. Duration and Sequence of Specific Activities for Test 1
[30 CFR Part 11, Subpart H, § 11.85, et seq]

Activity	Service Time							
	3 minutes	5 minutes	10 minutes	15 minutes	30 minutes	45 minutes	1 hour	2, 3 and 4 hours
Sampling and Readings	3			2	2	2	2	Perform 1 hour test 2, 3 or 4 times, respectively
Walks at 4.8 km (3 mi) per Hour		5	3	4	8	12	18	
Sampling and Readings			2	2	2	2	2	
Walks at 4.8 km (3 mi) per Hour			3	5	8	12	18	
Sampling and Readings			2	2	2	2	2	
Walks at 4.8 km (3 mi) per Hour					6	13	16	
Sampling and Readings					2	2	2	

Table XXXIII.   Duration and Sequence of Specific Activities for Test 2 [30 CFR Part 11, Subpart H, § 11.85, et seq]

Activity	Service Time							
	3 minutes	7½ minutes	10 minutes	15 minutes	30 minutes	45 minutes	1 hour	2, 3 and 4 hours[a]
Sampling and Readings				2	2	2	2	2
Walks at 4.8 km (3 mi) per Hour			1	1	3	4	6	10
Carries 23-kg (50-lb) Weight Over Overcast			1 time in 2 minutes	1 time in 2 minutes	2 times in 4 minutes	3 times in 6 minutes	4 times in 8 minutes	5 times in 10 minutes
Walks at 4.8 km (3 mi) per Hour				1	3	3	3	5
Climbs Vertical Treadmill[b] (or equivalent)	1	1	1	1	1	1	1	1
Walks at 4.8 km (3 mi) per Hour		1	1			2	3	5
Climbs Vertical Treadmill (or equivalent)		1				1	1	1
Sampling and Readings					2	2	2	2
Walks at 4.8 km (3 mi) per Hour				2	2	3	5	11
Climbs Vertical Treadmill (or equivalent)				1	1	1	1	1
Carries 23-kg (50-lb) Weight Over Overcast				1 time in 2 minutes	3 times in 6 minutes	4 times in 8 minutes	5 times in 10 minutes	5 times in 10 minutes

Activity					
Sampling and Readings			2	2	2
Walks at 4.8 km (3 mi) per Hour	1	3	3	2	2
Climbs Vertical Treadmill (or equivalent)	1	1	1	1	Then repeat above activities once
Walks at 4.8 km (3 mi) per Hour	2		3	2	
Climbs Vertical Treadmill (or equivalent)			1	1	
Carries 20-kg (45-lb) Weight and Walks at 4.8 km (3 mi) per Hour	1			2	2
Walks at 4.8 km (3 mi) per Hour	1	2	1	4	2
Sampling and Readings	2	2	2	2	2

[a] Total test time for test 2 for 2-hour, 3-hour and 4-hour apparatus is 2 hours.
[b] Treadmill shall be inclined 15° from vertical and operated at a speed of 1 fps.

Table XXXIV.   Duration and Sequence of Specific Activities for Test 3ª [30 CFR Part 11, Subpart H, § 11.85, et seq]

Activity	Service Time							
	3 minutes	75 minutes	10 minutes	15 minutes	30 minutes	45 minutes	1 hour	2, 3 and 4 hoursᵇ
Sampling and Readings				2	2	2	2	ᵇ
Walks at 4.8 km (3 mi) per Hour			1	1	2	2	3	
Runs at 9.7 km (6 mi) per Hour	1	1	1	1	1	1	1	
Pulls 20-kg (45-lb) Weight to 5 ft		15 times in 1 minute		30 times in 2 minutes	30 times in 2 minutes	30 times in 2 minutes	60 times in 6 minutes	
Lies on Side	½	1	1	2	3	4	5	
Lies on Back	½	1	1	2	2	3	3	
Crawls on Hands and Knees	1	1	1	2	2	2	2	
Sampling and Readings			2		2	2	2	
Runs at 9.7 km (6 mi) per Hour				1	1	1	1	
Walks at 4.8 km (3 mi) per Hour					2	8	10	
Pulls 20-kg (45-lb) Weight to 5 ft			30 times in 2 minutes	60 times in 6 minutes		60 times in 6 minutes	60 times in 6 minutes	
Sampling and Readings				2		2	2	

	1	3	4	10
Walks at 4.8 km (3 mi) per Hour	1			
Lies on Side			2	4
Lies on Back			2	1
Sampling and Readings		2	2	2

[a] Perform test No. 3 for 1-hour apparatus; then perform test No. 1 for 1-hour apparatus.
[b] Total test time for test 3 for 2-hour, 3-hour and 4-hour apparatus is 2 hours.

Table XXXV.   Duration and Sequence of Specific Activities for Test 4 [30 CFR Part 11, Subpart H, § 11.85, et seq.]

Activity	Service Time									
	3 minutes	5 minutes	10 minutes	15 minutes	30 minutes	45 minutes	1 hour	2 hours [a]	3 hours [b]	4 hours [c]
Sampling and Readings				2	2	2	2			
Walks at 4.8 km (3 mi) per Hour				1	2	2	2			
Climbs Vertical Treadmill (or equivalent)	1		1	1	1	1	1			
Walks at 4.8 km (3 mi) per Hour		1	1	1	2	2	2			
Pulls 20-kg (45-lb) Weight to 5 ft		30 times in 2 minutes	30 times in 2 minutes	30 times in 2 minutes	60 times in 5 minutes	60 times in 5 minutes	60 times in 5 minutes			
Walks at 4.8 km (3 mi) per Hour			1	1	1	2	3			
Carries 23-kg (50-lb) Weight Over Overcast				1 time in 1 minute	1 time in 1 minute	2 times in 3 minutes	4 times in 8 minutes			
Sampling and Readings			2		2	2	2			
Walks at 4.8 km (3 mi) per Hour				1	3	3	4			

Runs at 9.7 km (6 mi) per Hour	1	1	1	1	1
Carries 23-kg (50-lb) Weight Over Overcase		1 time in 1 minute	2 times in 3 minute	4 times in 6 minutes	6 times in 9 minutes
Pulls 20-kg (45-lb) Weight to 5 ft	15 times in 1 minute	60 times in 1 minute	30 times in 5 minutes	36 times in 2 minutes	3 minutes
Sampling and Readings		2	2	2	2
Walks at 4.8 km (3 mi) per Hour	1			2	6
Pulls 20-kg (45-lb) Weight to 5 ft			60 times in 5 minutes	60 times in 5 minutes	60 times in 5 minutes
Carries 20-kg (45-lb) Weight and Walks at 4.8 km (3 mi) per Hour				3	3
Sampling and Readings		2	2	2	2

[a] Perform test No. 1 for 30-minute apparatus; then perform test No. 4 for 1-hour apparatus; then perform test No. 1 for 30-minute apparatus.

[b] Perform test No. 1 for 1-hour apparatus; then perform test No. 4 for 1-hour apparatus; then perform test No. 1 for 1-hour apparatus.

[c] Perform test No. 1 for 1-hour apparatus; then perform test No. 4 for 1-hour apparatus; then perform test No. 1 for 1-hour apparatus twice (i.e., two 1-hour tests).

[d] Treadmill shall be inclined 15° from vertical and operated at a speed of 30 cm (1 foot) per second.

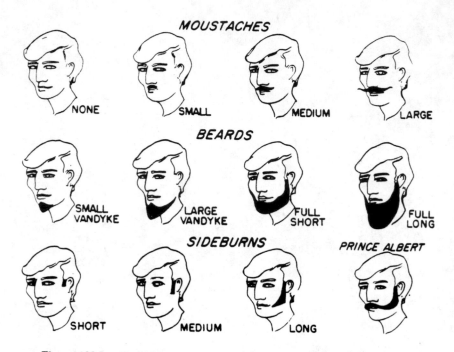

Figure 102.   Classification of moustaches, beards and sideburns [97].

indicated that excessive facial hair interferes with the respirator seal, causing the degree of respirator performance to drop.

OSHA [8] also recognizes the individual who wears glasses. Section 1910.134(e)(5)(ii) states: "Providing respiratory protection for individuals wearing corrective glasses is a serious problem. A proper seal cannot be established if the temple bars of eye glasses extend through the sealing edge of the full facepiece." Manufacturers have tried various methods of securing the glasses to the respirator. Figure 103 shows one type. Currently, the only problem with this is cost because special-type respirators cost more; however, this is not a problem that cannot be overcome.

In high noise areas, hearing protection is a problem. Figures 104 and 105 illustrate typical equipment with hearing protection, voice couplers and throat microphones. The "Loud Mouth" (Figure 104) is a rugged self-contained, 9-volt battery-operated voice amplification system. Designed to provide LOUD and CLEAR voice communications among persons wearing any type of respiratory protective device, the "Loud Mouth" accepts input from the SCBA voice coupler or the throat microphone. The "Loud Mouth" is designed with ample gain for noisy environments and features a versatile "clip-on mount." It has easily acces-

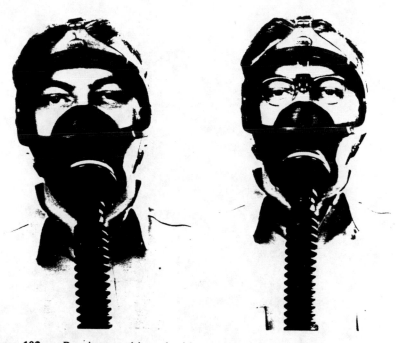

Figure 103.   Respirator with and without glasses on the wearer. Note special bridge adaptation on right photo.

sible on-off and volume controls. Lightweight but ruggedly constructed, it is dependable under extreme conditions. Batteries are replaced easily without tools.

Wireless communication on SCBA's and respirators protect breathing only to create another problem. The wearer cannot communicate! The SCBA voice coupler (Figure 105) comprises a miniature microphone capsule applied to the inside of the faceplate, electromagnetically coupled to a receiver module attached to the outside surface of the faceplate. The voice coupler does not violate the integrity of the faceplate. The HINT/COM throat microphone system utilizes a rugged dynamic-type throat microphone sealed in durable nontoxic vinyl. These systems are adapted easily to all HINT/COM communication systems, providing clear voice communication from within the mask.

FIT TESTING—GENERAL PROCEDURES

1.   All persons being tested should be screened medically first.

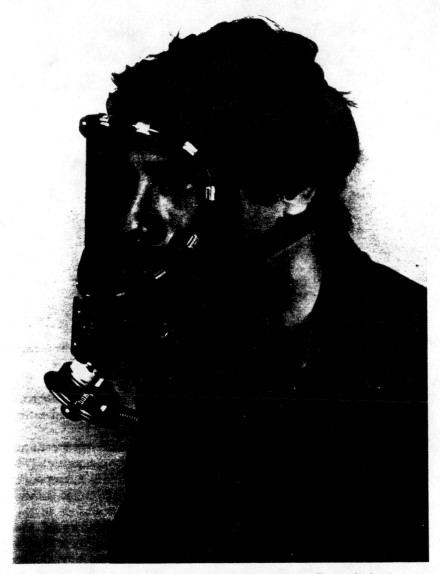

Figure 104.   Voice amplification system (courtesy Earmark, Inc.).

2. The procedure should be explained fully and, if possible, slides should explain the process.
3. The results should be explained to the wearer and emphasis placed on the proper fit, not the fit the company or union would like.

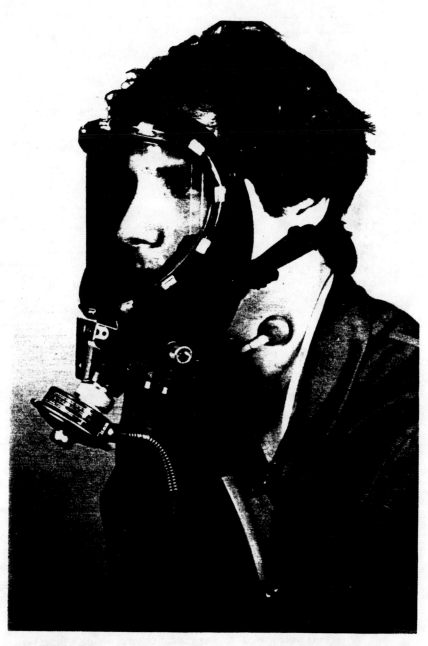

Figure 105.   The SCBA voice coupler (courtesy Earmark, Inc.).

DATE: _____ Location: __Philadelphia, PA__

NAME: _____ Soc. Sec. No. _____

Respirator: Manufacturer _____ Size: _____

            Model _____ Type: _____

            Approval No: __TC-__ _____

	Pass	Fail
PRE-TEST Positive/Negative Pressure	☐	☐
Isoamyl Acetate/Irritant Smoke	☐	☐

AVERAGE PENETRATION (%)

	Test 1	Test 2	Test 3
Initial Upstream	_____	_____	_____
Initial Clear	_____	_____	_____
Normal Breathing	_____	_____	_____
Deep Breathing	_____	_____	_____
Side to Side	_____	_____	_____
Up and Down	_____	_____	_____
Reading	_____	_____	_____
Grimaeing	_____	_____	_____
Bending	_____	_____	_____
Normal Breathing	_____	_____	_____
Final Clear	_____	_____	_____
Final Up Stream	_____	_____	_____
AVERAGE	_____	_____	_____
PROTECTION FACTOR	_____	_____	_____

REMARKS _____

_____

_____

TECHNICIAN _____ DATE: _____

Figure 106. Quantitative respirator fit test result.

4. In using booths, bags and test stands, all tube connections should be labeled. Oxygen and medical assistance shall be available as many people suffer heart attacks when being tested in hospitals, or suffer from fear of job loss.

5. If private testing is done for a large group of workers, the company should include a person dressed like a worker to ensure that the outside contractor explains all aspects to the people being tested, does all the tests and does not create a feeling of negative reaction against the company.

6. The results of individual testing should be recorded on a form such as given in Figure 106. The tests should be signed by the technician and dated, listing the equipment tested and the number of tests performed.

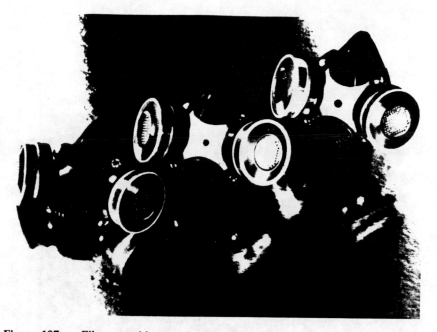

Figure 107. Filter cartridge respirators in three sizes with color-coded yokes for quick identification—small (black), medium (silver) and large (gold) (courtesy Mine Safety Appliance Co.).

7. As some test methods use flammable gases such as propane in the flame photometers and ethylene, the safe handling of these gases is vital.

Proper fit testing enables specification and purchase of respiratory equipment by sizes. Figures 107 and 108 show filter cartridge respirators and full facepieces in three sizes—small, medium and large.

RESPIRATOR CLEANING

Cleanup is a problem under normal working conditions, but for respirator users it is vital to good sanitary and health conditions. Therefore, the easiest, most efficient and safest method for management and personnel responsible for respirators is the convenient packaged cleaning system. Through education and operation, such systems can prevent skin disease and respiratory problems due to contaminated respirators, thus eliminating unnecessary absence and discomfort.

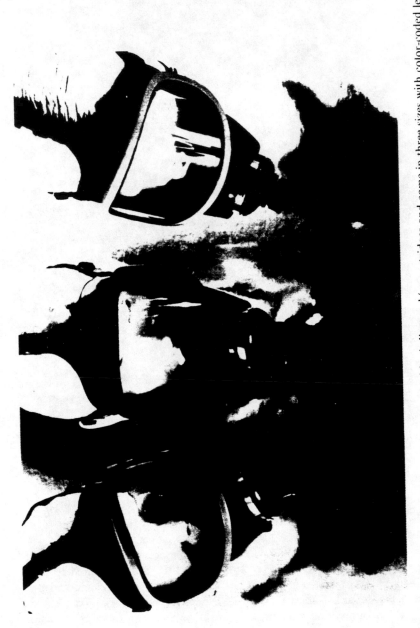

Figure 108. Full-face facepieces can be equipped with air line and/or cartridges and come in three sizes with color-coded lens-retaining rings for quick identification—small (gray), medium (black) and large (gold) (courtesy Mine Safety Appliance Co.).

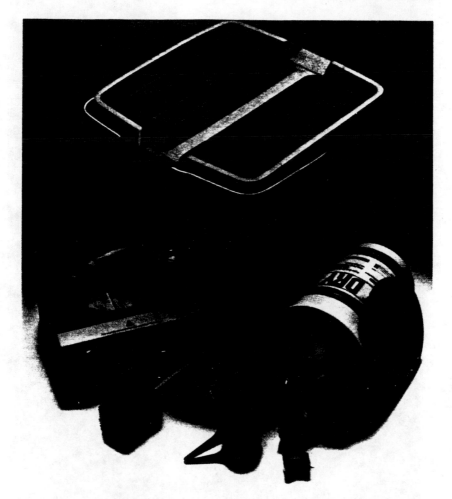

Figure 109.   Product contents of a cleaning kit for respirator systems (courtesy Georgia Steel & Chemical Co., Inc.).

Although such systems are designed to be used by the individual worker/respirator user, management can maintain control of the respirator cleaning function more easily through inventory and inspection. Once installed as part of the respiratory protection program, these systems provide personnel and management with a simple, easy-to-learn and use method for cleaning respirators. As replacements for cleaning packets and storage bags are necessary, inventory records indicate frequency of use. Also, because the storage bags must be annotated with the

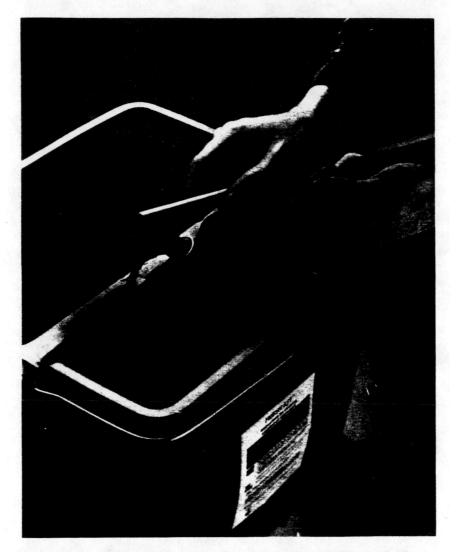

Figure 110.   Supplied-air respirator being disinfected in a large complete Fresh-Kit® system cleaning pail (courtesy Georgia Steel & Chemical Co., Inc.).

name of the person who cleaned the respirators and when (and can also be inspected through the clear plastic bag), management can spot-check stored respirators to determine efficiency of the program.

The use of SCBA units and similar devices has created further need for

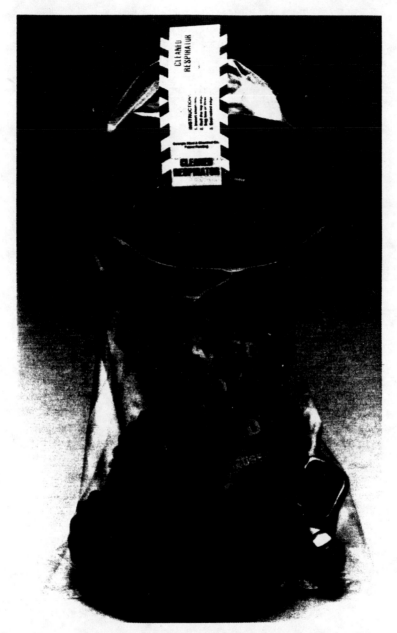

Figure 111.   Cleaned supplied-air respirator properly stored in sterile storage bag (courtesy Georgia Steel & Chemical Co., Inc.).

proper facemask cleaning. The Fire Service, among others, has spent thousands of dollars to ensure that their SCBA air is of the highest quality. Consequently, to pass this clean air through a dirty facemask constitutes a serious health hazard (Figures 109–111).

CHAPTER 10

CHOOSING THE APPROPRIATE RESPIRATOR

INTRODUCTION

Probably the most important question in respiratory protection is "what is the right respirator for me?" A typical small user calls the local safety equipment supply house or places a checkmark in a box in one of the dozen publications that a typical plant may receive. Then the plant receives a visit from the local sales representative of the respirator-safety and health equipment company manufacturer. A large firm may have a safety engineer or maintenance supervisor whose responsibility it is to specify this type of equipment. A large corporation would use the medical or insurance staff or industrial hygienist to specify the type of respirator that should be worn.

A more common occurrence since 1971 is that the OSHA inspector may have issued the company a citation (legal term requiring corrections of alleged unsafe activities) specifying possible monetary penalties and abatement dates (time limits by which the work must be completed or the condition corrected). The term "alleged" is used because violation of the OSHA Act is not a matter of record until the employer accepts it by paying the fine, making the corrections or settling the contested case. The employer has the right to disagree with the citation and can go to court to explain why he feels he has not violated the Act.

The OSHA Act is a complex law [2]. The best source of information on OSHA is the local OSHA office. Local offices are members of Regional offices, a list of which is provided in Table XXXVI. The importance of contacting OSHA regional offices is that a similar problem and answer issued to a user may have arisen previously, thereby saving time and money.

The single, most serious problem of the user's respiratory protection is

Table XXXVI.   OSHA Regional Offices

Region I
U.S. Department of Labor
Occupational Safety and Health Administration
JFK Building, Room 1804
Boston, Massachusetts 02203 .... Telephone: 617/223-6712/3

Region II
U.S. Department of Labor
Occupational Safety and Health Administration
1515 Broadway (1 Astor Plaza), Room 3445
New York, New York 10036 .... Telephone: 212/944-5941/2

Region III
U.S. Department of Labor
Occupational Safety and Health Administration
15220 Gateway Center, 3535 Market Street
Philadelphia, Pennsylvania 19104 .... Telephone: 215/596-1201

Region IV
U.S. Department of Labor
Occupational Safety and Health Administration
1375 Peachtree Street, N.E., Suite 587
Atlanta, Georgia 30309 .... Telephone: 404/526-3573/4 or 2281/2

Region V
U.S. Department of Labor
Occupational Safety and Health Administration
230 S. Dearborn, 32nd Floor
Chicago, Illinois 60604 .... Telephone: 312/353-4716/7

Region VI
U.S. Department of Labor
Occupational Safety and Health Administration
555 Griffin Square Building, Room 602
Dallas, Texas 75202 .... Telephone: 214/749-2477/8/9 or 2567

Region VII
U.S. Department of Labor
Occupational Safety and Health Administration
Federal Building, Room 3000, 911 Walnut Street
Kansas City, Missouri 64106 .... Telephone: 816/374-5861

Region VIII
U.S. Department of Labor
Occupational Safety and Health Administration
Federal Building, Room 15010, 1961 Stout Street
Denver, Colorado 80202 .... Telephone: 303/837-3883

Region IX
U.S. Department of Labor
Occupational Safety and Health Administration
9470 Federal Building, 450 Golden Gate Avenue

Table XXXVI, continued

Post Office Box 36017	
San Francisco, California 94102	Telephone: 415/556-0584
Region X	
U.S. Department of Labor	
Occupational Safety and Health Administration	
6048 Federal Office Building, 909 First Avenue	
Seattle, Washington 98174	Telephone: 206/442-5930

lack of knowledge. Most plant engineering, maintenance, insurance and safety people have only a faint idea of what respirator training is because few engineering colleges and universities have textbooks on respirators and few, if any, formal training courses were given until the late 1970s.

The way in which legislators present requirements is complex. Also, few respirator companies manufacture full lines of products or require the user to know what kind of hazards they may encounter.

In this chapter, we will present a guide to the regulatory agencies and material and a background method for selecting respirators.

MINE SAFETY AND HEALTH ADMINISTRATION

The Mine Safety and Health Administration (MSHA) is an agency under the U.S. Department of Labor. Its origin is the Bureau of Mines, Department of the Interior. The Department of the Interior had control over natural resources such as coal, gas, oil, etc. Respiratory protection required for coal mines and mineral miners was a long established fact. In 1974, the Bureau of Mines was changed (politically) to the Mine Enforcement & Safety Administration (MESA) and, in 1978, to the Mine Safety and Health Administration.

MSHA is important for very fundamental reasons. Historically, the Bureau of Mines published key research documents such as reports of investigations, research results, information circulars and various technical studies leading to the formation of the current respiratory protective apparatus standards. Problems, new advances and investigations are noted in various chapters of this book. MSHA standard 30 CFR 11 [1] refers to a publication on respiratory protective apparatus. This section specifies how a respirator is tested, the design requirements and the fees that must be paid for the respirator to carry MSHA approval.

OCCUPATIONAL SAFETY AND HEALTH ADMINISTRATION

The OSHA Act [2] is a law "to assure safe and healthful working conditions for working men and women." It provides medical criteria to assure, as much as practicable, that no employee will suffer diminished health, functional capacity or life expectancy as a result of his work experience. The Act also called for the Secretary of Health, Education and Welfare to conduct research and establish methods for dealing with safety and health problems. The National Institute of Occupational Safety and Health (NIOSH) was created to perform or assist in these various functions.

OSHA specifies respiratory protection in its three codes: (1) Maritime (shipbuilding), Ship Breaking, Ship Repair and Longshoring [98]; (2) Construction [99], and (3) General Industry [8].

The Construction Codes 1926–103, Respiratory Protection, include the General Industry Code for Abrasive Blasting (1910.94) and Respiratory Protection (1910.134) in their latest publication.

The General Industry [8] OSHA Standards require respiratory protection in several different sections. An outline is given in Table XXXVII.

THE NATIONAL INSTITUTE OF OCCUPATIONAL SAFETY AND HEALTH

NIOSH is currently under the U.S. Department of Health and Human Services, Public Health Science Center for Disease Control. NIOSH has three basic functions vital to respirator users:

- Research and publication of studies
- Training
- Approval of respiratory apparatus

In this book, several of the thousands of NIOSH criteria documents and studies conducted or contracted out have been used as examples and referenced. NIOSH also publishes a program plan by program areas for every fiscal year [7]. This publication explains the current respiratory and other research being conducted by NIOSH and allows various groups to be contacted for public comment.

Training in respiratory protection is provided by NIOSH course #593—Occupational Respiratory Protection—aimed at the individual responsible for any portion of a respirator program initiation or upgrad-

**Table XXXVII.   Respirator Requirements as Required
by Specific OSHA Standards**[a]

Several standards promulgated by OSHA require the use of specific respirator type:

A. Abrasive Blasting
    1. 1910.94   (a) (5-6)
                  (d) (iv)

B. Spray Finishing
    1. 1910.94   (c) (6)(iii)

C. Open Surface Tanks
    1. 1910.94   (d)(a)(vi)
                  (d)(11)(v)
                  (d)(11)(vi)

D. Storage and Handling of Anhydrous Ammonia
    1. 1910.111   (b)(10)(ii)

E. Welding, Cutting and Brazing
    1. 1910.252   (f)(1)
                  (f)(4)
                  (f)(5-10)

F. Pulp, Paper and Paperboard Mills

1. 1910.261		
(b)(2)	(g)(10)	
(d)(1)(i)	(g)(11)(ii)	
(f)(6)(iii)	(g)(15)(ii)	
(g)(2)	(g)(15)(v)	
(g)(4)	(h)(2)(iii-iv)	
(g)(6)	(ii-iii)	

G. Textiles
    1. 1910.262   (qq)(1-2)

H. Sawmills
    1. 1910.265   (c)(17)(ii-iii)

I. Pulpwood Logging
    1. 1910.266   (c)(1)(v)

J. Asbestos
    1. 1910.1001 (d(1-2)

K. Cotton Dust
    1. 1910.1043 (f)(2)
    2. 1910.1046 (d)

L. Carcinogens
    1. 1910.1003–1016 (c)(4)(iv)
                          (c)(5)(i)
                          (c)(6)(vii)(a)
    2. 1910.1017 (g)(4)
    3. 1910.1029 (g)(2)

M. General Respirator Requirements
    1. 1910.134

Table XXXVII, continued

N. Fire Brigades
        (f)(i)

O. Inorganic Arsenic
    1. 1910.1018 (h)(1)

P. Lead
    1. 1910.1025 (f)(1)

Q. Benzene
    1. 1910.1028 (g)(1)

R. Acrylonitrile
    1. 1910.1045 (h)(1)

[a] Any of the above specific requirements may be modified or deleted by OSHA in response to the legislative process. Additions to the list also are possible. The reader can find out the status of the above requirements by contacting the nearest OSHA regional office.

ing. Its goal is to have the trainee meet the minimum requirements set forth in OSHA Section 1910.134 [8]. The course is conducted by NIOSH, Division of Training and Manpower Development, Cincinnati. Other courses also are available on industrial hygiene sampling and Chemistry and Noise. A list can be furnished on written request.

NIOSH is also responsible for the Testing and Certification Branch (TCB), Division of Safety Research, located in Morgantown, West Virginia. The TCB was established to assure that certain devices and instruments used for control and evaluation of occupational hazards meet minimum performance requirements necessary to protect workers' health and safety.

The following are its functions:

1. Publish certification requirements.
2. Test and certify products meeting those requirements.
3. Publish lists of certified products.
4. Survey manufacturers' plants to determine acceptability of their quality assurance programs.
5. Sample products from the open market and test them for continued conformance to certification requirements.
6. Research and development (R&D) of new test methods and requirements for product improvement, where necessary, to assure worker protection.

The NIOSH publication supplement to the NIOSH Certified Equipment List [100] lists certification of:

- Coal mine dust personal sampler units
- Gas detector tube units
- Respiratory protection devices
- Obsolete respirators
- Sound level meter sets

A free copy may be obtained by sending a self-addressed mailing label to: Division of Standards Development and Technology Transfer, National Institute for Occupational Safety & Health, Robert A. Taft Laboratories, 4676 Columbia Parkway, Cincinnati, OH 45226.

THE AMERICAN NATIONAL STANDARDS INSTITUTE

The American National Standards Institute (ANSI) publishes various standards for industry. Its "Practices for Respiratory Protection" [101] is referenced by the OSHA standards in 1910.134—Respiratory Protection (c), Selection of Respirators [8]. Proper selection of respirators shall be made according to American National Standards Practices for Respiratory Protection Z 88.2-1969.

ANSI modifies its standards, and a new ANSI standard number Z 288.2-1980 [101] has been published but not been adopted by OSHA yet in the standard process. OSHA has incorporated many of the ANSI Safety and Health Standards into its own regulation manuals. The ANSI group is important because it represents a cross section of industrial [102], government and insurance groups. Some organized labor groups have criticized ANSI committees for being promanagement and not giving unions enough representation on standards formulation committees. Information on joining the committees and participation can be obtained by contacting ANSI, 1430 Broadway, New York, New York 10018.

RESPIRATOR TYPES

Respirators are of two basic types: air filtering and air supplying. Medically speaking, respirators also are used in hospitals and inhalation therapy work for treatment of disease. We have considered respirators for industrial usage only. Respirators restrict the atmosphere inhaled into the lungs by covering the nose and the mouth. Five different devices provide this covering:

- Single-use respirator
- Quarter-mask respirator
- Half-mask respirator
- Full-face respirator
- Protective hood or garment-style full suit

The relative merits of each system will be discussed now, noting the modifications that are made for specific applications.

The Single-Use Dust Respirator

Figure 112 illustrates the single-use dust respirator. This generally is sold in hardware-paint stores by the boxful and worn to prevent irrita-

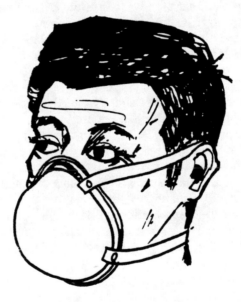

Figure 112.   Single-use respirator.

tion against a dust, mist or fumes by filtering out the irritant particulates. It generally was not taken seriously until some styles received NIOSH approval for use for various dusts. Its principal advantages are that it is inexpensive, disposable and requires no maintenance or cleaning. Its disadvantages are that it includes no method of measuring the protection factor, no method of fit testing and no method of estimating service life.

Disposable Mouth Bit Respirator

This type of disposable respirator also requires no maintenance. It is compact, lightweight, low in cost, and equipped with inhalation and exhalation valves and a one-piece polypropylene body with belt clip. It is designed for emergency escape protection against a variety of toxic gases, such as acid gas, ammonia, chlorine, organic vapors, etc., depending on the type of chemical fill used (Figure 113).

Depending on user preference, the respirator can be carried suspended from the neck on a neck strap or attached at the waist by means of an integral clip. Built-in inhalation and exhalation valves direct the flow of

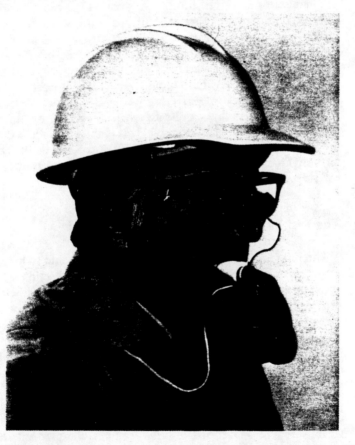

Figure 113.   Disposable mouth bit respirator (courtesy Scott Aviation, Div. of Figgie International Inc.).

air in one direction through the chemical cartridge. This low-cost respirator requires no cleaning, sanitizing, cartridge replacement or maintenance.

The respirator contains 180 cc of chemical fill to provide the required protection. The respirator must not be used where the oxygen content of the atmosphere is less than 19.5% or in atmospheres immediately dangerous to life or health. NIOSH Certification TC-23C-55 is issued to provide respiratory protection during escape only from atmospheres containing not more than 10 ppm of chlorine gas by volume.

Quarter-Mask and Half-Mask Respirators

The quarter-mask respirator mask covers the mouth and nose (Figure 114). It represented a first step in providing a better seal between the wearer's face and the respirator. The respirator was improved further to the half-mask style, which includes the nose, mouth and chin. The advantage is a more secure fit, and a better sealing capacity allows the respirator to be used where more toxic material exists.

The masks consist of purifying elements such as filters, chemical cartridges or canisters that can be attached directly or by use of a breathing hose, depending on the size and weight. Inhalation and exhalation valves are used to draw the air in from the filter and exhale the carbon dioxide air out. Figure 115 illustrates a typical half-face respirator fit with dual cartridges.

The Full Facepiece

The full facepiece covers the entire face from chin to hairline and from ear to ear. This respirator provides added eye protection and a better seal between the respirator body and the face. Not only is better protection provided against contaminants, but this respirator can be fit-tested and secured to the face for operations such as fire fighting and rescue. Figure 116 illustrates a full facepiece type with a supplied air line corrugated hose attached. This respirator offers a choice of three facepieces and two control valves, all approved by the U.S. Bureau of Mines for use in atmospheres not immediately hazardous to life or health. With this respirator, a continuous flow of breathable air is supplied to the facepiece and provides a cooling effect as it meets the respiratory requirements of the wearer. Figure 117 shows a full facepiece complemented by chemical cartridges and filters. Constructed of optically correct polycarbonate material, it gives a wide field of vision, designed to meet the impact and

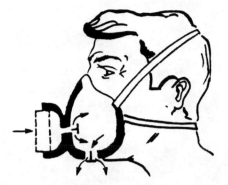

Figure 114.   Quarter-mask respirator.

penetration requirements of a face shield as specified in ANSI Z 87.1. The complete unit with pair of dust and mist filters weighs only 14.5 ounces.

The full-face respirator has many attachments that can be incorporated to make it more versatile. As a filter respirator, it can be equipped with filters, chemical cartridges, canisters, and powered air-purifier systems. As an air-supplied respirator, it can be equipped with an air line arrangement or a tank-supplied compressed air/oxygen system, either for closed or open operation.

Figure 118, a tank supplied system, shows a positive-pressure self-contained breathing apparatus that features a lightweight, long-term (up to 60 minutes) oxygen/air supply. It recirculates the major portion of the user's exhaled gas, permitting the unit to be much smaller and lighter than open circuit equipment, in which all of the user's exhaled breath is vented. Properly used, the minimum duration will be 60 minutes, regardless of the user's size or level of activity. Oxygen is supplied to the breathing chamber continuously. In addition, the unit will add oxygen automatically to compensate for heavy workloads or outward mask leakage.

The emergency escape breathing device shown in Figure 119 is a lightweight escape hood and life support apparatus designed to provide breathing protection from oxygen-deficient, smoke-laden or other toxic atmospheres. This device is sold under the trade name of SCRAM. SCRAM is a semiclosed-circuit, 15-minute, completely disposable emergency escape breathing device consisting of four major components:

1.   a solid state oxygen supply source;
2.   a chemical carbon dioxide and water vapor scrubber;

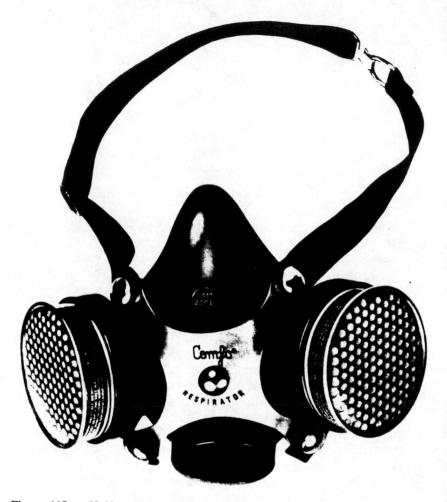

Figure 115. Half-mask respirator with dual filter cartridges (courtesy Mine Safety Appliance Co.).

3. a loose-fitting hood with a head harness and neck seal to enclose the head and provide the respirable environment for the user; and

4. a venturi "pumping" arrangement powered by the oxygen generator, which provides makeup oxygen and recirculates the breathing gas within the system loop consisting of the scrubber and the hood.

The hood serves as a counter lung to the user's respiratory system. Surplus system gas is vented through a protected relief valve to preclude overinflation of the hood.

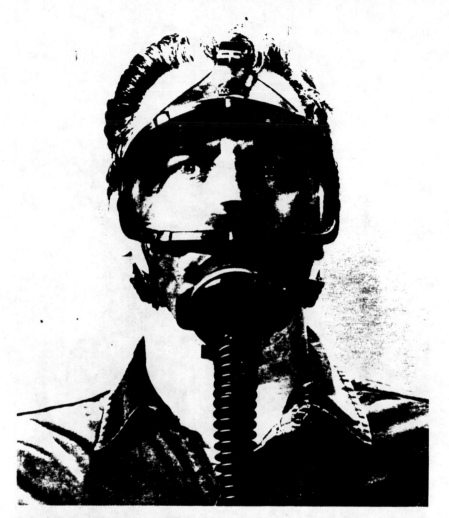

Figure 116.   Ultraview full-face respirator (courtesy Mine Safety Appliance Co.).

Protective Hood or Garment-Style Full Suit

A protective hood or garment-style full suit is the ultimate in protection for the worker exposed to hazardous chemicals and other media, such as abrasive blasting, heat, and cold, at one time. The concept is a method most companies will use to protect workers exposed to hazardous materials. It originated as the hard hat diver's suit and was modified to an abrasive blasting-air line breathing-supplied system. The

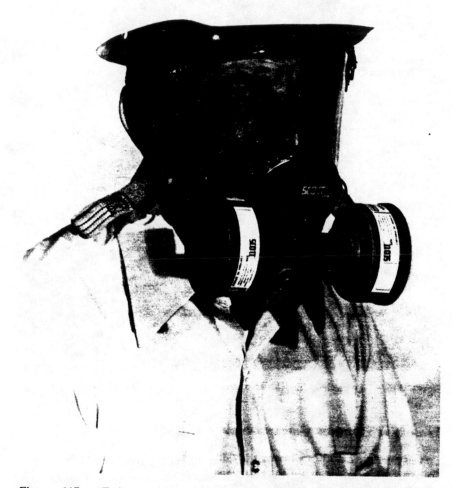

Figure 117. Twin-cartridge respirator with full facepiece (courtesy Scott Aviation, Lancastesr, New York).

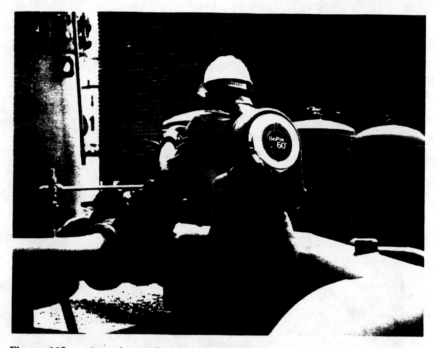

Figure 118.   A tank-supplied system that can be used both in atmospheres that are totally oxygen deficient and, because of the positive pressure in the facepiece, in toxic gas or vapor atmospheres (courtesy Rexnord-Electronic Products Div.).

design was modified further by vortex cooling tubes to produce not only ventilation but cooling as well (see Chapter 7). Further modifications of the suit protect the respirator suit wearer totally from a hostile environment. Figure 120 shows an all-clear vinyl window with green antiglare rear panel and clear top for overhead visibility. This type equipment also allows beards, spectacles and low hairlines worn by workers without problems of fitting.

HOW NIOSH SELECTS THE PROPER RESPIRATOR

This section contains the "Joint NIOSH-OSHA Standards Completion Program—Respirator Decision Logic." It is offered only as a guide to the reader because compliance with OSHA can be assured only through the guidance of OSHA, and limitations of the equipment must

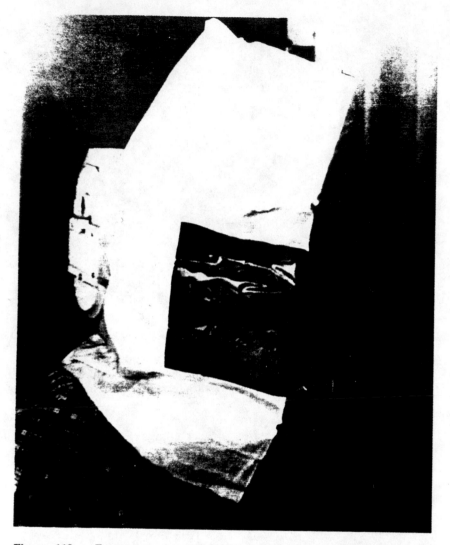

Figure 119. Emergency escape breathing device (courtesy Scott Aviation, Lancaster, New York).

be explained by the manufacturer, who bears the responsibility of its product. In selecting the proper respiratory protection device, the physiology of the wearer, the toxicity of the hazards encountered by leakage or misuse and the hazard of sampling all must be considered carefully.

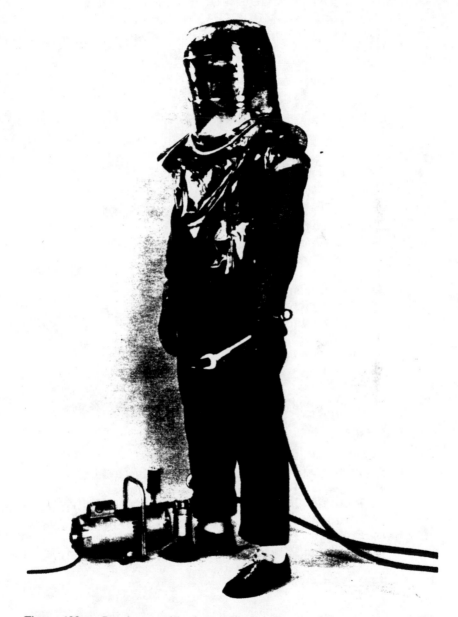

Figure 120.   Respirator with clear top, allowing overhead visibility (courtesy E. D. Bullard Co.).

JOINT NIOSH/OSHA STANDARDS COMPLETION PROGRAM
Nelson A. Leidel and SCP Respirator Committee
2 August 1976
Table of Contents

Introduction

The purpose of the Respirator Decision Logic is to assure technical accuracy and uniformity between substances in the selection of respirators and to provide necessary criteria to support this selection. The decision logic is a step-by-step elimination of inappropriate respirators until only those that are acceptable remain. Judgment by persons knowledgeable of inhalation hazards and respiratory protection equipment is essential to ensure appropriate selection of respirators.

The primary technical criteria for what constitutes a permissible respirator is based on the technical requirements of 30 CFR Part 11 (Department of the Interior, Bureau of Mines, Respiratory Protective Devices and Tests for Permissibility). The proposed health standards will allow only respirators approved by the Bureau of Mines [or Mining Enforcement and Safety Administration (MESA)]* and NIOSH under 30 CFR 11. Classes of respirators are only included when at least one device has been approved.

Protection factors are criteria used in determining what limiting concentrations are to be permitted for each respirator type that will afford adequate protection to the wearer. The referenced Subparts of 30 CFR 11 give technical descriptions concerning each type or class of respirators referenced in the decision logic. 30 CFR 11 should be used with the decision logic to properly understand the criteria for the specification of allowable respirators.

General Decision Logic Flowchart

Step 1—Assemble Information on Substance

One must assemble necessary toxicological, safety and research information for the particular contaminant. Typically, the following are required:

1. permissible exposure limits specified in 29 CFR 1910.1000 (Tables Z-1, Z-2, and Z-3), the former 29 CFR 1910.93 tables;
2. warning properties if the substance is a gas or a vapor (refer to Part IV(B) of this logic);
3. eye irritation potential of the substance (refer to Part IV(D) of this logic);
4. LFL (lower flammable limit) for the substance (refer to Part IV(F) of this logic);
5. IDLH (immediately dangerous to life or health) concentration for the substance (refer to Part IV(E) of this logic);
6. any possibility of poor sorbent efficiency at IDLH concentration and below (refer to Part IV(C) of this logic);

---

*Currently Mine Safety and Health Administration (MSHA).

7. any possibility of systemic injury or death resulting from absorbance of the substance (as a gas or vapor) through the skin (refer to Part IV(A) of this logic);

8. any possibility of severe skin irritation resulting from contact of the skin with corrosive gases, vapors or particulates (refer to Part IV(A) of this logic);

9. the vapor pressure of the substance (and equivalent ppm);

10. any possibility of high heat of reaction with sorbent material in cartridge or canister; and

11. any possibility of shock sensitivity of substance sorbed on sorbent of cartridge or canister.

Step 2—Determine Physical State of Substance

One must determine the physical state(s) of the substance as it is likely to be encountered in the occupational environment. It will be either (1) gas or vapor; (2) particulate (dust, fume or mist), or (3) a combination of these.

Step 3—Assemble a Table of Permissible Respiratory Protection for Substance

This is done using the material from Step 1 and the appropriate Specific Decision Logic Chart from Part III of this logic and the Respirator Protection Factors in Appendix I.

Classes of respirators are included only where at least one device has been approved.

Specific Decision Logic Charts

Respiratory Protection Against Gases or Vapors

Condition	Selection Sequence
Routine Use	1. Consider skin irritation and sorption of the material through the skin.
	2. Poor warning properties—eliminate all air-purifying respirators.
	3. Eye irritation—eliminate or restrict use of half-mask respirators.

4. IHLH or LFL—above this concentration eliminate all but positive-pressure self-contained breathing apparatus and combination positive-pressure supplied-air respirator with auxiliary positive-pressure self-contained breathing apparatus.

5. List all allowed respirators by condition of use and type.

Entry and escape from unknown concentrations

Use positive-pressure self-contained breathing apparatus or combination positive-pressure supplied-air respirator with auxiliary positive-pressure self-contained breathing apparatus.

Firefighting

Use positive-pressure self-contained breathing apparatus.

Escape

Use gas mask or escape self-contained breathing apparatus.

Respiratory Protection Against Particulates

Condition	Selection Sequence
Routine Use	1. Consider skin irritation or sorption of the material through the skin.
	2. Eye irritation—eliminate or restrict the use of half-mask respirators.
	3. Systemic poison—eliminate single-use respirators.
	4. For permissible exposures less than 0.05 mg/m^3, eliminate DFM respirators, except with high-efficiency particulate filter.
	5. IDLH or LFL—above this concentration eliminate all but positive-pressure self-contained breathing apparatus and combination positive-pressure supplied-air

respirator with auxiliary positive-pressure self-contained breathing apparatus.

6. List all allowed respirators by condition of use and type.

Entry and escape from unknown concentration

Use positive-pressure self-contained breathing apparatus or combination positive-pressure supplied-air respirator with positive-pressure self-contained breathing apparatus.

Firefighting

Use positive pressure self-contained breathing apparatus.

Escape

Use any dust, fume or mist respirator, except single-use, or any escape self-contained breathing apparatus.

Respiratory Protection Against Combination of Gas or Vapor and Particulates

Condition	Selection Sequence

Routine Use

1. Consider skin irritation or sorption of the material through the skin.

2. Poor warning properties or inadequate sorbent efficiency—eliminate all air-purifying respirators.

3. Eliminate all respirators except with combination sorbent/particulate filter.

4. Eye irritation—eliminate or restrict use of half-mask respirator.

5. For permissible exposures less than 0.05 mg/m^3, eliminate all respirators except with sorbent/high-efficiency particulate filter.

6. IDLH or LFL—above this concentration eliminate all but positive-pressure self-contained breathing apparatus and combination positive-pressure supplied-air

respirator with auxiliary positive-pressure self-contained breathing apparatus.

7. List all allowed respirators by condition of use and type.

Entry and escape from unknown concentration

Use-positive-pressure self-contained breathing apparatus or combination positive-pressure supplied-air respirator with auxiliary positive-pressure self-contained breathing apparatus.

Firefighting

Use positive-pressure self-contained breathing apparatus.

Escape

Use gas mask or escape self-contained breathing apparatus.

Decision Logic Criteria

Skin Absorption and Irritation

Personal protection requirements for protection against exposure to substances that may cause injury by absorption through the skin from materials splashed or spilled on the skin are covered in Section (f) of each substance standard. Respirator selection criteria are based primarily on the inhalation hazard of the substance. A supplied-air suit may provide skin protection for extremely toxic substances, which may be absorbed through the skin, or for substances that may cause severe skin irritation or injury.

Supplied-air suits are not covered in 30 CFR 11. Data are not available on which to make recommendations for supplied-air suits for all types of exposures.

Where information is available indicating systemic injury or death resulting from absorbance of a gas or vapor through the skin or where severe skin irritation or injury may occur from exposure to a gas, corrosive vapor or particulate, the following statement is included as a footnote to the respirator tables. Both employee and employer are cautioned in the appendixes concerning their use:

"Use of supplied-air suit may be necessary to prevent skin contact and respiratory exposure from airborne concentrations of (specific substance). Supplied-air suits should be selected, used, and maintained under the immediate supervision of persons knowledgeable in the limitations and potential life endangering characteristics of supplied-air suits. Where supplied-air suits are used above a concentration which may be immediately dangerous to life and health, (concentration) an auxiliary positive-pressure self-contained breathing apparatus must also be worn."

The supplied-air suit statement is an advisory footnote. The decision whether to include the footnote is made by the NIOSH/OSHA Review Committees based on available information. As most information concerning skin irritation is not quantitative, but rather presented in commonly used descriptive terms, such as "a strong skin irritant, highly irritating to the skin," "corrosive to the skin," etc., the decision by the committees concerning skin irritation is judgmental, often based on non-quantitative information. As a guideline for inclusion of the supplied-air suit statement for substances sorbed through the skin, a single skin penetration LD_{50} of 2 g/kg for any species is used.

The footnote is advisory in nature and its inclusion does not make the use of supplied-air suits mandatory. Further, employers may use supplied-air suits in any situation in which they provide adequate protection, regardless whether there is an advisory footnote in the respirator table. To assure the health and safety of persons using supplied-air suits, it is imperative that they be used under the immediate supervision of persons knowledgeable in the limitations and potential life endangering characteristics of supplied-air suits.

Poor Warning Properties

It is important to realize that 30 CFR 11 [1] NIOSH/MESA* approvals for air-purifying (organic vapor) devices prohibit use of organic vapors with poor warning properties. Specifically, 30 CFR 11.90(b) (note 4) covers gas masks (canister respirators) and 30 CFR 11.150 (note 7) covers chemical cartridge respirators. Thus, these approvals are only for those organic vapors with adequate warning properties and not all organic vapors.

Warning properties include odor, eye irritation and respiratory irritation. Warning properties relying on human senses are not foolproof;

---

*NIOSH/MSHA.

however, they provide some indication to the employee of possible sorbent exhaustion or of poor facepiece fit or other respirator malfunction.

Adequate warning properties can be assumed when the substance odor, taste or irritation effects are detectable and persistent at concentrations "at" or "below" the permissible exposure limit.

It is expected that environmental concentrations will vary considerably and, therefore, warning of a respirator failure soon would be perceived at contaminant concentrations somewhat above the permissible exposure limit.

If the odor or irritation threshold of a substance is more than three times greater than the permissible exposure limit, this substance should be considered to have poor warning properties. If the substance odor or irritation threshold is somewhat above the permissible exposure limit (not in excess of three times the limit) and there is no ceiling limit, consideration is given to whether undetected exposure in this concentration range could cause serious or irreversible health effects. If not, the substance is considered to have adequate warning properties. Some substances have extremely low thresholds of odor and irritation in relation to the permissible exposure limit. Because of this, these substances can be detected by a worker within the facepiece of the respirator, even when the respirator is functioning properly. Therefore, these substances are considered to have poor warning properties.

Although 30 CFR 11 [1] does not specify eliminating air-purifying respirators for pesticides with poor warning properties, the Standards Completion Program Respirator Review Committee believes the SCP should not allow pesticide respirators for gases and vapors with poor warning properties.

Sorbents

Where supporting evidence exists or immediate (less than three minutes) breakthrough time at the IDLH concentration and below for a cartridge or canister sorbent, air-purifying devices shall not be allowed for any use, escape or otherwise.

Where there is reason to suspect that commonly used sorbents (e.g., activated charcoal) do not provide adequate sorption efficiency against a specific contaminant, use of such sorbents shall not be allowed. However, where another sorbent material has been demonstrated to be effective against a specific contaminant, approved respirators utilizing the effective sorbent material shall be allowed. The statement in the respirator table shall read, "Any chemical cartridge respirator providing protection against (specific substance)," and "Any gas mask providing protection against (specific substance)."

Where there is reason to suspect that a sorbent has a high heat of reaction with a substance, use of that sorbent is not allowed. In such cases, only sorbents providing safe protection against (specific substance) may be used. For such substances, a footnote is added to the respirator table that reads as follows: "(Specific substance) is a strong oxidizer and should be kept away from oxidizable material. Some cartridges and canisters may contain activated charcoal and shall not be used to provide protection against (specific substance). Only nonoxidizable sorbents are allowed." Where the oxidizable material may be an oxidizable filter, the footnote reads: "(Specific substance) is a strong oxidizer and should be kept away from oxidizable substances. Only air-purifying respirators with nonoxidizable filters are allowed.

Where there is reason to suspect that a substance sorbed on a sorbent of a cartridge or canister is shock sensitive, use of air-purifying respirators is disallowed.

Eye Irritation

For routine work operations, any perceptible eye irritation is considered unacceptable. Therefore, only full facepiece respirators are permissible in contaminant concentrations that produce eye irritation. Note that 30 CFR 11.90(b) (note 6) specifies that eye protection may be required in certain concentrations of gases and vapors. For escape, some eye irritation is permissible if it is determined that such irritation would not inhibit escape and is reversible.

Where quantitative eye irritation data cannot be found in the literature and theoretical considerations indicate the substance should not be an eye irritant, half facepiece respirators are allowed.

Where a review of the literature indicates a substance causes eye irritation but where no eye irritation threshold is specified, the data will be evaluated to determine whether quarter- or half-facepiece respirators are to be included in the respirator tables. When a table is developed for such substances, the respirators with quarter- and half-facepieces shall be footnoted as follows: "When an employee informs his employer that he is experiencing eye irritation from **Name** while wearing a respirator allowed in Table 2, the employer shall provide and ensure that the employee use an equivalent respirator with a full facepiece, helmet or hood.

IDLH

The definition of IDLH provided in 30 CFR [1] 11.3(t) is as follows:

> "Immediately dangerous to life or health" means conditions that pose an immediate threat to life or health or conditions that pose an immediate threat of severe exposure to contaminants, such as radioactive materials, which are likely to have adverse cumulative or delayed effects on health.

The purpose of establishing an IDLH exposure concentration is to ensure that the worker can escape without injury or irreversible health effects from an IDLH concentration in the event of failure of the respiratory protective equipment. The IDLH is considered a maximum concentration above which only highly reliable breathing apparatus providing maximum worker protection is permitted. As IDLH values are set conservatively, any approved respirator may be used up to its maximum use concentration below the IDLH.

In establishing the IDLH concentration the following factors are considered:

1. escape without loss of life or irreversible health effects (30 minutes is considered the maximum permissible exposure time for escape); and
2. severe eye or respiratory irritation or other reactions that would prevent escape without injury.

IDLH should be determined from the following sources:

1. specific IDLH provided in the literature, such as the AIHA Hygienic Guides;
2. human exposure data;
3. acute animal exposure data;
4. acute toxicological data from analogous substances (where such above mentioned data are lacking).

The following guidelines should be used to interpret toxicological data reported in the literature for animal species:

1. Where acute exposure animal data are available (30-minute to 4-hour exposures), the lowest exposure concentration causing death or irreversible health effects in any species is determined to be the IDLH concentration.
2. Chronic exposure data may have no relevance to the acute effects and

should be used in determining the IDLH concentration only on competent toxicological judgment.

3. Where there is no toxicological evidence of an IDLH concentration, 500 times the permissible exposure limit shall determine the upper limit above which is used only highly reliable breathing apparatus providing maximum worker protection.

Lower Flammable Limit and Firefighting

Contaminant concentrations in excess of the LFL are considered to be immediately dangerous to life or health. At or above the LFL, the use of respirators is limited to those devices that provide the maximum protection, i.e., positive-pressure SCBA and the combination positive-pressure supplied-air respirators with auxiliary positive-pressure SCBA.

Firefighting is defined by ANSI Z88.5-1971 [102] as being immediately dangerous to life. For firefighting, the only device providing adequate protection is the positive-pressure SCBA.

Protection Factors

Protection factors are a measure of the overall effectiveness of a respirator. Filtering efficiency is a part of the protection factor and becomes a significant consideration for less-efficient air-purifying respirators.

The protection factors used in the preparation of the standards are based on quantitative fit tests performed at Los Alamos Scientific Laboratory and elsewhere and, in some instances, on professional judgment. Appendix I shows the protection factors for each class of respirators listed in the checklists. The entries in each list are for an entire class of respirators.

Variations With 30 CFR 11

1. The Type A supplied-air respirator is allowed in 30 CFR 11 [1] for use in immediately dangerous to life or health atmospheres. However, the airflow requirement of 50 l/min is insufficient to maintain a positive pressure in the facepiece under all working conditions. Therefore, this device should have the same protection factor as applied to other air-purifying and atmosphere-supplying respirators having a negative pressure in the facepiece (see Appendix I). 30 CFR 11 [1] will require a revision to eliminate approval of Type A supplied-air respirators for IDLH atmospheres.

2. 30 CFR 11 [1] does not contain protection factor requirements. Protection factors are used in the decision logic. An amendment to 30 CFR 11 is planned to include protection factor requirements for DFM respirators. Future amendments are contemplated for other types of respirators.
3. 30 CFR 11 [1] does not permit the use of an escape gas mask against acid gases or organic vapors with poor warning properties. A change to 30 CFR 11 is necessary to permit the use of an escape gas mask against substances with poor warning properties.

Escape

Where escape respirators are provided they shall be selected from the escape category in Table 2. The employer shall provide and ensure that employees carry an escape respirator where exposure may occur to extremely toxic substances. (An extremely toxic substance is defined as a gas or vapor having a rat LC_{50} of less than 10 ppm.)

The following statement is added to the introduction to the respirator table for these substances:

Employers shall provide each employee working in areas where **NAME** may be released into the workplace air with an approved escape respirator as specified in Table 2. The employer shall ensure that each employee carry the escape respirator in the area where **NAME** may be released into the workplace.

"Entry into Tanks or Closed Vessels or ..."

Item (d)(4)(iv) is a variable provision in the introductory statements to the respirator tables that lists the specific operations in which a respirator is considered to be an acceptable means of control. Examples of situations in which this may occur are for operations that require occasional entry into tanks or other closed vessels.

Appendix I

A. Protection Factors for Particulate Filter Respirators

Protection Factor	Permissible Respiratory Protection [1]
5X	Any dust and mist respirator (30 CFR 11.130)
5X	Any dust and mist respirator, except single use (30 CFR 11.130

10X	Any dust and mist respirator, except single-use or quarter-mask respirator (30 CFR 11.130)
10X	Any fume respirator (30 CFR 11.130)
10X	Any high-efficiency particulate filter respirator (30 CFR 11.130)
100X	A high-efficiency particulate filter respirator with a full facepiece (30 CFR 11.130)
1000X	A powered air-purifying respirator with a high-efficiency particulate filter (30 CFR 11.130)

B. Protection Factors for Chemical Cartridges and Gas Masks

Protection Factor	Permissible Respiratory Protection [1]
10X	Any chemical cartridge respirator with a **Name** cartridge(s) (30 CFR 11.150)
100X	A chemical cartridge respirator with full facepiece and **Name** cartridge(s) (30 CFR 11.150)
100X	A gas mask with a full facepiece and **Name** canister (30 CFR 11.90(a))
1000X	A powered air-purifying chemical cartridge respirator with a **Name** cartridge (unlisted device)*
Escape	Any gas mask providing protection against **Name** vapors (30 CFR 11.90)

* Classes of respirators are only included in situations in which at least one device has been approved.

NOTE: The approval **Name** may consist of acid gases or organic vapors as a class or specific acid gases, ammonia or organic vapors. It also may consist of combinations of acid gases, organic vapors and other gases and vapors.

C. Protection Factors for Combination Chemical Cartridges and Particulate Filters and Gas Masks and Particulate Filters

Protection Factors	Permissible Respiratory Protection [1]
10X	Any chemical cartridge respirator with **Name** cartridge(s) and **Name** filter(s) (30 CFR 11.150 and 11.130)
100X	A chemical cartridge respirator with a full facepiece, **Name** cartridge(s) and high-efficiency filter(s) (30 CFR 11.150 and 11.130)
150X	A gas mask with a full facepiece and **Name** canister and high-efficiency filter (30 CFR 11.90(a) and 11.130)
1000X	A powered air-purifying chemical cartridge respirator with a **Name** cartridge and high-efficiency particulate filter
Escape	Any gas mask providing protection against **Name** and particulates (30 CFR 11.90 and 11.130)

Name refers to any acid gas, alkaline gas, organic vapor or other specific gas or vapor.

Type refers to dust and mist, fume or high-efficiency particulate.

NOTE: A pesticide respirator is a special type of chemical cartridge respirator or gas mask with a combination sorbent and particulate filter. Where a substance is a pesticide, the following phrase is added as a footnote to the respirator tables. "Including pesticide respirators which meet the requirements of this class."

D. Protection Factors for Supplied-Air Respirators

Protection Factor	Permissible Respiratory Protection [1]
10X	Any supplied-air respirator (30 CFR 11.110(a))
50X	Any supplied-air respirator with a full facepiece, helmet or hood (30CFR 11.110(a))
1000X	*A Type C supplied-air respirator operated in pressure-demand or other positive-pressure or continuous-flow mode (30 CFR 11.110(a))
2000X	A Type C supplied-air respirator with a full facepiece operated in pressure-demand or other positive pressure mode or with a full facepiece, hood or helmet operated in continuous flow mode (30 CFR 11.110(a))

*This category is not covered fully by preceding category.

E. Protection Factors for Self-Contained Breathing Apparatus

Protection Factor	Permissible Respiratory Protection [1]
10X	Any self-contained breathing apparatus (30 CFR 11.70(a))
50X	Any self-contained breathing apparatus with a full facepiece (30 CFR 11.70(a))
10,000 + X	Self-contained breathing apparatus with a full facepiece operated in pressure-demand or other positive-pressure mode (30 CFR 11.70(a))
10,000 + X	A combination respirator, which includes a Type C supplied-air respirator with a full facepiece operated in pressure-demand or other positive-pressure or continuous-flow mode and auxiliary self-contained breathing apparatus operated in pressure-demand or positive pressure mode (30 CFR 11.70(b))
Escape	Any escape self-contained breathing apparatus (30 CFR 11.70(a))

Appendix II—Bibliography

The following are the primary reference sources used in this Decision Logic.

1. Chemical Safety Data Sheets, Manufacturing Chemists Association, Washington, DC.
2. Sax, N. I. *Dangerous Properties of Industrial Materials,* 3rd ed (New York: Van Nostrand Reinhold Company, 1968).
3. American Industrial Hygiene Association. "Hygienic Guide Series," Detroit, MI.
4. Chemical Company Guides: a) Allied Chemical; b) Commercial Solvents Co.; c) Dow Chemical; d) Eastman Kodak; e) Exxon,

f) FMC; g) Monsanto; h) Olin chemicals; i) Rohm & Haas; j) Shell; k) Union Carbide Company.

5. American National Standards Institute, Inc. "American National Standard Acceptable Concentrations," New York, NY.

6. Browning, E. *Toxicity and Metabolism of Industrial Solvents* (New York: Elsevier-North Holland, Inc., 1965).
   Browning, E. *Toxicity of Industrial Metals* (London: Butterworths, 1961).

7. American Conference of Governmental Industrial Hygienists, *Documentation of the Threshold Limit Values for Substances in Workroom Air,* 3rd ed., Cincinnati, OH (1971).

8. Gleason, M. N., R. E. Gosselin, H. C. Hodge and R. P. Smith. *Clinical Toxicology of Commercial Products,* 3rd ed. (Baltimore: Williams & Wilkins Co., 1969).

9. Thienes, O. H., and T. J. Haley. *Clinical Toxicology* 5th ed. (Lea and Febiger, 1972).

10. Spector, W. S., W. O. Negherbon, R. M. Grebe, and D. S. Dittmer, Eds. *Handbook of Toxicology* (Philadelphia, W. B. Saunders Co., 1956–1959).

11. Paget, G. E. Blackwell Scientific Publications. *Methods in Toxicology* (Oxford: 1970).

12. Stolman, A., ed. *Progress in Chemical Toxicology,* Vol 2 and 4, (New York: Academic Press, Inc., 1969).

13. Patty, F. A., Ed. *Industrial Hygiene and Toxicology,* vol. 2 (New York: Interscience Publishers, 1963).

14. Hunter, D. *The Diseases of Occupations,* (Boston: Little, Brown and Company, 1969).

15. Stauden, A., Ed. *Kirk-Othmer Encyclopedia of Chemical Technology,* 2nd ed. (New York: Interscience Publishers, 1972).

16. Glick, D., ed. *Methods of Biochemical Analysis* (New York: Interscience Publishers, 1969).

17. Altman, P. L., and D. S. Dittmer, Eds. *Biology Data Book,* Federation of American Societies for Experimental Biology (1964).

18. Deichmann, W. B., and H. W. Gerarde. *Toxicology of Drugs and Chemicals* (New York: Academic Press, Inc., 1969).

19. Stecher, P. G., Ed. *The Merck Index,* 8th ed. Merck & Co., Inc., New Jersey (1968).

20. International Labour Office. *Encyclopaedia of Occupational Health and Safety* (New York: McGraw-Hill Book Company, 1971).

21. "Hygienic Information Guides," Commonwealth of Pennsylvania, Department of Environmental Resources, Bureau of Occupational Health.

22. Christensen, H. E., and T. L. Luginbyhl, Eds. *NIOSH Toxic Substance List,* 1974 edition, HEW Publication No. 74-134 (1974).

23. Survey of Compounds Which Have Been Tested for Carcinogenic Activity,'' U.S. Public Health Service Publication No. 149, Original, Supplements 1 and 2 (1961-1967; 1968-69; 1970-71).

24. Spencer, E. Y. *Guide to the Chemicals Used in Crop Protection,* 6th ed., Publication 1093, Research Branch, Agriculture Canada (1973).

25. National Safety Council. "National Safety Council Industrial Data Sheets,'' Chicago, IL.

26. Baskin, A. D., Ed. "Handling Guide for Potentially Hazardous Commodities, Railway Systems and Management Association,'' Chicago, IL (1972).

27. American Mutual Insurance Alliance. *Handbook of Organic Industrial Solvents,* Technical Guide No. 6, 4th ed., Chicago, IL (1972).

28. Committee on Hazardous Materials, Division of Chemistry & Chemical Technology National Research Council, National Academy of Science. "Fire Hazard Classification of Chemical Vapors Relative to Explosion-Proof Electrical Equipment,'' Report III, a supplementary report prepared by the Electrical Hazards Panel, Washington, DC (May 1973).

29. National Fire Protection Association. *National Fire Codes,* Volume 1, *Flammable Liquids,* NFPA 325, Boston, MA (1969).

30. National Fire Protection Association. *National Fire Codes,* Volume 7, *Alarm and Special Extinguishing Systems,* NFPA 69, Boston (1973).

31. National Fire Protection Association. *National Fire Codes, Manual of Hazardous Chemical Reactions,* NFPA 491M, Boston (1971).

32. National Fire Protection Association. *National Fire Codes,* Volume 3, *Combustible Solids, Dusts and Explosives,* NFPA 49, Boston (1973).

33. National Fire Protection Association. Bahme, C. W. *NFPA Fire Officer's Guide to Emergency Action,* Appendix A, Boston, MA (1974).

34. Factory Mutual Engineering Corporation. *Handbook of Industrial Loss Prevention,* 2nd ed. (New York: McGraw-Hill Book Company, 1967).

35. Armistead, G., Jr. *Safety in Petroleum Refining and Related Industrial* (Appendix A), 2nd ed. (New York: John C. Simmonds and Co., Inc., 1959).

36. Doolittle, A. K. "Laquer Solvents in Commercial Use,'' *Ind. Eng. Chem.* 27: 1169-1179 (1935).

37. Grant, W. M. *Toxicology of the Eye,* 2nd ed. (Springfield, IL: Charles C. Thomas, Publisher, 1974).

38. American Petroleum Institute. *API Toxicological Reviews,* New York, NY.

39. Gleason, M. N., R. E. Gosselin, H. C. Hodge and R. P. Smith. *Bulletin of Supplementary Material for Clinical Toxicology of Commercial Products,* University of Rochester (1969–1975).

40. May, J. "Odor Thresholds of Solvents for Assessment of Solvent Odors in the Air," *Staub* 26: 34–38 (September 1966).

41. Oelert, H. H., and T. Florian. "Detection and Evaluation of Odor Nuisance from Diesel Exhaust Gases," *Staub* 32: 20–31 (October 1972).

42. Summer, W. *Odour Pollution of Air,* (Cleveland: CRC Press, 1971).

43. Hyatt, E. C. "Respirator Protection Factors," Los Alamos Scientific Laboratory, New Mexico, LA-6084-MS (January 1976).

CHAPTER 11

THE ASBESTOS PROBLEM

No book on respiratory protection would be complete without some mention of asbestos. Asbestos has been, and continues to be, widely used as an article of construction and insulation. Due to its inherent nature as a health hazard and potential carcinogen, asbestos has received much notoriety in the mass media, at technical meetings, and in the scientific literature. An overview of this material has been excerpted from *A Guide to the Work Relatedness of Disease* [14].

INTRODUCTION

Asbestos is a mineral fiber and encompasses about 30 silicate compounds. Of these, only the following 5 are of significance in industry:

- Chrysotile (white asbestos)
- Amosite
- Tremolite
- Crocidolite (blue asbestos)
- Anthophyllite

Chrysotile accounts for about 97% of all the asbestos used in this country.

Asbestos is widespread in the environment because of its extensive use in industry and the home. More than 3000 products contain asbestos. Because of this wide usage, it may be difficult at times to determine whether a disease resulting from exposure to asbestos is occupational in origin. For example, the air of some relatively new apartment buildings has been found to contain more asbestos fibers than the maximum recommended levels in industry. The source of the fibers in the apartment buildings is the insulating materials used in the ventilating system.

Exposure to asbestos can produce a lung fibrosis called *asbestosis*. Its onset is gradual, usually developing over a period of 10–30 years of exposure to significant concentrations of asbestos. Occasionally, massive exposures may cause the disease to develop more quickly.

Asbestos is also a *cancer*-producing agent (bronchogenic carcinoma, mesothelioma) and can cause certain specific skin diseases (asbestotic subcutaneous granulomatosis and asbestotic cutaneous verruca). Heavy exposure to dust containing asbestos can cause *skin irritation*. Epidemiological (experience with groups of people) and animal studies have shown that increased exposure to any of the types of asbestos increases the risk of lung cancer (bronchial carcinoma). This carcinoma appears to be related to the degree of exposure to asbestos, the type of asbestos and cigarette smoking. It is also significant that cigarette smoking in men and women greatly increase the risk of lung cancer in those who are exposed to asbestos. Smoking is a factor that should be considered when determining whether lung cancer is caused, wholly or in part, by an occupational exposure to asbestos.

Mesothelioma, a rare malignant tumor of the membrane that lines the chest and abdominal cavities, is occurring with increasing frequency in workers exposed to asbestos. The development of this tumor apparently is not related to the amount of asbestos inhaled, and it is found in persons not having asbestosis. Levels of exposure that are within accepted standards for protection against asbestosis may not protect against mesothelioma.

An increased incidence of malignancy of the stomach and colon has been reported among insulation workers using asbestos.

The following occupations involve potential exposure to asbestos:

Acoustical product makers	Crushers (asbestos)
Acoustical product installers	Fiberizers (asbestos)
Air filter makers	Fireproofers
Asbestos-cement products makers	Firemen
Asbestos-cement products users	Furnace filter makers
Asbestos-coatings makers	Gasket makers
Asbestos-coatings users	Heat-resistant clothing makers
Asbestos-grout makers	Insulation workers
Asbestos-grout users	Inert filter media workers
Asbestos-millboard makers	Ironing board cover workers
Asbestos-millboard users	Laboratory hood installers

Asbestos-mortar makers
Asbestos-mortar users
Asbestos millers
Asbestos miners
Asbestos-paper makers
Asbestos-paper users
Asbestos-plaster makers
Asbestos-plaster users
Asbestos sprayers
Asbestos workers
Asphalt mixers
Automobile repair garage workers
Brake lining makers
Building demolition workers
Carders (asbestos)
Caulking compound makers
Caulking compound users
Clutch facing makers
Cobbers (asbestos)
Construction workers

Laggers
Paint makers
Pipe insulators
Plastics makers
Pump packing makers
Roofers
Roofing materals makers
Rubber compounders
Single makers
Ship builders
Ship demolition workers
Spinners (asbestos)
Talc miners
Talc workers
Textile flameproofers
Textile workers
Undercoaters
Vinyl-asbestos tile makers
Vinyl-asbestos tile installers
Weavers (asbestos)

MEDICAL EVALUATION

In addition to the usual medical history, the following should be considered:

1. Any history of diseases of the heart or lung or abnormal tissue growth should be evaluated carefully to determine the relationship between the previous disease and the claimant's present condition.
2. A questionnaire can be useful in evaluating the extent and importance of such respiratory symptoms as:
   - Breathlessness
   - Phlegm (sputum) production
   - Chest pain
   - Cough
   - Wheezing

Asbestosis

Shortness of breath on exertion is usually the first symptom, frequently accompanied by a dry cough. This symptom develops after several years of progressive pulmonary fibrosis. As asbestosis progresses, the following signs and symptoms are observed:

- Cough with production of sputum
- Anorexia (loss of appetite)
- Secondary respiratory infections that are difficult to control
- Rapid breathing
- Repetitive end-inspiratory crackles (crackling sounds heard in the lower part of the lungs through stethoscope when employee completes each of a series of inhaled breaths)
- Orthopnea (breathing difficulty in a recumbent postiion)
- Cyanosis (change in skin color to bluish, grayish, slatelike or dark purple
- Decrease of chest expansion
- Digital clubbing (rounding of the ends and swelling of the fingers and/or toes)
- Sequelae (other resultant diseases) including corpulmonale (right heart failure), bronchogenic carcinoma (lung cancer), stomach or intestinal cancer or pleural carcinoma (cancer of the membrane lining the chest)

Fibrosis results in alveolo-capillary block (impaired ability of the lungs to transfer oxygen into the blood). This impairment is often more severe than is indicated by chest X-rays.

Mesothelioma

In cases of mesothelioma, there may be a long latency period, as much as 40 years, between initial exposure to asbestos and development of the tumor. Mesothelioma of the *peritoneum* (membrane surrounding the abdominal organs) usually is accompanied by abdominal swelling and pain that is not concentrated in a particular area. Signs and symptoms of this type of tumor (that *may* be associated with asbestos exposure) include:

- Weight loss
- Obstruction of the bowel
- Excessive accumulation of fluid in the abdominal cavity (ascites)

This malignant tumor of the peritoneum may spread to the chest cavity. With mesothelioma of the *pleura,* complaints include chest pain and breathlessness. Signs and symptoms of pleural mesothelioma include:

- Pleural effusion (accumulation of fluid in the space around the lungs)

- Growth of the tumor outward through the chest wall in the form of a lump beneath the skin (subcutaneous lump)

The tumor may spread to involve bone, lymph glands (nodes), mediastinum (area between the right and left lungs) and pericardium (the sac enclosing the heart). As a result, the supraclavicular nodes may become enlarged, ribs may develop tumors and obstruction of the superior vena cava (major vein draining the upper portion of the body) may occur. In addition, pericardial effusion (fluid in the heart cavity) may occur, causing tamponade.

Laboratory

The following tests will assist in arriving at a correct diagnosis:

Chest X-Rays

Findings should be classified according to the ILO/UC 1971 Classification of the Radiographs of the Pneumoconioses. Findings for asbestosis vary, but the usual picture shows a density in both lungs, with the lower one-third of the lungs involved. In the affected area there is a "ground glass" appearance.

As asbestosis progresses, more and more of the lung is involved, except the apices (tips of the lungs). The X-rays will show gradual obscuring of the border between the lungs and the diaphragm. It may show shadows from the presence of nodules.

As the asbestosis progresses, X-ray findings usually will show reduced radiographic volume and formation of cysts combined with increased size of the heart and dilation (enlargement) of the proximal pulmonary arteries (arteries that lead from the heart to the lungs)

Lung Function Tests

Reduced lung capacity and other lung changes do not differ from those resulting from other forms of lung fibrosis, both occupational and nonoccupational. Therefore, the results of lung function tests or chest X-ray findings alone do not lead to diagnosis. Asbestos bodies in lymph nodes indicate exposure, but not necessarily asbestosis.

Asbestosis causes a reduction in the vital capacity (VC) of the lungs and a reduction in total lung capacity (TLC). These capacities are further reduced as the disease progresses. The residual volume (RV) of the lungs will be normal or slightly increased. The lungs' diffusing capacity for carbon monoxide (D_L) will be reduced.

Other lung function test results found in those suffering from asbestosis include:

- Increased minute ventilation (amount of air breathed in 1 minute)
- Reduced oxygenation of the arterial blood (arterial hypoxemia)
- Increased static transpulmonary pressures
- Decreased lung compliance

An exercise test will show that an increased amount of air is required during physical effort, and it also will show decreased oxygen in the blood, leading to cyanosis.

Sputum Examination

Asbestos fibers or bodies may be found in the sputum. These indicate asbestos exposure, but not necessarily asbestosis. Where cancer cells are present in the sputum and chest X-ray findings are normal, bronchoscopy may be necessary to confirm and locate the lung tumor.

Skin Tests

The following tests should be performed by the physician to exclude possible infectious diseases:

- PPD (tuberculin test)
- Blastomycin
- Histoplasmin
- Coccidioidin

EPIDEMIOLOGICAL DATA

Various epidemiological studies have demonstrated the relationship between asbestos and lung disease, including mesothelioma, in such trades and occupations as mining, insulation installation, textiles, paint and electrical industries, as a result of the widespread use of this substance.

The available information indicates a dose-response relationship for asbestos exposure and the risk of asbestosis and/or bronchogenic carcinoma. However, much of this information is epidemiological in nature and there is little correlation between epidemiological data and environmental exposure data. For this reason and others, including the long latency period for the development of carcinomas, it is difficult to develop a specific dose-response relationship. This should be taken into consideration when referring to the following material.

Enterline [103] has reported an exposure-response relationship between asbestos exposure (evaluated as millions of particles per cubic foot years) and the risk of malignant and nonmalignant respiratory disease. Enterline's data indicates that the risk of respiratory cancer increased from 166.7 (standardized mortality ratio) at minimum exposure to 555.6 at cumulative exposures exceeding 750 million particles per cubic foot years. Enterline's data are summarized by NIOSH [104].

Murphy [105] reported that asbestosis was 11 times more common among pipe coverers in new ship construction than in a control group. The first asbestosis was found after 13 years of exposure to an estimated cumulative dose of about 60 mppcf years. After 20 years, asbestosis prevalence was 38%. Murphy reported no asbestosis for men exposed to 60 mppcf years but 20% asbestosis in men exposed to 75–100 mppcf years. Murphy reports that atmospheric dust concentrations ranged from 0.8 to 10.0 mppcf years depending on the different operations evaluated. Asbestosis was considered present if the worker had at least three of the following: vascular rales in two or more sites, clubbing of the fingers, vital capacity of less than 80% predicted, roentgenography consistent with moderately advanced or advanced asbestosis, shortness of breath on climbing one flight of stairs.

The Pennsylvania Department of Health [106] reported a study of asbestos dust concentrations in two plants (one from 1930–1967 and the other from 1948–1968); 64 cases of asbestosis were reported. In the two plants, the study indicates that the air concentrations of particulates were generally less than 5 mppcf and, in many cases, less than 2 mppcf.

Epidemiological evidence is also available relating the development of mesothelioma with exposure to asbestos. Selikoff [107,108] reported 14 deaths from mesothelioma in 532 asbestos insulation workers from 1943–1968. No deaths from mesothelioma would be expected from the same number of individuals in the general population.

EVIDENCE OF EXPOSURE

Historically, there have been two air sampling and analysis methods to determine the quantity of asbestos in the workplace. The earlier light field impinger count method allowed only a measure of the overall dust level in the air rather than focusing on the amount of asbestos fibers in the air. The current fiber count method satisfactorily determines the amount of asbestos fibers in the air. It is performed by collecting airborne materials on a membrane filter and then counting the fibers using a phase contrast microscope at a 400–450X magnification ratio.

Asbestos fibers occur in varying lengths and diameters. The Occupational Safety and Health Act establishes maximum allowable limits for asbestos fibers greater than 5 μm in length. OSHA limits such asbestos fibers to no more than 5/cc of air (based on an 8-hour time-weighted average exposure. OSHA further requires that no workers be exposed to more than 10 asbestos fibers (greater than 5 μm in length) during any 15-minute period.

For samples collected by the field impinger count method, results may be compared to the pre-1970 limit (TLV) of five million particles per cubic foot of air.

Occupational exposure to asbestos fibers 5 μm in length or greater at quantities averaging more than 5 fibers/cc of air, or frequent exposures to more than 10 such fibers during a 15-minute period of time is evidence of a possible causal relationship between disease and occupation.

CONCLUSION

The diagnosis of occupational asbestosis is based on meeting the following criteria:

1. confirmed history of occupational exposure to asbestos;
2. X-ray findings compatible with those indicating asbestosis according to ILO/UC 1971 "Classification of Radiographs of the Pneumoconioses;" and
3. pulmonary impairment, particularly a decrease in lung-diffusing capacity and an increase in alveolar-arterial oxygen difference, as demonstrated by lung function tests.

The diagnosis of occupational mesothelioma is based on meeting the following criteria:

1. confirmed history of occupational exposure to asbestos; and
2. pathological evidence of mesothelioma.

ASBESTOS REMOVAL SYSTEM

A proven system to remove asbestos fibers from renovation or demolition sites is available that provides the maximum possible protection from contamination. The backbone of the system is a truck-mounted, vacuum filtration system called a Vactor® (Figures 121 and 122). This unit remains outside the job location and services it through a single vacuum line. The work area itself is sealed off and entered by Peabody personnal wearing completely disposable safety clothing. The personnel are highly trained in handling hazardous materials, and the complete service provides for removal, air monitoring (both in the removal area and in the clean zone), transportation and disposal of the material. Limited use of water spray, in a technique pioneered by Peabody International

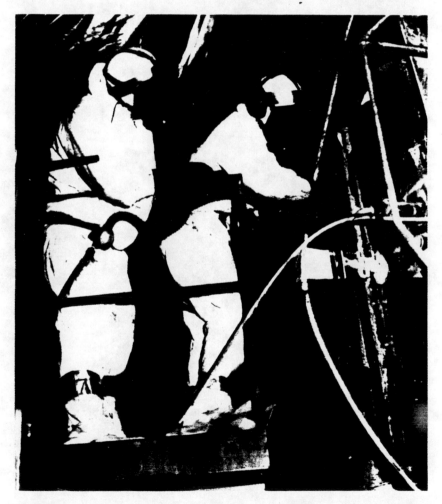

Figure 121. Asbestos removal system (courtesy Peabody International Corp., Stamford, Connecticut).

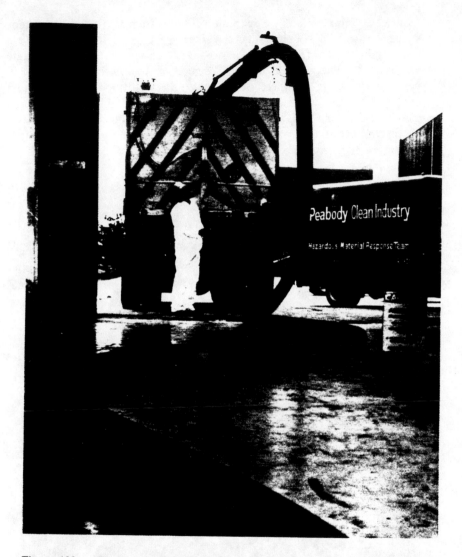

Figure 122. Peabody's Vactor, a huge wet-dry truck-mounted vacuum system, can be located as much as 1000 feet from the work area. Only the hose need be given access. Material is handled, removed and disposed of according to U.S. Environmental Protection Agency (EPA) regulations (courtesy Peabody International Corp., Stamford, Connecticut).

Corp. can keep airborne fiber levels low and still not interfere with electrical and mechanical equipment. The Peabody asbestos removal plan has been designed as a start-to-finish operation providing skilled personnel and sophisticated equipment that can reduce exposure claims. The plan allows complete control of the entire program, eliminating the need for subcontractors, while ensuring compliance with all regulations.

CHAPTER 12

AREAS OF SPECIAL INTEREST

INTRODUCTION

To complete the view of respiratory protection, we will examine briefly the special areas of fire fighters, confined spaces and new developments in garments worn when handling propellants. For fire fighters, little information has been published on respiratory protection due to the difficulty in correlating the different types of fires. Confined spaces are subtle killers that are most often taken for granted. New development in propellant handlers garments show how all types of protective equipment can be combined into a complete protective garment. This approach probably will be the engineering control method of the future.

Research will show and require total protection rather than separate gloves, boots, hats, glasses or respirators in dealing with hazardous and highly toxic materials.

FIRE FIGHTERS

As a fireman works for a municipality, he is not covered by OSHA, MSHA or other federal standards. The National Fire Protection Association [109] Standard 19B-1971 specifies that only self-contained breathing apparatus approved by the U.S. Bureau of Mines meets the provisions of the standard. The apparatus shall have a one-half hour minimum service life. The apparatus is to be inspected at regular intervals, and defective equipment is to be replaced immediately.

The International Association of Fire Fighters (IAFF) [110] stated in 1977 that 1 out of every 150 fire fighters in the United States dies or is forced to retire or change occupations each year because of occupational diseases (heart or lung).

Since December 15, 1980, employees assigned to Fire Brigades under OSHA section 1910.156(f) [8] are required to meet the general requirements of section 1910.134 [1]. The standard also recognizes the difference between interior structural fires and exterior fires. Section f(2)(i) [8] states: "The employer shall assure that self-contained breathing apparatus ordered or purchased after July 1, 1981 for use by fire brigade member performing interior structural fire fighting are of the pressure demand or other positive pressure type." Section f(2)(iii) [8] states "that negative-pressure self-contained breathing apparatus with a rated service life of more than 2 hours and which have a minimum protection factor of 5,000, as determined by an acceptable quantitative fit test performed on each individual is acceptable for use only during those interior structural fire fighting situations for which the employer demonstrates that long duration breathing apparatus is necessary."

This is noteworthy because OSHA uses the terms *quantitative fit test* and *protection factor*, which never were discussed in the main respirator sections. Appendix A to Subpart L of OSHA standard [8] also defines Protection Factor (sometimes called Fit Factor) as the ratio of the contaminant concentrations outside the respirator to the contaminant concentrations inside the facepiece of the respirator. This is a big step for OSHA to define respirator protection factors and require use of fit testing for these types of respirators. Hopefully, municipal fire companies will move more closely to examine their own rules.

The NIOSH study of Boston Fire Fighters [111] with Harvard University probably has been one of the most comprehensive. It began in 1969 when the Boston Fire Department reviewed its respiratory protection program and decided to eliminate the use of air-purifying respirators and rely on self-contained breathing apparatus. The fire department asked the Harvard School of Public Health to evaluate the respiratory protection needs of the fire service. Although it has been illustrated clearly that high carbon monoxide concentrations exist and low oxygen levels are present, the amount of carboxyhemoglobin (COHB) in the fire fighter's blood after a fire is the main question. A study of members of the Denver Fire Department pointed out the risk of carbon monoxide to fire fighters by demonstrating blood carboxyhemoglobin (COHB) levels of up to 43% after fighting a fire [112]. The respiratory minute volume during active fire fighting was measured using spirometry during actual fire fighting conditions. Oxygen levels were recorded by a membrane sensor in the range of 0 to 21%. A combustible gas detector was modified to be specific for carbon monoxide in the range of 0.02 to 10.0%. A series of incidents were studied in cooperation with the Boston Fire Department.

The results took into consideration that they were based on one municipal fire department and that industrial fires can produce unique toxic air contaminants at exceedingly high concentrations. The personal air sampling conducted for carbon monoxide and oxygen during this study revealed maximum air concentrations of carbon monoxide of approximately 2% (20,000 ppm) and minimum oxygen levels as low as 15.5% [112].

Spirometry on working fire fighters indicated a median minute volume of 60 l/min. If 30 minutes is required for open circuit, self-contained breathing apparatus, 1800 liters minimum must be stored but 2100 liters would be more appropriate.

A method for detecting carboxyhemoglobin exposure by examining exhaled breath samples up to 2½ hours after exposure to a fire were discussed. The effects of smoking and carbon monoxide levels were examined, and a method of considering the additive factors of each was considered.

Basically, the report ended with recommendations for further research to study the problems in greater detail. Possibly, the firemen of the future will wear combination fire suit respirators. New lightweight, water-resistant and heat-reflecting materials will be combined with oxygen sensor electronic circuits to switch from a powered air purifier to compressed air supply system. This would allow the firemen to switch from smoke hazard to oxygen hazard automatically.

CONFINED SPACES—THE SUBTLE KILLERS

Confined spaces are the subtle killer that most maintenance workers face daily. The NIOSH definition [113] of *confined space* is that which, by design, has limited openings for entry and exit and unfavorable natural ventilation, which could contain or produce dangerous air contaminants and which is not intended for continuous employee occupancy. Confined spaces include, but are not limited to, storage tanks, compartments of ships, process vessels, pits, silos, vats, degreasers, reaction vessels, boilers, ventilation and exhaust ducts, sewers, tunnels, underground utility vaults and pipelines.

They are subtle because they exist all around us and usually can result in more than one fatality if respiratory protection is not provided to the rescue team member or members. A typical case results when an employee climbs into a subsurface area, such as a vault, and passes out. The employee who accompanies him assumes that the first man has had a heart attack and goes to help him, resulting in a double fatality.

A typical example of exposure to hydrogen sulfide has been outlined by Bio-Marine Industries [114]. For example, two employees of a fertilizer company descended into an old 35-foot well to repair a pump. The well was covered with a concrete slab and entry was made through a covered manhole. About 6 feet below the opening was a plank platform. When the first worker dropped to the platform he was immediately overcome and fell unconscious into the water below. His partner sought help quickly. When the two helpers entered the well, they too fell unconscious to the water below.

A passerby, in an attempt to save the drowning men, jumped into the water and drowned also. By this time, the fire department had arrived. The fire chief, wearing a self-contained breathing apparatus, went to rescue the victims. On the platform he removed his face mask to give instructions to those above and was overcome. Subsequent tests revealed that the well atmosphere contained a lethal concentration of hydrogen sulfide. The firemen died as a result of pulmonary paralysis.

The National Safety Council [115] has documented other such stories. The hazard is not recognized until tests are made for atmospheres containing hazadous materials, and respiratory protection (self-contained) must be worn to ensure that those readings will not be the last the sampler takes.

Most people think confined spaces are small and hard to reach, but they also can exist in the opening of floating roof-type petroleum storage tanks. As flammable and combustible liquids have a high evaporation rate, they change from a liquid to a gas easily. Large petroleum storage tanks are fixed or floating roof-type design. The floating roof was designed to raise or lower itself with the level of liquid in the storage tank. A hinged rolling bottom ladder is used to gain access to the top of the roof for maintenance or manual gauge procedure. As these tanks can be 134 feet in diameter and more than 60 feet high, a considerable concentration of gas vapors can build up during hot, atmospherically calm weather. Figure 123 illustrates a Horton Double-Deck Roof [116] design, with the ladder way to the top of the floating roof. The maintenance man with manual gauging or check equipment could be overcome easily and pass out without the proper protection. A typical large refinery could have several large tanks, and the time required to manually gauge them could be sufficient in length for the individual to die before help arrives, perhaps even claiming a second victim.

The designer and installler cannot be responsible for these problems encountered in everyday operation. The National Safety Council Sheet #563 [117] must be followed. Section #30 states that "Unless tests definitely indicate the atmosphere above a floating roof is uncontami-

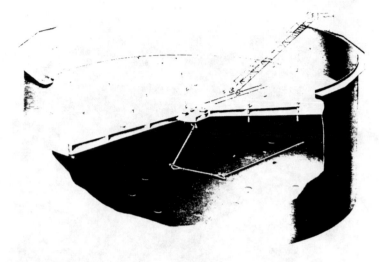

Figure 123. A double-deck floating roof for large-volume storage tanks (courtesy Chicago Bridge & Iron Co.).

nated by suffocating or toxic vapors, the gauger who descends to the roof shall wear personal protective equipment."

Tank work done inside tanks can involve added hazards of material behind rust or scaling. For example, a tank was ventilated during the night with cool air. The next morning, the test was made at 7:00 A.M. The sun's heat was intense and concentration was not checked again. Large amounts of scale and rust were removed, exposing wet areas of solvents and vapors. This is a typical situation in which an explosion or a fatality can occur due to asphyxiation.

The solution to these problems is the use of proper instruments by a trained individual and a confined space entry form of some type. Figure 124 shows a combination oxygen and combustible gas indicator. This instrument measures oxygen in a range of 0 to 25%, and combustible gas in a range of 0 to 100% of the lower explosive limit (LEL). The indicator operates on an integral rechargeable 2.4-volt battery pack. The combustible gas and oxygen indicator can be used wherever there is a need for inspecting any area for combustible gas build up or oxygen deficiency, such as gas and electrical utilities, vaults, etc. It is not to be used for measuring combustibles in otherwise pure oxygen or in atmospheres containing oxygen concentrations greater than 25% by volume. The NIOSH document [113] recommends a typical form such as Figures 125a and b.

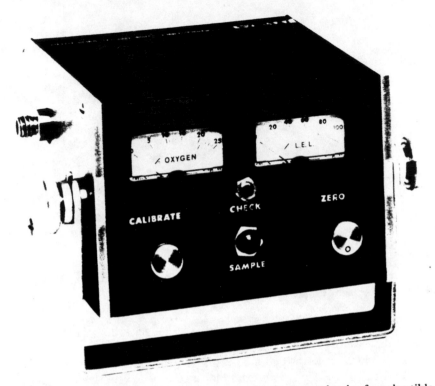

Figure 124.   Sampling of an air atmosphere for dangerous levels of combustible gas and/or oxygen deficiency by placing two detection units in a single, rugged aluminum housing (courtesy Mine Safety Appliance Co.).

In reality, industry would and does use a form similar to this in many areas; however, in the construction trades a calibrated meter is a considerable achievement.

Designers of equipment that must be cleaned manually or that requires entry during maintenance always should make the opening large enough for a worker to wear protective equipment and provide a method for the worker to be removed if injured.

Morse and Swift [118] discussed the key elements in evaluating an unknown atmosphere:

1. Know the major hazard types present in any confined space (oxygen deficiency, combustibility, toxicity). Test for all three.
2. Know the specific hazards likely in the space to be entered.
3. Consider special hazards that might arise. Are contaminants lighter/heavier than air? Are there chances for static electricity?
4. Maintain and check instruments used to monitor confined spaces.

CLASS ____

Location of Work: _____

Description of Work (Trades): _____

Employees Assigned: _____

Entry Date: _____ Entry Time: _____

Outside Contractors: _____

Isolation Checklist:

    Blanking and/or Disconnecting
    Electrical
    Mechanical
    Other

Hazardous Work:

    Burning
    Welding
    Brazing
    Open Flame
    Other

Hazards Expected:

    Corrosive Materials
    Hot Equipment
    Flammable Materials
    Toxic Materials
    Drains Open
    Cleaning (Ex: chemical or water lance)
    Spark Producing Operations
    Spilled Liquids
    Pressure Systems
    Other

Vessel Cleaned:

    Deposits _____
    Method _____
    Inspection _____
    Neutralized with _____

Fire Safety Precautions: _____
_____

Personal Safety:

    Ventilation Requirements
    Respirators
    Clothing
    Head, Hand, and Foot Protection
    Shields
    Life Lines and Harness
    Lighting
    Communications

```
    Employee Qualified
    Buddy System
    Standby Person
    Emergency Egress Procedures
    Training Sign Off (Supervisor or Qualified Person)_____
    Remarks: _____
```

Atmospheric Gas Tests

```
        Tests Performed    -    Location    -    Reading

Example: (Oxygen)_____       _____        (19.5%)
Example: (Flammability)          _____        (Less than 10% LFL)
         _____              _____        _____
         _____              _____        _____
         _____              _____        _____
```

Remarks: _____

Test Performed By: _____
                                    Signature

Time: _____ .

Authorizations:

```
    Supervisor: _____
    Prod Supervisor: _____
    Line Supervisor: _____
    Safety Supervisor: _____
    Etc.: _____
```

Entry and Emergency Procedures Understood:

```
    Standby Person _____
    Rescue _____
    Telephone _____
```

Permit Expires: _____

Classification: _____

Figure 125.   Sample permit, confined space entry [113].

5. *Always assume a hazard exists.*
6. Never assume a space will remain safe because it tested safe before
    entry. Monitor and periodically check the environment during the
    working period.

These authors give three rules to govern every entrance into a confined
space:

1. An observer should be stationed near the entrance of the space. He should be equipped with protective equipment that will allow him to enter the space in an emergency.
2. The observer must be connected physically to the worker inside by a lifeline and harness assembly, and they should be able to communicate with each other.
3. The worker inside must wear equipment that will protect him from the worst possible anticipated hazard.

The American National Standards Institute (ANSI) standard Z 117.1–1977 [119] also outlines recommendations.

PROTECTIVE GARMENT ENSEMBLE

"A Protective Garment Ensemble," described in National Aeronautics and Space Administration Tech Briefs [120] is basically a composite of several types of respiratory and protective measures. The wearer can be provided with air from an air line (air line respirator) or an environmental control unit (powered air filter respirator) with a self-contained emergency air supply (self-contained respirator). The individual is totally protected during filling operations with toxic propellants.

Figure 126 illustrates the suit with the enclosed environmental control unit and emergency air supply mounted on the wearer's back as well as a front view of the umbilical quick disconnects for air line-supplied air or the external mounting of the environmental control unit. The protective fabric was designed to provide the following permeability to the propellants listed in Table XXXVIII for a two-hour test period.

1. Noise inside the unit shall not exceed 85 dBA on the "A"-weighted, slow-response scale.
2. The sealing effect of the suit is accomplished by having the sleeves of the coverall form a liquid- and vaporproof seal with the gloves. A similar seal is provided with the garment legs and boots.

It is suggested that the garment have the following advantages over existing protective garments:

1. Variety of configurations:
    • Environmental control unit, back mounted
    • Environmental control unit, hand carried
    • Air line supply
2. Lightweight design, vortex heating and cooling.

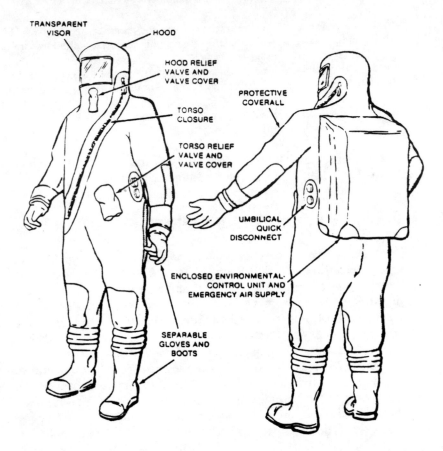

Figure 126.   Protective garment ensemble with an internally mounted environmental control unit, which contains its own air supply. Alternatively, a remote environmental control unit or an air line is attached at the umbilical quick disconnect [120].

Table XXXVIII.   Exposure Limit of Propellants [118]

Propellant	Exposure Limit (ppm)
Monomethylhydrazine (MMH)	0.04
Unsymmetrical Dimethylhydrazine (UDMH)	0.06
Hydrazine (N_2H_4)	0.03
Nitrogen Dioxide (NO_2)	1.0

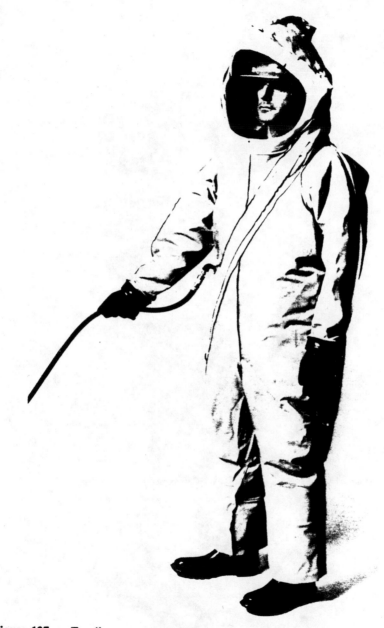

Figure 127.   Totally encapsulating chemical protective suit with umbilical air supply (courtesy Safety Clothing & Equipment Co., Div. of Safety First Industries Inc.).

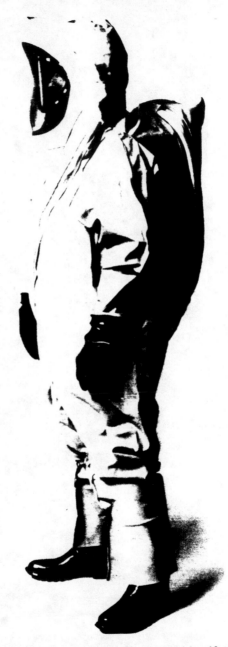

Figure 128.   Totally encapsulating protective suit with self-contained breathing apparatus (courtesy Safety Clothing & Equipment Co., Div. of Safety First Industries Inc.).

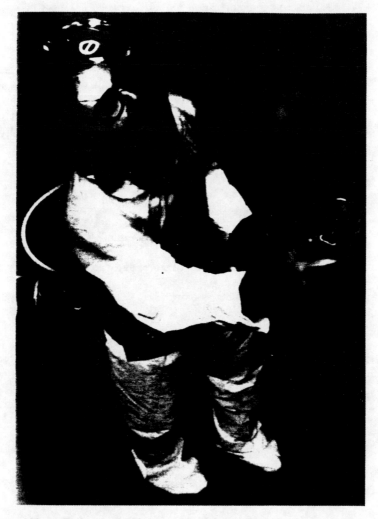

Figure 129. Full suit features an overhead 360° vision (courtesy Safety & Supply Co., Radsafe Div.).

3. The environmental control unit has a low level alarm to provide the operator with a warning of impending depletion of the breathing air supply.
4. The entry closure has two methods of sealing it.
5. Emergency breathing air supply (4 minutes) is an integral part of the ensemble.
6. The system has a flow diverter to provide air primarily to the head section when the garment becomes torn.

7. A universal communication harness has been provided that may be readily removed from the garment to facilitate cleaning or impedence changes.

The importance of this garment ensemble is that respiratory protection can be integrated into a fully protective garment with mobility and little loss in ability to achieve work.

Some other examples of carefully designed and researched suits are shown in Figures 127–129. Figures 127 and 128 show a totally encapsulating protective suit, which provides protection, comfort and safety in hazardous chemicals handling. These suits feature:

- Use with umbilical air supply (Figure 127), or self-contained breathing apparatus (Figure 128)
- Easy front entry—double sealing closure
- Internal pressure control through two exhaust valves
- Weight of approximately 4 lb
- Chemically inert fabric (easy to store, and decontaminate)
- Visual area of 180°
- Optional liquid cooling system

It is not suitable for fire entry.

Figure 129 features an overhead 360° vision, optically clear face section of pressed polished PVC. The low-noise, compact air system is under 80 decibels at 15 cfm. The flexible hood material allows the wearer to maneuver in close quarters. Safety accessories include low-pressure alarms, hard cap, recoil hose and filter systems.

APPENDIX A*

1910.134—RESPIRATORY· PROTECTION

(a) Permissible practice.

(1) In the control of those occupational diseases caused by breathing air contaminated with harmful dusts, fogs, fumes, mists, gases, smokes, sprays or vapors, the primary objective shall be to prevent atmospheric contamination. This shall be accomplished as far as feasible by accepted engineering control measures (for example, enclosure or confinement of the operation, general and local ventilation and substitution of less toxic materials). When effective engineering controls are not feasible, or while they are being instituted, appropriate respirators shall be used pursuant to the following requirements.

(2) Respirators shall be provided by the employer when such equipment is necessary to protect the health of the employee. The employer shall provide the respirators which are applicable and suitable for the purpose intended. The employer shall be responsible for the establishment and maintenance of a respiratory protective program which shall include the requirements outlined in paragraph (b) of this section.

(3) The employee shall use the provided respiratory protection in accordance with instructions and training received.

(b) Requirements for a minimal acceptable program.

(1) Written standard operating procedures governing the selection and use of respirators shall be established.

(2) Respirators shall be selected on the basis of hazards to which the worker is exposed.

*Reprinted from: *General Industry: OSHA Safety and Health Standards* (*29 CFR 1910*), U.S. Department of Labor, Occupational Safety and Health Administration, OSHA 2206, Revised June 1981 [8].

(3) The user shall be instructed and trained in the proper use of respirators and their limitations.

(4) Where practicable, the respirators should be assigned to individual workers for their exclusive use.

(5) Respirators shall be regularly cleaned and disinfected. Those issued for the exclusive use of one worker should be cleaned after each day's use, or more often if necessary. Those used by more than one worker shall be thoroughly cleaned and disinfected after each use.

(6) Respirators shall be stored in a convenient, clean, and sanitary location.

(7) Respirators used routinely shall be inspected during cleaning. Worn or deteriorated parts shall be replaced. Respirators for emergency use such as self-contained devices shall be thoroughly inspected at least once a month and after each use.

(8) Appropriate surveillance of work area conditions and degree of employee exposure or stress shall be maintained.

(9) There shall be regular inspection and evaluation to determine the continued effectiveness of the program.

(10) Persons should not be assigned to tasks requiring use of respirators unless it has been determined that they are physically able to perform the work and use the equipment. The local physician shall determine what health and physical conditions are pertinent. The respirator user's medical status should be reviewed periodically (for instance, annually).

(11) Approved or accepted respirators shall be used when they are available. The respirator furnished shall provide adequate respiratory protection against the particular hazard for which it is designed in accordance with standards established by competent authorities. The U.S. Department of Interior, Bureau of Mines, and the U.S. Department of Agriculture are recognized as such authorities. Although respirators listed by the U.S. Department of Agriculture continue to be acceptable for protection against specified pesticides, the U.S. Department of the Interior, Bureau of Mines, is the agency now responsible for testing and approving pesticide respirators.

(c) Selection of respirators.

Proper selection of respirators shall be made according to the guidance of American National Standard Practices for Respiratory Protection Z88.2—1969.

(d) Air quality.

(1) Compressed air, compressed oxygen, liquid air, and liquid oxygen used for respiration shall be of high purity. Oxygen shall meet the requirements of the United States Pharmacopoeia for medical or breathing oxygen. Breathing air shall meet at least the requirements of the specification for Grade D breathing air as described in Compressed Gas Association Commodity Specification G—7.1—1966. Compressed oxygen shall not be used in supplied-air respirators or in open circuit self-contained breathing apparatus that have previously used compressed air. Oxygen must never be used with air line respirators.

(2) Breathing air may be supplied to respirators from cylinders or air compressors.

   (i) Cylinders shall be tested and maintained as prescribed in the Shipping Container Specification Regulations of the Department of Transportation (49 CFR Part 178).

   (ii) The compressor for supplying air shall be equipped with necessary safety and standby devices. A breathing air-type compressor shall be used. Compressors shall be constructed and situated so as to avoid entry of contaminated air into the system and suitable in-line air purifying sorbent beds and filters installed to further assure breathing air quality. A receiver of sufficient capacity to enable the respirator wearer to escape from a contaminated atmosphere in event of compressor failure, and alarms to indicate compressor failure and overheating shall be installed in the system. If an oil-lubricated compressor is used, it shall have a high-temperature or carbon monoxide alarm, or borh. If only a high-temperature alarm is used, the air from the compressor shall be frequently tested for carbon monoxide to insure that it meets the specifications in subparagraph (1) of this paragraph.

(3) Air line couplings shall be incompatible with outlets for other gas systems to prevent inadvertent servicing of air line respirators with non-respirable gases or oxygen.

(4) Breathing gas containers shall be marked in accordance with American National Standard Method of marking Portable Compressed Gas Containers to Identify the Material Contained, Z48.1—1954; Federal Specification BB—A—1034a, June 21, 1968, Air, Compressed for Breathing Purposes; or Interim Federal Specification GG—B—00675b, April 27, 1965, Breathing Apparatus, Self-Contained.

(e) Use of respirators.

(1) Standard procedures shall be developed for respirator use. These should include all information and guidance necessary for their proper selection, use, and care. Possible emergency and routine uses of respirators should be anticipated and planned for.

(2) The correct respirator shall be specified for each job. The respirator type is usually specified in the work procedures by a qualified individual supervising the respiratory protective program. The individual issuing them shall be adequately instructed to insure that the correct respirator is issued. Each respirator permanently assigned to an individual should be durably marked to indicate to whom it was assigned. This mark shall not affect the respirator performance in any way. The date of issuance should be recorded.

(3) Written procedures shall be prepared covering safe use of respirators in dangerous atmospheres that might be encountered in normal operations or in emergencies. Personnel shall be familiar with these procedures and the available respirators.

(i) In areas where the wearer, with failure of the respirator, could be overcome by a toxic or oxygen-deficient atmosphere, at least one additional man shall be present. Communications (visual, voice, or signal line) shall be maintained between both or all individuals present. Planning shall be such that one individual will be unaffected by any likely incident and have the proper rescue equipment to be able to assist the other(s) in case of emergency.

(ii) When self-contained breathing apparatus or hose masks with blowers are used in atmospheres immediately dangerous to life or health, standby men must be present with suitable rescue equipment.

(iii) Persons using air line respirators in atmospheres immediately hazardous to life or health shall be equipped with safety harnesses and safety lines for lifting or removing persons from hazardous atmospheres or other and equivalent provisions for the rescue of persons from hazardous atmospheres shall be used. A standby man or men with suitable self-contained breathing apparatus shall be at the nearest fresh air base for emergency rescue.

(4) Respiratory protection is no better than the respirator in use, even though it is worn conscientiously. Frequent random inspections shall be conducted by a qualified individual to assure that respirators are properly selected, used, cleaned, and maintained.

(5) For safe use of any respirator, it is essential that the user be properly instructed in its selection, use, and maintenance. Both supervisors and workers shall be so instructed by competent persons. Training shall provide the men an opportunity to handle the respirator, have it fitted properly, test its face-piece-to-face seal, wear it in normal air for a long familiarity period, and, finally, to wear it in a test atmosphere.

(i) Every respirator wearer shall receive fitting instructions including demonstrations and practice in how the respirator should be worn, how to adjust it, and how to determine if it fits properly. Respirators shall not be worn when conditions prevent a good face seal. Such conditions may be a growth of beard, sideburns, a skull cap that projects under the facepiece, or temple pieces on glasses. Also, the absence of one or both dentures can seriously affect the fit of a facepiece. The worker's diligence in observing these factors shall be evaluated by periodic check. To assure proper protection, the facepiece fit shall be checked by the wearer each time he puts on the respirator. This may be done by following the manufacturer's facepiece fitting instructions.

(ii) Providing respiratory protection for individuals wearing corrective glasses is a serious problem. A proper seal cannot be established if the temple bars of eye glasses extend through the sealing edge of the full facepiece. As a temporary measure, glasses with short temple bars or without temple bars may be taped to the wearer's head. Wearing of contact lenses in contaminated atmospheres with a respirator shall not be allowed. Systems have been developed for mounting corrective lenses inside full facepieces. When a workman must wear corrective lenses as part of the facepiece, the facepiece and lenses shall be fitted by qualified individuals to provide good vision, comfort, and a gas-tight seal.

(iii) If corrective spectacles or goggles are required, they shall be worn so as not to affect the fit of the facepiece. Proper selection of equipment will minimize or avoid this problem.

(f) Maintenance and care of respirators.

(1) A program for maintenance and care of respirators shall be adjusted to the type of plant, working conditions, and hazards involved, and shall include the following basic services:

(i) Inspection for defects (including a leak check),

(ii) Cleaning and disinfecting,

(iii) Repair,

(iv) Storage

Equipment shall be properly maintained to retain its original effectiveness.

(2)

(i) All respirators shall be inspected routinely before and after each use. A respirator that is not routinely used but is kept ready for emergency use shall be inspected after each use and at least monthly to assure that it is in satisfactory working condition.

(ii) Self-contained breathing apparatus shall be inspected monthly. Air and oxygen cylinders shall be fully charged according to the manufacturer's instructions. It shall be determined that the regulator and warning devices function properly.

(iii) Respirator inspection shall include a check of the tightness of connections and the condition of the facepiece, headbands, valves, connecting tube, and canisters. Rubber or elastomer parts shall be inspected for pliability and signs of deterioration. Stretching and manipulating rubber or elastomer parts with a massaging action will keep them pliable and flexible and prevent them from taking a set during storage.

(iv) A record shall be kept of inspection dates and findings for respirators maintained for emergency use.

(3) Routinely used respirators shall be collected, cleaned, and disinfected as frequently as necessary to insure that proper protection is provided for the wearer. Each worker should be briefed on the cleaning procedure and be assured that he will always receive a clean and disinfected respirator. Such assurances are of greatest significance when respirators are not individually assigned to workers. Respirators maintained for emergency use shall be cleaned and disinfected after each use.

(4) Replacement or repairs shall be done only be experienced persons with parts designed for the respirator. No attempt shall be made to replace components or to make adjustment or repairs beyond the manufacturer's recommendations. Reducing or admission valves or regulators shall be returned to the manufacturer or to a trained technician for adjustment or repair.

(5)

(i) After inspection, cleaning, and necessary repair, respirators shall be stored to protect against dust, sunlight, heat, extreme cold, excessive moisture, or damaging chemicals. Respirators placed at stations and work areas for emergency use should be quickly accessible at all times and should be stored in compartments built for the purpose. The compartments should be clearly marked. Routinely used respirators, such as dust respirators, may be placed in plastic bags. Respirators should not be stored in such places as lockers or tool boxes unless they are in carrying cases or cartons.

(ii) Respirators should be packed or stored so that the facepiece and exhalation valve will rest in a normal position and function will not be impaired by the elastomer setting in an abnormal position.

(iii) Instructions for proper storage of emergency respirators, such as gas masks and self-contained breathing apparatus, are found in "use and care" instructions usually mounted inside the carrying case lid.

(g) Identification of gas mask canisters.

(1) The primary means of identifying a gas mask canister shall be by means of properly worded labels. The secondary means of identifying a gas mask canister shall be by a color code.

(2) All who issue or use gas masks falling within the scope of this section shall see that all gas mask canisters purchased or used by them are properly labeled and colored in accordance with these requirements before they are placed in service and that the labels and colors are properly maintained at all times thereafter until the canisters have completely served their purpose.

(3) On each canister shall appear in bold letters the following:

(i)

Canister for . . . .

(Name for atmospheric contaminant)

or

Type N Gas Mask Canister

(ii) In addition, essentially the following wording shall appear beneath the appropriate phase on the canister label: "For respiratory protection in atmospheres containing not more than . . . . percent by volume of . . . ."

(4) Canisters having a special high-efficiency filter for protection against radionuclides and other highly toxic particulates shall be labeled with a statement of the type and degree of protection afforded by the filter. The label shall be affixed to the neck end of, or to the gray stripe which is around and near the top of, the canister. The degree of protection shall be marked as the percent of penetration of the canister by a 0.3-micron-diameter dioctyl phthalate (DOP) smoke at a flow rate of 85 liters per minute.

Table I-1

Atmospheric contaminants to be protected against	Colors aassigned*
Acid gases	White.
Hydrocyanic acid gas	White with ½-inch green stripe completely around the canister near the bottom.
Chlorine gas	White with ½-inch yellow stripe completely around the canister near the bottom.
Organic vapors	Black.
Ammonia gas	Green.
Acid gases and ammonia gas	Green with ½-inch white stripe completely around the canister near the bottom.
Carbon monoxide	Blue.
Acid gases and organic vapors	Yellow.
Hydrocyanic acid gas and chloropicrin vapor	Yellow with ½-inch blue stripe completely around the canister near the bottom.
Acid gases, organic vapors, and ammonia gases	Brown.
Radioactive materials, excepting tritium and noble gases	Purple (Magenta).
Particulates (dusts, fumes, mists, fogs, or smokes) in combination with any of the above gases or vapors	Canister color for contaminant, as designated above, with ½-inch gray stripe completely around the canister near the top.
All of the above atmospheric contaminants	Red with ½-inch gray stripe completely around the canister near the top.

*Gray shall not be assigned as the main color for a canister designed to remove acids or vapors.

NOTE: Orange shall be used as a complete body, or stripe color to represent gases not included in this table. The user will need to refer to the canister label to determine the degree of protection the canister will afford.

(5) Each canister shall have a label warning that gas masks should be used only in atmospheres containing sufficient oxygen to support life (at least 16 percent by volume), since gas mask canisters are only designed to neutralize or remove contaminants from the air.

(6) Each gas mask canister shall be painted a distinctive color or combination of colors indicated in Table I-1. All colors used shall be such that they are clearly identifiable by the user and clearly distinguishable from one another. The color coating used shall offer a high degree of ressistance to chipping, scaling, peeling, blistering, fading, and the effects of the ordinary atmospheres to which they may be exposed under normal conditions of storage and use. Appropriately colored pressure sensitive tape may be used for the stripes.

APPENDIX B

HAZARDOUS MATERIALS DEFINITIONS

The following definitions have been abstracted from the Code of Federal Regulations, Title 49-Transportation, Parts 100 to 199. Refer to the referenced sections for complete details. *NOTE:* Rule-making proposals are outstanding or are contemplated concerning some of these definitions.

Hazardous Material—means a substance or material that has been determined by the Secretary of Transportation to be capable of posing an unreasonable risk to health, safety and property when transported in commerce, and that has been so designated (Sec. 171.8).

Multiple Hazards—a material meeting the definitions of more than one hazard class is classed according to the sequence given in Sec. 173.2.

Hazard Class	Definitions
	Explosive—Any chemical compound, mixture or device, the primary or common purpose of which is to function by explosion, i.e., with substantially instantaneous release of gas and heat, unless such compound, mixture or device is otherwise specifically classified in Parts 170–189 (Sec. 173.50).
Class A Explosive	Detonating or otherwise of maximum hazard. The nine types of Class A explosives are defined in Sec. 173.53.
Class B Explosive	In general, it functions by rapid combustion rather than detonation and includes some explo-

331

Hazard Class	Definitions
	sive devices such as special fireworks, flash powders, etc. **Flammable hazard** (Sec. 173.88).
Class C Explosive	Certain type of manufactured articles containing Class A or Class B explosives, or both, as components, but in restricted quantities, and certain type of fireworks. **Minimum hazard** (Sec. 173.100).
Blasting Agents	A material designed for blasting and that has been tested in accordance with Sec. 173.114a(b) and found to be so insensitive that there is very little probability of accidental initiation to explosion or of transition from deflagration to detonation (Sec. 173.114a(a).
Combustible Liquid	Any liquid having a flash point above 100°F and below 200°F as determined by tests listed in Sec. 173.115(d). Exceptions to this are found in Sec. 173.115(b).
Corrosive Material	Any liquid or solid that causes visible destruction of human skin tissue or a liquid that has a severe corrosion rate on steel (see Sec. 173.240(a) and (b) for details.)
Flammable Liquid	Any liquid having a flash point below 100°F as determined by tests listed in Sec. 173.115(d). Exceptions are listed in Sec. 173.115(a). **Pyroforic Liquid**—any liquid that ignites spontaneously in dry or moist air at or below 130°F (Sec. 173.115(c)). **Compressed Gas**—any material or mixture having in the container a pressure *exceeding* 40 psia at 70°F or 104 psia at 130°F or any liquid flammable material having a vapor pressure exceeding 40 psia at 100°F (Sec. 173.300(a)).
Flammable Gas	Any compressed gas meeting the requirements for lower flammability limit, flammability limit range, flame projection or flame propagation criteria, as specified in Sec. 173.300(b).

Hazard Class	Definitions
Nonflammable Gas	Any compressed gas other than a flammable compressed gas.
Flammable Solid	Any solid material, other than an explosive, that is liable to cause fires through friction, retained heat from manufacturing or processing, or that can be ignited readily and, when ignited, burns so vigorously and persistently as to create a serious transportation hazard (Sec. 173.150).
Organic Peroxide	An organic compound containing the bivalent –O–O structure that may be considered a derivative of hydrogen peroxide where one or more of the hydrogen atoms have been replaced by organic radicals. (See Sec. 173.151(a) for details about exceptions.)
Oxidizer	A substance such as chlorate, permanganate, inorganic peroxide or a nitrate that yields oxygen readily to stimulate the combustion of organic matter (see Sec. 173.151).
Poison A	**Extremely Dangerous Poisons**—poisonous gases or liquids of such nature that a very small amount of the gas or vapor of the liquid mixed with air is *dangerous to life* (Sec. 173.326).
Poison B	**Less Dangerous Poisons**—substances, liquids or solids (including pastes and semisolids), other than Class A or Irritating materials, that are known to be so toxic to man that they afford a hazard to health during transportation, or that, in the absence of adequate data on human toxicity, are presumed to be **toxic to man** (Sec. 173.343).
Irritating Material	A liquid or solid substance that on contact with fire or when exposed to air, gives off dangerous or intensely irritating fumes, but **not including any poisonous material, Class A** (Sec. 173.381).
Etiologic Agent	An "etiologic agent" means a viable microorganism or its toxin that causes or may cause

Hazard Class	Definitions
	human disease (Sec. 173.386). (Refer to the Department of Health, Education and Welfare Regulations, Title 42, CFR, Sec. 72.25(c) for details.)
Radioactive Material	Any material, or combination of materials, that spontaneously emits ionizing radiation and that has a specific activity greater than 0.002 μCi/g (Sec. 173.389). *NOTE:* See Sec. 173.389(a) through (l) for details.
	ORMA-A, B or C (Other Regulated Materials)— any material that does not meet the definition of a hazardous material, other than a combustible liquid in packaging having a capacity of 110 gallons or less, and is specific in Sec. 172.101 as an ORM material or that possesses one or more of the characteristics described in ORM-A through D below (Sec. 173.500). *NOTE:* An ORM with a **flash point of 100–200°F** when transported with more than 110 gallons in one container **shall be classed as a combustible liquid.**
ORM-A	A material that has an anesthetic, irritating, noxious, toxic or other similar property and that can cause extreme annoyance or discomfort to passengers and crew in the event of leakage during transportation (Sec. 173.500(a)(1)).
ORM-B	A material (including a solid when wet with water) capable of causing significant damage to a transport vehicle or vessel from leakage during transportation. Materials meeting one or both of the following criteria are ORM-B materials: (1) a liquid substance that has a corrosion rate exceeding 0.250 inch per year (IPY) on aluminum (nonclad 7075-T6) at a test temperature of 130°F. (An acceptable test is described in NACE Standard TM-01-69); and (2) specifically designated by name in Sec. 172.101 (Sec. 173.500(a)(2)).

Hazard Class	Definitions
ORM-C	A material that has other inherent characteristics not described as an ORM-A or ORM-B but that make it unsuitable for shipment, unless properly identified and prepared for transportation. Each ORM-C material is specifically named in Sec. 172.101 (Sec. 173.500(a)(4).
ORM-D	A material such as a consumer commodity that although otherwise subject to the regulations of this subchapter, presents a limited hazard during transportation due to its form, quantity and packaging. They must be materials for which exceptions are provided in Sec. 172.101. A shipping description applicable to each ORM-D material or category of ORM-D materials is found in Sec. 172.101 (Sec. 173.500(a)(4).
Consumer Commodity (see ORM-D)	A material that is packaged or distributed in a form intended and suitable for sale through retail sales agencies or instrumentalities for consumption by individuals for purposes of personal care or household use. This term also includes drugs and medicines.
Flash Point	The minimum temperature at which a substance gives off flammable vapors that will ignite in contact with spark or flame (Sec. 173.115 and 173.150).
Forbidden	The hazardous material is one that must **not be offered or accepted** for transportation (Sec. 172.100(d)).
Limited Quantity	The maximum amount of a hazardous material, as specified in those sections applicable to the particular hazard class, for which there are **specific exceptions** from the requirements of this subchapter. See Sec. 173.118, 173.118a, 173.153, 173.244, 173.306, 173.345 and 173.364.
Spontaneously Combustible	A solid substance (including sludes and pastes) that may undergo spontaneous heating or self-

Hazard Class	Definitions
Material (Solid)	ignition under conditions normally incident to transportation or that may, on contact with the atmosphere, undergo an increase in temperature and ignite.
Water-Reactive Material (Solid)	Any solid substance (including sludges and pastes) that, by interaction with water, is likely to become spontaneously flammable or to give off flammable or toxic gases in dangerous quantities.

REFERENCES

1. Mine Safety and Health Administration. "Code of Federal Regulations," 30 CFR, Subchapter B, Respiratory Protective Apparatus, U.S. Government Printing Office, Washington, DC (1981).
2. "The Occupational Safety and Health Act," Public Law 91-596—91st Congress, General Industry Standards, Department of Labor, U.S. Government Printing Office, Washington, DC (December 1970).
3. Drinker, P., and T. Hatch. *Industrial Dust.* (New York: McGraw-Hill Book Co., 1936).
4. Pritchard, J.A. "A Guide to Industrial Respiratory Protection," NIOSH Publication No. 76-189, U.S. Department of Health, Education and Welfare, Cincinnati, OH, U.S. Government Printing Office, Washington, DC (1976).
5. Naval Sea Systems Command. *U.S. Navy Diving Manual,* U.S. Government Printing Office, Washington, DC (1975).
6. ACGIH. "Threshold Limit Values for Chemical Substances in Workroom Air," Cincinnati, OH (1981).
7. NIOSH. "Program Plan by Program Areas for Fiscal Year 1981," Publication No. 81-112, Department of Health and Welfare, Cincinnati, OH, U.S. Government Printing Office, Washington, DC (1980).
8. U.S. Department of Labor. "OSHA General Industry Standards," 29 CFR 1910 (1981).
9. Horvath, E.P. *NIOSH, Manual of Spirometry in Occupational Medicine,* U.S. Department of Health and Human Services, Cincinnati, OH (1981).
10. Oregon Thoracic Society. "Chronic Obstructive Pulmonary Disease," National Tuberculosis and Respiratory Disease Association (1966).
11. "Evaluating Commercially Available Spirometers," *Am. Rev. Resp. Dis.* 121:73-82 (1980).
12. Morris, J. F., et al. *Am. Rev. Resp. Dis.* 103:57-67 (1971).
13. Knudson, R. J. *Am. Rev. Resp. Dis.* 113 (1976).
14. Hutchinson, M. K., Ed. *A Guide to the Work-Relatedness of Disease,* U.S. Department of Health, Education and Welfare, NIOSH Publication No. 77-123 (1976).
15. International Business Machines Corporation. Automated Breathing Metabolic Simulator, Gaitherburg, MD (1973).

16. DeRosa, M., and R. Levin. "Simulation of Man's Respiratory and Metabolic Functions by the Automated Breathing Metabolic Simulator," Bureau of Mines, Information Circular, Pittsburgh, PA (1978).

17. Bergersen, B. *Pharmacology in Nursing.* 12th ed. (St. Louis, MO: C. V. Mosby Company, 1973).

18. Meek, W. J. "The Gentle Art of Poisoning," Medicohistorical Papers, University of Wisconsin, Madison, WI (1954).

19. Thomson, C. J. S. *Poisons and Poisoners* (London: H. Shaylow, 1931).

20. Loomis, T. *Essentials of Toxicology.* 2nd ed. (Philadelphia: Lea & Febiger, 1974).

21. Casarett, L., and J. Doull. *Toxicology, The Basic Science of Poisons.* (New York: Macmillan Publishing Co., Inc., 1975).

22. Peterson, J. *Industrial Health.* (Englewood Cliffs, NJ: Prentice-Hall, Inc., 1977).

23. NIOSH Public Health Service. *Respiratory Protection: An Employer's Manual,* Cincinnati, OH (1978).

24. "Exposure Chambers for Research in Animal Inhalation," Public Health Monograph No. 57, U.S. Department of Health, Education and Welfare, U.S. Government Printing Office, Washington, DC (1959).

25. Cook, W. A. "Maximum Allowable Concentrations of Industrial Atmospheric Contaminants," *Ind. Med.* (November 1945).

26. American Medical Association. "Threshold Limit Values," *Arch. Ind. Hyg. Occup. Med.* 2:98–100 (1950).

27. Patty, F. A., and W. P. Yant. "Acute Response of Guinea Pigs to Vapor of Vinyl Chloride," Public Health Report No. 45 (August 1930).

28. "NIOSH Registry of Toxic Effects of Chemical Substances," U.S. Department of Health, Education and Welfare, Cincinnati, OH (1979).

29. "A Guide to Industrial Respiratory Protection," NIOSH, U.S. Department of Health, Education and Welfare, Cincinnati, OH (1976).

30. Hodge, H. C., and J. H. Sterner. "Tabulation of Toxicity Classes," *Am. Ind. Health Assoc. Quart.* 10:93–96 (1949).

31. American Conference on Governmental Industrial Hygienists. *Air Sampling Instruments—for Evaluation of Atmospheric Contaminants,* 5th ed., Cincinnati, OH (1978).

32. *NIOSH Manual of Sampling Data Sheets,* U.S. Department of Health, Education and Welfare, Cincinnati, OH (1977).

33. American Board of Industrial Hygiene. "License Procedures," Akron, OH.

34. NIOSH. "Health Hazard Evaluation Summaries," U.S. Department of Health and Human Services," Cincinnati, OH (January 1982).

35. NIOSH. *Occupational Exposure Sampling Strategy Manual,* Publication No. 77-173, U.S. Department of Health, Education and Welfare, Cincinnati, OH (1977).

36. Hatch, T. F. "Respiratory Dust Retention and Elimination," *Proc. Pneumoconiosis Conf.,* Johannesburg, (London: J. & A. Churchill Ltd., 1959), pp. 113–132.

37. Hamilton, R. J., and R. J. Walton. "The Selective Sampling of Airborne Dust," Report No. 139 National Coal Board, Scientific Department, Central Research Establishment (1952).

38.   Hatch, T. F. "Developments in the Sampling of Airborne Dust," *Arch. Ind. Hyg. Occup. Med.* 11:212–217 (1955).

39.   Wells, W. F. *Airborne Contagion and Air Hygiene.* (Cambridge, MA: Harvard University Press, 1955), p. 106.

40.   Brown, J. H., K. M. Cooke, F. G. Ney and T. F. Hatch. "Influence of Particle Size upon the Retention of Particulate Matter in the Human Lung," *J. Am. Public Health Assoc.* 40:450–458 (1950).

41.   Harper, G. J., and J. D. Morton. "The Respiratory Retention of Bacterial Aerosols: Experiment with Radioactive Spores," *J. Hyg.* 51: 372–385 (1953).

42.   Hamilton, R. J. "The Falling Speed and Particle Size of Airborne Dusts in Coal Mines," Report No. 137, National Coal Board, Scientific Department, Central Research Establishment (1952).

43.   Morrow, P. E. "Evaluation of Inhalation Hazards Based upon the Respirable Dust Concept and the Philosophy and Application of Selective Sampling," *Am. Ind. Hyg. Assoc. J.* 25:213 (May-June 1964).

44.   Andersen, A. A. "New Sampler for the Collection, Sizing and Enumeration of Viable Airborne Particles," *J. Bacteriol.* 76:471–484 (1958).

45.   Andersen, A. A. "Sampler for Respiratory Health Hazard Assessment," *AIHAJ.* 27 (March-April 1966).

46.   *ASHRAE Handbook 1981 Fundamentals* American Society of Heating, Refrigeration and Air-Conditioning Engineers, Inc., (Atlanta: 1981).

47.   "OSHA Safety and Health Standards for General Industry," OSHA No. 2206, Superintendent of Documents, U.S. Government Printing Office, Washington, DC (1981), pp. 631–637.

48.   May, J. W. *The Physics of Air.* (Louisville, KY: American Air Filter Company Inc., 1968), p. 13.

49.   Reigel, S. A., and C. D. Doyle. "Using the Psychrometric Chart," *Poll. Eng.* 5(8): (1973).

50.   Cheremisinoff, P. N., and R. A. Young. *Pollution Engineering Practice Handbook.* (Ann Arbor, MI: Ann Arbor Science Publishers, Inc., 1975).

51.   Cheremisinoff, P. N. "Fans and Blowers," *Poll. Eng.* 6(7): (1974).

52.   Rosen, K. M. "Practical Ducting Design, Part I—Basic Principles and Technology," *Plant Eng.* 26(20) (October 5, 1972).

53.   Rosen, K. M. "Practical Ducting Design, Part II—Calculating Duct Losses," *Plant Eng.* 26(22) (November 2, 1972).

54.   Wales, R. O. "Simplified Duct Sizing," *Poll. Eng.* 3(1) (January/February 1971).

55.   Molnar, J. "Duct Weight Calculator," *Poll. Eng.* 2(5) (November/December 1970).

56.   Cheremisinoff, P. N. "Sizing Roof Ventilators," *Plant Eng.* 27(19) (September 20, 1973).

57.   Schrenk, H. H. "Testing and Design of Respiratory Protective Devices," U.S. Department of Interior, Bureau of Mines, Washington, DC, Information Circular 7086 (1939).

58.   *Respiratory Protective Devices Manual.* (American Industrial Hygiene Association and American Conference of Governmental Industrial Hygienists, 1963).

59.   Stein, S. C., H. W. Zeller, and A. Schekman. "The Aerosol Efficiency

and Pressure Drop of a Fibrous Filter at Reduced Pressures," *J. Colloid Science,* 15:546–562 (December 1960).

60. Davies, C. N. "The Separation of Airborne Dust and Particles," *Inst. Mech. Eng., Brit. Proc.* (1952–1953), pp. 185–213.

61. Jordan, H., and L. Silverman. "Effect of Pulsating Airflow on Fiber Filter Efficiency," Report NYO 4814, Air Cleaning Laboratory, School of Public Health, Harvard University, Boston, MA (December 1961).

62. Smith, W. T., and E. Stafford. "Dry Fibrous Filters for Dust-Free Air," paper presented at the U.S. Technical Conference on Air Pollution, Washington, DC (May 1950).

63. Silverman, L. "Filtration Through Porous Materials," *Am. Ind. Hyg. Assoc. Quart.* 11:11–20 (March 1950).

64. Thomas, W. J., and R. E. Yoder. "Aerosol Size for Maximum Penetration Through Fiberglass and Sand Filters," *Am. Med. Assoc. Arch. Ind. Health* 13:545–549 (1956).

65. "Development of Improved Respirator Cartridge and Canister Test Method," NIOSH Publication No. 77-209, U. S. Department of Health, Education and Welfare, Cincinnati, OH (July 1977), p. 3.

66. Nelson, G. O., and A. Correia. "Respirator Cartridge Efficiency Studies: VII, Summary and Conclusions," *Am. Ind. Hyg. Assoc. J.* (September 1976).

67. Freedman, R. W., B. I. Ferber and A. M. Hartstein. "Service Lives of Respirator Cartridges versus Several Classes of Organic Vapors," *Am. Ind. Hyg. Assoc. J.* 34:55 (1973).

68. Dubinin, M. M. "The Potential Theory of Adsorption of Gases and Vapors for Adsorbents with Energetically Nonuniform Surfaces," *Chem. Rev.* 235 (1960).

69. Jonas, L. A., and J. A. Rehrmann. "The Rate of Gas Adsorption by Activated Carbon," *Carbon* 12:95 (1974).

70. Burrage, L. J., and A. J. Allmand. "The Effects of Moisture on the Sorption of Carbon Tetrachloride from an Air Stream by Activated Charcoal," *J. Soc. Chem. Ind.* 57:424 (1938).

71. Nelson, G. E., A. Correia and A. Harder. "Respirator Cartridge Efficiency Studies: VII—Effect on Relative Humidity and Temperature," Lawrence Livermore Laboratory, Report UCRL-77390 (1975).

72. Nelson, G., A. Correia and A. Harder. "Respirator Cartridge Efficiency Studies VIII—Summary and Conclusions," *Am. Ind. Hyg. Assoc. J.* 514 (September 1976).

73. Burgess, W. "An Improved Air-Purifying Respirator," *Arch. Environ. Health* 16 (May 1968).

74. Cecala, A. and J. Volkwein. "Protection Factors of the Airstream Helmet," Bureau of Mines, Report of Investigation 8591, Pittsburgh Research Center, Pittsburg, PA (1981).

75. Compressed Gas Association. "Commodity Specification for Air," G-7.1, New York (1966).

76. Department of Transportation, Hazardous Material Section. "Part 178—Shipping Container Specifications," U.S. Department of Transportation, U.S. Government Printing Office, Washington, DC.

77. Compressed Gas Association. "Compressed Air for Human Respiration," Pamphlet G-7, New York (1976).

78. Gibs, C. W., ed. "Compressed Air and Gas Data," Ingersoll-Rand Company, Woodcliff Lake, NJ (1971).

79. "Man Cooling Systems," Vortec Corporation, Cincinnati, OH (1978).

80. Deltech Engineering, Inc. "Bulletin 216A Del-Monex Purifiers," Letter to Barry White, OSHA, Washington, New Castle, DE.

81. Blair, A. "Abrasive Blasting Respiratory Protective Practices Survey," NIOSH Publication Contract #HSM099-71-47, U.S. Department of Health, Education and Welfare, U.S. Government Printing Office, Washington, DC (1973).

82. NIOSH. "Industrial Health and Safety Criteria for Abrasive Blast Cleaning Operations," U.S. Department of Health, Education and Welfare, U.S. Government Printing Office, Washington, DC (1974).

83. Draeger, B. "The Historical Development of Breathing Apparatus," Dragerwerk, Lubeck, Germany (1911).

84. Morrow, A., and W. Demkowicz. "Mine Rescue Apparatus and Auxiliary Equipment," U.S. Department of Interior, Bureau of Mines, U.S. Government Printing Office, Washington, DC (1961).

85. "Self-Contained Oxygen Breathing Apparatus," Bureau of Mines, Department of the Interior, U.S. Government Printing Office, Washington, DC (1941).

86. Silverman, L., et al. "Fundamental Factors in Design of Protective Equipment," ORSD Report No. 5732, U.S. Government Printing Office, Washington, DC (1945).

87. Mine Safety Appliance Co. "Basic Elements of Respiratory Protection," Pittsburgh, PA (1975).

88. Kloos, E. T., and T. A. Lamonica. "A Machine-Test Method for Measuring Carbon Dioxide in the Inspired Air of Self-Contained Breathing Apparatus," U.S. Department of Interior, Bureau of Mines, Report of Investigation #6865, U.S. Government Printing Office, Washington, DC (1966).

89. Kloos, E. T., L. D. Raymond and L. Spinetti. "Performance of Open-Circuit Self-Contained Breathing Apparatus at $-25°F$," U.S. Department of Interior, Bureau of Mines, Report of Investigation #7077, U.S. Government Printing Office, Washington, DC (1968).

90. NIOSH. "Anthropometry for Respirator Sizing," U.S. Department of Health, Education and Welfare (1972).

91. McConville, J. T., and E. Churchill. "Human Variability and Respirator Sizing," U.S. Department of Health, Education and Welfare, NIOSH (1976).

92. Hack, A. "Selection of Respirator Test Panels Representative of U.S. Adult Facial Sizes," Los Alamos Scientific Laboratory of the University of California, Los Alamos, NM (1974).

93. Reist, P., and F. Rex. "Odor Detection and Respirator Cartridge Replacement," *Am. Ind. Hyg. Assoc. J.* 38 (October 1977).

94. Kolesar, E. "Respirator Qualitative/Quantitative Fit Test Method Analysis," *Aeromed. Rev.*, USAF School of Aerospace Medicine, Brooks Air Force Base, TX (August 1980).

95. Hyatt, E. "Respirator Protection Factors," Los Alamos Scientific Laboratories, University of California, Los Alamos, NM (1975).

96. "NIOSH Training Course: Occupational Respiratory Protection—Course #593" Joint NIOSH/OSHA Standard Completion Program, Respirator Decision Logic (August 1976).

97. Hyatt, E. C., et al. "Effect of Facial Hair on Respirator Performance," *Am. Ind. Hyg. Assoc. J.* 135 (April 1973).

98. "OSHA Maritime Codes 1915, 1916, 1917, 1918 Ship Building, Ship Breaking, Ship Repair and Longshoring," U.S. Department of Labor, U.S. Government Printing Office, Washington, DC.

99. "OSHA Construction Code 1926," U.S. Department of Labor, U.S. Government Printing Office, Washington, DC (1979).

100. "Supplement to the NIOSH Certified Equipment List," NIOSH Publication No. 82-106, U.S. Department of Health and Human Services, Cincinnati, OH, U.S. Government Printing Office, Washington, DC (1981).

101. American National Standards Institute. "Practices for Respiratory Protection," ANSI Z 88.2-1969, New York (1969).

102. American National Standards Institute. "Practice for Respiratory Protection for the Fire Service," ANSI Z 88.5-1971, New York (1971).

103. Enterline, P., et al. "A Study of the Dose-Response Relationship Asbestos Dust and Lung Cancer," Unpublished results.

104. NIOSH. "Criteria for a Recommended Standard—Occupational Exposure to Asbestos," Cincinnati, OH (1972).

105. Murphy, R. L. H., et al. *New England J. Med.* 285:1271 (1971).

106. Pennsylvania Department of Public Health. Unpublished results.

107. Selikoff, I. J., et al. *J. Am. Med. Assoc.* 204:106 (1968).

108. Selikoff, I. J., et al. *J. Am. Med. Assoc.* 188:22 (1964).

109. National Fire Protection Association. "Respiratory Protective Equipment for Firefighters," Boston, MA (1971).

110. International Association of Fire Fighters. "1977 Annual Death and Injury Survey," Washington, DC (1978).

111. Burgess, W. A., et al. "Design Specifications for Respiratory Breathing Devices for Firefighters," NIOSH Publication No. 76-121, U.S. Department of Health, Education and Welfare, Cincinnati, OH (1975).

112. Gordon, G. S., and R. L. Rodgers. "Project Monoxide," International Association of Fire Fighters, Washington, DC (1969).

113. NIOSH. "Criteria for a Recommended Standard Working in Confined Spaces," Publication No. 80-106, U.S. Department of Health, Education and Welfare, Cincinnati, OH (1980).

114. Bio Marine Industries. *A Primer on Confined Area Entry.* Malvern, PA.

115. "Work in Confined Areas, Part I and II," *Nat. Safety News* 114(5) (February/April 1976).

116. "Horton Floating Roofs," Bulletin No. 3200, Chicago Bridge & Iron Co. (1971).

117. "Manual Gauging and Sampling of Petroleum Tanks," National Safety Council Data Sheet #563, Chicago (1975).

118. Morse, G. L., and R. L. Swift. "Working Safely in Confined Spaces," *Plant Eng.* (April 29, 1982).

119. American National Standards Institute. "Safety Requirements for Working in Tanks and Other Confined Spaces," ANSI Z 117.1-1977, New York (1977).

120. "Protective Garment Ensemble," *NASA Tech Briefs* 6(2):KSC-11203 (1981).

BIBLIOGRAPHY

Advisory Committee on Asbestos Cancers. "The Biological Effects of Asbestos," paper presented to the World Health Organization, Lyon, France, October 5–6, 1972.

Arena, J. M. *Poisoning, Toxicology, Symptoms, Treatments* (Springfield: Charles C. Thomas, Publisher, 1970).

Beard, R. R. and N. W. Grandstaff. *Proc. Ann. Conf. Environ. Toxicol.* 1:93 (1970).

Beard, R. R. and G. Wertheim. *Am. J. Public Health* 57:2012 (1967).

Breaker, W. and A. L. Mossman. "Toxic Gases: First Aid and Medical Treatment," Matheson Gas Products (1970).

Council on Occupational Health. *Arch. Environ. Health* 7:130 (1963).

Gafafer, W. M. "Occupational Diseases—A Guide to their Recognition," U.S. Government Printing Office, Washington, DC (1966).

Halperin, M. H. et al. *J. Physiol.* 146:583 (1959).

Hamilton, A. and H. L. Hardy. *Industrial Toxicology*, 3rd ed. (Akron, OH: Publishing Sciences Group, 1974).

Horvath, S. M. *Arch. Environ. Health* 23:343 (1972).

Hunter, D. *The Diseases of Occupations*, 4th ed. (Boston: Little, Brown & Company, 1969).

McFarland, R. A. *J. Aviation Med.* 15:381 (1944).

Morgan, W. K. C. and A. Seaton. *Occupational Lung Diseases* (Philadelphia: W. B. Saunders & Co., 1975).

NIOSH. "Criteria for a Recommended Standard—Occupational Exposure to Asbestos," Cincinnati, OH (1972).

NIOSH. "Criteria for a Recommended Standard—Occupational Exposure to Carbon Monoxide," Cincinnati, OH (1972).

Plunkett, E. R. *Handbook of Industrial Toxicology* (New York: Chemical Publishing Co., 1966).

Sayers, R. R. et al. *USPHS Bull.* 186 (1929).

Schulte, J. H. *Arch. Environ. Health* 7:524 (1963).

Trouton, D. and H. J. Eysewck. *Handbook of Abnormal Psychology* (New York: Basic Books, 1961).

Yater, W. M. and W. F. Oliver. Symptom Diagnosis, 5th ed. (New York: Appleton, Century, Crofts, 1961).